Cardiology

Pocket Consultant

Cardiology

R.H. Swanton MA, MD, FRCP, FESC
Consultant Cardiologist
The Middlesex Hospital, Mortimer Street, London W1N 8AA

Fourth Edition

Presented as a service to medical education
by Boehringer Ingelheim Hospital Division,
suppliers of Actilyse (alteplase, rt-PA)

Blackwell
Science

© 1984, 1989, 1994, 1998 by
Blackwell Science Ltd
Editorial Offices:
Osney Mead, Oxford OX2 0EL
25 John Street, London WC1N 2BL
23 Ainslie Place, Edinburgh EH3 6AJ
350 Main Street, Malden
  MA 02148 5018, USA
54 University Street, Carlton
  Victoria 3053, Australia

Other Editorial Offices:
Blackwell Wissenschafts-Verlag GmbH
Kurfürstendamm 57
10707 Berlin, Germany

Blackwell Science KK
MG Kodenmacho Building
7–10 Kodenmacho Nihombashi
Chuo-ku, Tokyo 104, Japan

First published 1984
Reprinted 1986
Italian edition 1986
Spanish edition 1986
Second edition 1989
Reprinted (twice) 1990, 1991
Yugoslav edition 1990
Italian edition 1991
German edition 1994
Third edition 1994
Reprinted 1994
Polish translation 1994
Fourth edition 1998

Set by Semantic Graphics, Singapore
Printed and bound in Great Britain
at the University Press, Cambridge

The Blackwell Science logo is a
trade mark of Blackwell Science Ltd,
registered at the United Kingdom
Trade Marks Registry

DISTRIBUTORS

Marston Book Services Ltd
PO Box 269
Abingdon, Oxon OX14 4YN
(Orders: Tel: 01235 465500
          Fax: 01235 465555)

USA
Blackwell Science, Inc.
Commerce Place
350 Main Street
Malden, MA 02148 5018
(Orders: Tel: 800 759 6102
              781 388 8250
         Fax: 781 388 8255)

Canada
Copp Clark Professional
200 Adelaide St West, 3rd Floor
Toronto, Ontario M5H 1W7
(Orders: Tel: 416 597-1616
              800 815-9417
         Fax: 416 597-1617)

Australia
Blackwell Science Pty Ltd
54 University Street
Carlton, Victoria 3053
(Orders: Tel: 3 9347 0300
         Fax: 3 9347 5001)

A catalogue record for this title
is available from the British Library

ISBN 0-632-04839-5

Library of Congress
Cataloging-in-publication Data

Swanton, R. H.
    Cardiology / R.H. Swanton. — 4th ed.
         p.   cm. — (Pocket consultant)
    Includes bibliographical references and
index.
    ISBN 0-632-04839-5
    1. Cardiology — Handbook, manuals, etc.
    I. Title.   II. Series.
    [DNLM: 1. Heart Diseases — handbooks.
    WG 39 S972c 1998]
RC682.S837 1998
616.1'2 — dc21
DNLM/DLC
for Library of Congress   91-29781
                                      CIP

Contents

Appendices

Preface to the Fourth Edition

It is hoped that this book will be of practical help to doctors and nurses confronted by typical management problems in the cardiac patient. As a practical guide it is necessarily dogmatic and much information is given in list format or in tables, especially in the sections dealing with drug therapy.

Some subjects in cardiology are often not well covered in clinical training and it is intended that some sections will help fill any gaps in the doctors' or nurses' clinical course, e.g. sections on congenital heart disease, pacing and cardiac investigations.

Practical procedures such as cardiac catheterization cannot be learnt from a book and technical aspects of catheterization are not covered here. However, interpretation of catheter laboratory data is discussed and it is hoped that the book will be of value to the doctor learning invasive cardiology. A practical subject like echocardiography cannot be covered in depth in a book of this size, but the fundamentals and common cardiac conditions are discussed.

Since the publication of the third edition 3 years ago there have been enormous advances in many aspects of cardiology and I have tried to highlight these. Many sections have been extensively revised: particularly those on coronary disease, pacing, infective endocarditis and treatment of heart failure. New sections have been added: including the surgical treatment of heart failure, the follow up of the patient following heart transplantation and the long QT syndrome. The place of the implantable cardioverter defibrillator is becoming clearer and its use is rising in the UK. A more detailed section on ICD therapy is now included. Transoesophageal echocardiography has become a routine investigation in many units with cardiac anaesthetists and ITU specialists getting trained in its use. Its advantages and indications are discussed. Genetics and heart disease is a rapidly expanding subject. I have added basic information on this where known – particularly in the cardiomyopathies, long QT and Marfan syndromes.

The huge increase in trials in cardiology cannot be done justice to here. The reference section has been expanded to include what I feel are the most important trials whose acronyms are now part of the language of cardiology. Space prevents discussion of each but their

....

I am very grateful to colleagues who have suggested improvements or the inclusion of new material and would encourage the reader to contact me with further suggestions of subjects that are not covered, or dealt with inadequately. To my great regret, a separate chapter on nuclear cardiology remains excluded owing to the expense of colour diagrams. However, the use of nuclear cardiological investigations is discussed in relevant sections.

Acknowledgements

I would like to thank my wife Lindsay and my secretary Tracy Harvey for their enormous help in preparing the manuscript.

The work of a large number of authors has contributed to the body of knowledge in this book and it would be impossible to thank them individually or to provide detailed references to their work in a pocket book. The list of further reading and the references I have been able to incorporate cover their work and my thanks to them all. My thanks also to my many colleagues who have helped with suggestions and alterations. I am indebted to Dr R. Sutton and Medtronic Ltd for permission to modify their pacing code diagrams, to Dr S. Horner for the figure on ventricular tachycardia provocation and to Dr P.E. Gower for permission to include the nomogram for body surface area. My thanks also to AVE (Arterial Vascular Engineering Inc.) for permission to use their coronary stent diagram, and to CPI/Guidant corporation (and particularly to Cheryl Friedland) for their invaluable tuition with ICDs.

Finally I am particularly grateful to many of my cardiology registrars and cardiac technical staff for their enthusiastic help in providing me with so many ECGs, pressure tracings and echocardiograms.

1 Cardiac Symptoms and Physical Signs

1.1 Common cardiac symptoms

Angina

Typical angina presents as a chest tightness or heaviness brought on by effort and relieved by rest. The sensation starts in the retrosternal region and radiates across the chest. Frequently it is associated with a leaden feeling in the arms. Occasionally it may present in more unusual sites, e.g. pain in the jaws or teeth on effort, without pain in the chest. It may be confused with oesophageal pain, or may present as epigastric or even hypochondrial pain. The most important feature is its relation to effort. Unilateral chest pain (submammary) is not usually cardiac pain, which is generally symmetrical in distribution.

Angina is typically exacerbated by heavy meals, cold weather (just breathing in cold air is enough) and emotional disturbances. Arguments with colleagues or family and watching exciting television are typical precipitating factors.

Stable angina

Angina induced by effort and relieved by rest. Not increasing in frequency or severity, and predictable in nature. Associated with ST segment depression on ECG.

Decubitus angina

Angina induced by lying down at night or during sleep. It may be due to an increase in LVEDV (and hence wall stress) on lying flat, associated with dreaming, or getting into cold sheets. Coronary spasm may occur in REM sleep. It may respond to a diuretic, calcium antagonist or nitrate taken in the evening.

Unstable (crescendo) angina

Angina of increasing frequency and severity. Not only induced by effort but coming on unpredictably at rest. It may progress to myocardial infarction.

Variant angina (Prinzmetal's angina)

Angina occurring unpredictably at rest associated with transient ST segment elevation on the ECG. It is not common. It is associated with coronary spasm often in the presence of additional arteriosclerotic lesions.

Other types of retrosternal pain

- *Pericardial pain*. Described in **8.1**, page 361. It is usually retrosternal or epigastric, lasts much longer than angina and is often stabbing in quality. It is related to respiration and posture (relieved by sitting forward). Diaphragmatic pericardial pain may be referred to the left shoulder.

• *Aortic pain* (page 412). Acute dissection produces a sudden tearing intense pain retrosternally radiating to the back. Its radiation depends on the vessels involved. Aortic aneurysms produce chronic pain especially if rib or vertebral column erosion occurs.

• *Non-cardiac pain*. May be oesophageal or mediastinal with similar distribution to cardiac pain but not provoked by effort. Oesophageal pain may be provoked by ergonovine, making it a useless test for coronary spasm. Chest wall pain is usually unilateral. Stomach and gall bladder pain may be epigastric and lower sternal, and be confused with cardiac pain.

Dyspnoea

An abnormal sensation of breathlessness on effort or at rest. With increasing disability, orthopnoea and PND occur. Pulmonary oedema is not the only cause of waking breathless at night: it may occur in non-cardiac asthma. A dry nocturnal cough is often a sign of impending PND. With acute pulmonary oedema, pink frothy sputum and streaky haemoptysis occur. With poor LV function Cheyne–Stokes ventilation makes the patient feel dyspnoeic in the fast cycle phase.

Effort tolerance is graded by New York Heart Association criteria as follows:

Class 1

Patients with cardiac disease but without resulting limitations of physical activity. Ordinary physical activity does not cause undue fatigue, palpitation or angina.

Class 2

Patients with cardiac disease resulting in slight limitation of physical activity. They are comfortable at rest. Ordinary physical activity results in fatigue, palpitation, dyspnoea or angina (e.g. walking up two flights of stairs, carrying shopping basket, making beds, etc.). By limiting physical activity patients can still lead a normal social life.

Class 3

Patients with cardiac disease resulting in marked limitation of physical activity. They are comfortable at rest, but even mild physical activity causes fatigue, palpitation, dyspnoea or angina (e.g. walking slowly on the flat). Cannot do any shopping or housework.

Class 4
Patients with cardiac disease who are unable to do any physical activity without symptoms. Angina or heart failure may be present at rest. They are virtually confined to bed or a chair and are totally incapacitated.

Syncope
Syncope may be due to several causes.
• *Vasovagal* (vasomotor, simple faint). The commonest cause. Sudden dilatation of venous capacitance vessels associated with vagal-induced bradycardia. Induced by pain, fear, emotion.
• *Postural hypotension*. This is usually drug induced (by vasodilators). May occur in true salt depletion (by diuretics) or hypovolaemia.
• *Carotid sinus syncope*. A rare condition with hypersensitive carotid sinus stimulation (e.g. by tight collars) inducing severe bradycardia (see page 303).
• *Cardiac dysrhythmias*. Commonest causes are sinus arrest, complete AV block, ventricular tachycardia. Twenty-four-hour ECG monitoring is necessary.
• *Obstructing lesions*. Aortic or pulmonary stenosis, left atrial myxoma or ball-valve thrombus, HCM, massive pulmonary embolism. Effort syncope is commonly secondary to aortic valve or subvalve stenosis in adults and Fallot's tetralogy in children.
• *Cerebral causes*. Sudden hypoxia, transient cerebral arterial obstruction, spasm or embolism.
• *Cough syncope*. This may be due to temporarily obstructed cerebral venous return.
• *Micturition syncope*. This often occurs at night, and sometimes in men with prostatic symptoms. It may be in part due to vagal overactivity and partly due to postural hypotension.

The commonest differential diagnosis needed is sudden syncope in the adult with no apparent cause. Stokes–Adams attacks and epilepsy are the main contenders.

Stokes–Adams attacks	Epilepsy
No aura or warning	Aura often present
Transient unconsciousness (often only a few seconds)	More prolonged unconsciousness
Very pale during attack	Tonic/clonic phases
Rapid recovery	Prolonged recovery. Very drowsy
Hot flush on recovery	Absent

A prolonged Stokes–Adams episode may produce an epileptiform attack from cerebral hypoxia. It is not always possible to distinguish the two clinically.

Cyanosis

Central cyanosis should be detectable when arterial saturation is < 85% and when there is > 5 g reduced haemoglobin present. It is more difficult to detect if the patient is also anaemic. Cardiac cyanosis may be caused by poor pulmonary blood flow (e.g. pulmonary atresia), by right-to-left shunting (e.g. Fallot's tetralogy) or common mixing situations with high pulmonary blood flow (e.g. TAPVD).

Cyanosis from pulmonary causes should be improved by increasing the FiO_2. The child breathes 100% O_2 for 5 min. The arterial Po_2 should increase to > 160 mmHg if the cyanosis is pulmonary in origin. Cyanosis due to right-to-left shunting should change little in response to 100% O_2 and certainly < 160 mmHg.

Peripheral cyanosis in the absence of central cyanosis may be due to peripheral vasoconstriction, poor cardiac output or peripheral sludging of red cells (e.g. polycythaemia).

Embolism

Both systemic and pulmonary embolism are common in cardiac disease. Predisposing factors in cardiology are shown in the table:

Pulmonary emboli	Systemic emboli
Prolonged bed rest	Atrial fibrillation (5.5%/year)
High venous pressure	Aortic stenosis (calcium)
Central lines	Mitral stenosis AF > SR
Femoral vein catheterization	Infective endocarditis
Pelvic disease (tumour, inflammation)	LA myxoma
Tricuspid endocarditis	HCM
Deep vein thrombosis	Prosthetic aortic or mitral valves
	Floppy mitral valve
	Closed mitral valvotomy or valvuloplasty
	Mitral annulus calcification

Either or both
Myocardial infarction
Dilated cardiomyopathy
CCF
Polycythaemia
Diuretics
Procoagulable state
Eosinophilic heart disease

Oedema

Factors important in cardiac disease are: elevated venous pressure (CCF pericardial constriction), increased extracellular volume (salt and water retention), secondary hyperaldosteronism, hypoalbuminaemia (liver congestion, anorexia and poor diet), venous disease and secondary renal failure.

Acute oedema and ascites may develop in pericardial constriction. Protein-losing enteropathy can occur, with a prolonged high venous pressure exacerbating the oedema.

Other symptoms

These are discussed under relevant chapters:

Palpitation: principles of paroxysmal tachycardia diagnosis **7.10**, page 314.

Haemoptysis: mitral stenosis **3.2**, page 70.

Cyanotic attack: catheter complications **12.4**, page 492.

Physical examination

Hands

It is important to check for the following.

• Dilated hand veins with CO_2 retention.

• Temperature (? cool periphery with poor flows, hyperdynamic circulation).

• Peripheral cyanosis.

• Clubbing: cyanotic congenital heart disease, infective endocarditis.

• Capillary pulsation, aortic regurgitation, PDA.

• Osler's nodes, Janeway lesions, splinter haemorrhages: infective endocarditis.

• Nail-fold telangiectases: collagen vascular disease.

• Arachnodactyly: Marfan's syndrome.

• Polydactyly, syndactyly, triphalangeal thumbs: ASD.

• Tendon xanthomata: hypercholesterolaemia.

Facial and general appearance

Down's syndrome (AV canal), elf-like facies (supravalvar aortic stenosis), Turner's syndrome (coarctation, AS), moon-like plump facies (pulmonary stenosis), Noonan's syndrome (pulmonary stenosis, peripheral pulmonary artery stenosis), mitral facies with pulmonary hypertension, central cyanosis, differential cyanosis in PDA + pulmonary hypertension or interrupted aortic arch, xanthelasma, teeth: must be checked as part of general CVS examination, dyspnoea at rest? Accessory muscles of respiration.

Jugular venous pulse (JVP)

Waveform examples are shown in Figure 1.1. It should fall on inspiration. Inspiratory filling of the neck veins occurs in pericardial constriction (Kussmaul's sign). The waves produced are as follows:

'a' wave. Atrial systole. It occurs just before the carotid pulse. It is lost in AF. Large 'a' waves indicate a raised RVEDP (e.g. PS, PHT). Cannon 'a' waves occur in: junctional tachycardia, complete AV block, ventricular ectopics (atrial systole against a closed tricuspid valve).

'c' wave. Not visible with the naked eye. Effect of tricuspid valve closure on atrial pressure.

'x' descent. Fall in atrial pressure during ventricular systole due to downward movement of base of heart.

'v' wave. Atrial filling against a closed tricuspid valve.

'y' descent. Diastolic collapse following opening of the tricuspid valve.

's' wave occurs in tricuspid regurgitation. Fusion of 'x' descent and 'v' wave into a large systolic pulsation with rapid 'y' descent.

The normal range of jugular venous pressure is −7 to +3 mmHg. The patient sits at 45° and sternal angle is used as a reference point. Distinction of the JVP from the carotid pulse involves the following five features: timing, the ability to compress and obliterate the JVP, the demonstration of hepatojugular reflux, the alteration of the JVP with position, and the site of the pulsation itself.

The carotid pulse

Waveform examples are shown in Figure 1.2. There are three components to the carotid pulse: percussion wave, tidal wave, and dicrotic notch.

Percussion wave: a shock wave transmitted up the elastic walls of the arteries.

Tidal wave: reflection of the percussion wave with forward moving column of blood. It follows the percussion wave and is not usually palpable separately.

Dicrotic notch: times with aortic valve closure.

All the pulses are felt, radials and femorals simultaneously (coarctation). Any pulse may disappear with dissection of the aorta. Right arm and carotid pulses are stronger than left in supravalvar aortic stenosis (p. 94).

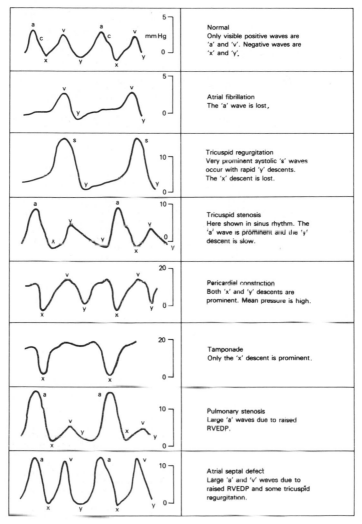

Figure 1.1 Examples of waveforms seen on jugular venous pulse.

An absent radial pulse may occur:
• following a peripheral embolus
• following a Blalock shunt on that side
• following brachial artery catheterization with poor technique on that side
• invariably following a radial artery line for pressure monitoring
• with subclavian artery stenosis.

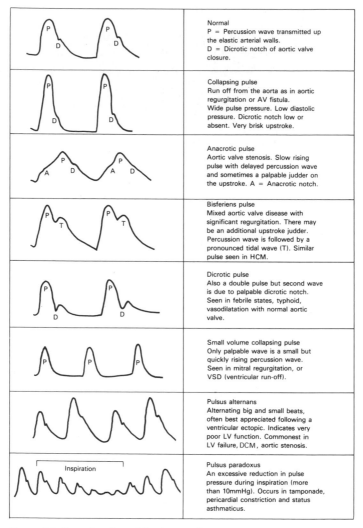

	Normal P = Percussion wave transmitted up the elastic arterial walls. D = Dicrotic notch of aortic valve closure.
	Collapsing pulse Run off from the aorta as in aortic regurgitation or AV fistula. Wide pulse pressure. Low diastolic pressure. Dicrotic notch low or absent. Very brisk upstroke.
	Anacrotic pulse Aortic valve stenosis. Slow rising pulse with delayed percussion wave and sometimes a palpable judder on the upstroke. A = Anacrotic notch.
	Bisferiens pulse Mixed aortic valve disease with significant regurgitation. There may be an additional upstroke judder. Percussion wave is followed by a pronounced tidal wave (T). Similar pulse seen in HCM.
	Dicrotic pulse Also a double pulse but second wave is due to palpable dicrotic notch. Seen in febrile states, typhoid, vasodilatation with normal aortic valve.
	Small volume collapsing pulse Only palpable wave is a small but quickly rising percussion wave. Seen in mitral regurgitation, or VSD (ventricular run-off).
	Pulsus alternans Alternating big and small beats, often best appreciated following a ventricular ectopic. Indicates very poor LV function. Commonest in LV failure, DCM, aortic stenosis.
	Pulsus paradoxus An excessive reduction in pulse pressure during inspiration (more than 10mmHg). Occurs in tamponade, pericardial constriction and status asthmaticus.

Figure 1.2 Examples of carotid pulse waveforms.

Palpation

This checks for: thrills, apex beat, abnormal pulsation, and palpable sounds. Systolic thrill in the aortic area suggests aortic stenosis. Feel for thrills in other sites:

Left sternal edge: VSD or HCM.

Apex: ruptured mitral chordae.

Pulmonary area: pulmonary stenosis.

Subclavicular area: subclavian artery stenosis.

Diastolic thrills are less common: feel for apical diastolic thrill in mitral stenosis with patient lying on left side and breath held in expiration. Left sternal edge diastolic thrill occasionally in aortic regurgitation.

Apex beat and cardiac pulsations

Heart is displaced, not enlarged (e.g. scoliosis, pectus excavatum?) Normal apex beat is in the fifth left intercostal space in the mid-clavicular line. It is palpable but does not lift the finger off the chest. In abnormal states distinguish between:

• normal site but thrusting, e.g. HCM, pure aortic stenosis, hypertension, all with good LV

• laterally displaced and hyperdynamic, e.g. mitral and/or aortic regurgitation, VSD

• laterally displaced but diffuse, e.g. DCM, LV failure

• high dyskinetic apex, e.g. LV aneurysm

• double apex (enhanced by 'a' wave), in HCM, hypertension

• left parasternal heave; RV hypertrophy, e.g. pulmonary stenosis, cor pulmonale, ASD

• dextrocardia with apex in fifth right intercostal space

Abnormal pulsations are very variable. e.g. ascending aortic aneurysm pulsating in aortic area, RVOT aneurysm in pulmonary area, collateral pulsation round the back in coarctation. Pulsatile RVOT in ASD.

Palpable heart sounds represent forceful valve closure, or valve situated close to the chest wall, e.g. palpable S_1 (mitral closure) in mitral stenosis; P_2 in pulmonary hypertension; A_2 in transposition; both S_1 and S_2 in thin patients with tachycardia.

1.3) Auscultation

Heart sounds

First and second heart sounds are produced by valve closure. Mitral (M1) and aortic (A_2) are louder than and precede tricuspid (T_1) and pulmonary (P_2). Inspiration widens the split.

Widely split second sound in mitral regurgitation and VSD is

....

First sound (S₁) = M₁ + T₁

Loud	Soft	Variable	Widely split
Short PR interval	Long PR interval	3° AV block	RBBB
Tachycardia	Heart block	AF	LBBB
Mitral stenosis	Delayed ventricular contraction (e.g. AS, infarction)	Nodal tachycardia or VT	VPBs VT

Second sound (S₂) = A₂ + P₂

Loud A₂	Widely split	Reversed split	Single
Tachycardia	RBBB	LBBB	Fallot
Hypertension	PS (soft P₂)	Aortic stenosis	Severe PS
Transposition	Deep inspiration	PDA	Pulmonary atresia
	Mitral regurgitation	RV pacing	Eisenmenger
	VSD		Large VSD
			Hypertension

Loud P₂	Fixed split
PHT	ASD

due to early ventricular emptying and consequent early aortic valve closure. However, the widely split sound is rarely heard as the loud pansystolic murmur usually obscures it.

Third sound (S₃)

This is pathological over the age of 30 years. It is thought to be produced by rapid LV filling, but the exact source is still debated. Loud S_3 occurs in a dilated LV with rapid early filling (mitral regurgitation, VSD) and is followed by a flow murmur. It also occurs in a dilated LV with high LVEDP and poor function (postinfarction, DCM). A higher pitched early S_3 occurs in restrictive cardiomyopathy and pericardial constriction.

Fourth sound (S₄)

The atrial sound is not normally audible but is produced at end diastole (just before S_1) with a high end-diastolic pressure or with a long PR interval. It disappears in AF. It is commonest in systemic hypertension, aortic stenosis, HCM (LV.S_4), pulmonary stenosis (RV.S_4), or following acute myocardial infarction.

Triple rhythm

A triple/gallop rhythm is normal in children and young adults but is usually pathological over the age of 30 years. S_3 and S_4 are summated in SR with a tachycardia.

S_3 and S_4 are low-pitched sounds. Use the bell of the stethoscope and touch the chest lightly.

Added sounds

Ejection sound. In bicuspid aortic or pulmonary valve (not calcified), i.e. young patients.

Mid-systolic click. Mitral leaflet prolapse.

Opening snap, mitral. Rarely tricuspid (TS, ASD, Ebstein).

Pericardial clicks (related to posture).

Innocent murmurs

Probably 30% of healthy young children have a heart murmur but < 1% will have congenital heart disease. They are usually due to a pulmonary flow murmur heard best at the left sternal edge radiating into the pulmonary area.

Characteristics of innocent murmur

- Ejection systolic. Diastolic or pansystolic murmurs are pathological. The only exceptions are a venous hum or mammary souffle.
- No palpable thrill.
- No added sounds (e.g. ejection click).
- No signs of cardiac enlargement.
- Left sternal edge to pulmonary area. May be heard at apex.
- Normal ECG. CXR or echocardiogram may be necessary for confirmation.

The venous hum is a continuous murmur, common in children, reduced by neck vein compression, turning the head laterally, bending the elbows back or lying down. They are at their loudest in the neck and around the clavicles. They may reappear in pregnancy.

Pathological murmurs

These are organic (valve or subvalve lesion) or functional (increased flow, dilated valve rings, etc.). They are discussed under individual conditions in subsequent chapters.

They should be graded as just audible, soft, moderate or loud. Grading on a 1–6 basis is unnecessary and unhelpful. The murmur should also be classified as to site, radiation, timing (systolic or diastolic, and which part of each), and behaviour with respiration and position. Many murmurs can be accentuated with effort. Alteration of the murmur with position (e.g. squatting) is important in HCM, mitral prolapse and Fallot's tetralogy. The quality of the murmur itself should also be described, e.g. low- or high-pitched, rasping, musical or honking in quality.

Some systolic murmurs can be accentuated by particular manoeuvres. Pansystolic murmurs of VSD and mitral regurgitation are increased by hand grip, and decreased by amyl nitrate inhalation. The systolic murmur of hypertrophic obstructive cardiomyopathy is typically accentuated during the Valsalva manoeuvre and by standing suddenly from a squatting position. The murmur in HCM is reduced by passive leg elevation, hand grip and by squatting from a standing position. (See **4.2**, page 130.)

Accurate documentation of the murmur is important because murmurs may change over time. With a closing VSD the murmur shortens from a pansystolic to an ejection systolic murmur (pages 19–22). With a floppy mitral valve, a soft late systolic mitral murmur may lengthen to become a pansystolic murmur as the mitral leak becomes worse (page 82).

Finally it is important to remember that the loudness of a murmur bears no relation to the severity of the valve lesion.

In summary any of the following features suggest that the murmur is organic/pathological:

- symptoms
- cyanosis
- thrill
- large heart clinically or on CXR
- a diastolic murmur
- a very loud murmur
- added sounds: ejection clicks, opening snaps, etc. (not S_3 which is normal in young people).

Special points in neonates and infants

- A murmur heard immediately after birth is usually due to a stenotic lesion. Murmurs from a small VSD or a PDA are usually heard a few days later, and from a large VSD still later, as the pulmonary vascular resistance falls. The absence of a murmur does not exclude congenital heart disease. Undersized neonates may have an innocent murmur that arises from relatively hypoplastic pulmonary arteries waiting to grow. This sort of murmur usually disappears by the age of 6 months.

- Does the child have other features? e.g.

Turner's syndrome:	coarctation, or atretic aortic arch
Noonan's syndrome:	pulmonary stenosis
Down's syndrome:	AV canal
Williams' syndrome:	supravalvar aortic stenosis, pulmonary artery stenoses

- Clubbing will not be apparent until the child has been cyanosed for ≥ 6 months. Cyanosis in a neonate always needs investigation.
- Pectus excavatum rarely causes any cardiac embarrassment, but may cause slight displacement of heart on CXR. Sometimes associated later with a straight-back syndrome and floppy mitral valve. Pectus carinatum (pigeon chest) is not due to cardiac enlargement. It may sometimes be due to a large main pulmonary artery in large left-to-right shunts.
- Tachypnoea, hepatomegaly, sweating forehead and Harrison's sulci all suggest cardiac failure that is most likely to be due to a left-to-right shunt
- Midline liver, aspenia, polysplenia, etc. suggest complex congenital heart disease.
- Poor pulses in the legs suggest coarctation or hypoplastic left heart syndrome. Bounding pulses in the legs: PDA, truncus arteriosus or aortic regurgitation.

2   Congenital Heart Disease

Congenital heart disease occurs in approximately 8 per 1000 live births. Although divided into cyanotic and acyanotic, there are several conditions that start acyanotic and become cyanotic with time, e.g. Fallot's tetralogy, Ebstein's anomaly and left-to-right shunts developing the Eisenmenger syndrome (1897).

The table below shows the commonest lesions presenting in a neonate and those presenting in the infant and older child.

Most congenital heart disease should be detected by a good neonatal examination or at a 6-week check-up.

	Neonate	Infant and older child
Cyanotic	TGA	TGA
	Tricuspid atresia	Fallot's tetralogy
	Obstructed TAPVD	
	Severe PS	
	Pulmonary atresia	
	Severe Ebstein with ASD	
	Hypoplastic left heart	
Acyanotic	Congenital aortic stenosis	VSD
	Coarctation + VSD/PDA	ASD
		PDA
		Congenital aortic stenosis
		Coarctation
		Pulmonary stenosis
		Partial APVD + ASD

Cyanotic congenital heart disease

Pulmonary plethora	Pulmonary oligaemia
TGA	Fallot's tetralogy
Single atrium	DORV + PS
AV canal	Single ventricle + PS
Truncus arteriosus	Ebstein + PS + ASD
TAPVD	Pulmonary atresia with
DORV	poor collaterals
Primitive ventricle	
Tricuspid atresia with no PS	

With RV hypertrophy	With LV hypertrophy
Fallot's tetralogy	Tricuspid atresia
DORV + PS	Pulmonary atresia with no VSD
Single ventricle + PS/subPS	Single ventricle
TGA + PS (LVOTO)	
Pulmonary atresia + VSD	
TAPVD	
Severe pulmonary stenosis	

The table on the previous page shows the cyanotic group divided into those conditions with pulmonary plethora or oligaemia, and those with LV or RV hypertrophy.

The addition of pulmonary stenosis to a lesion causes oligaemic lung fields and RV hypertrophy.

2.1 Ventricular septal defect (VSD)

The most common congenital heart lesion is an isolated VSD (2 per 1000 births). It also occurs as part of more complex lesions, e.g.

Fallot's tetralogy ⎫
DORV   ⎬ VSD an integral part of the syndrome
Truncus arteriosus ⎭

Tricuspid atresia ⎫
Pulmonary atresia ⎪ often associated with a VSD
TGA   ⎬
Coarctation   ⎭

Pathophysiology and symptoms

The immediate effects of a VSD in the neonate depend on its size and the pulmonary vascular resistance (PVR). The site of the VSD becomes important later.

As the PVR falls in the first few days of life, and RV pressure falls below systemic LV pressure, the VSD results in a gradually increasing left-to-right shunt. If the defect is large (> 1 cm^2/m^2 body surface area) the PVR does not fall with the large left-to-right shunt. The neonatal LV cannot cope with the large volume load and pulmonary oedema develops. These are the typical features of heart failure in infancy:

- tachypnoea
- failure to thrive, feeding difficulties, failure to suck adequately
- sweating on feeding
- intercostal recession (increased respiratory work with stiff lungs)
- hepatomegaly

Persisting high pulmonary blood flow results in frequent chest infections, retarded growth and chronic ill health in the untreated case.

Irreversible pulmonary changes start from about the age of 1 year with initial hypertrophy and secondary thrombotic obstruction of pulmonary arterioles.

Physical signs

These are summarized in the next table. Cases in which the VSD murmur is not pansystolic are either very small or very large. With increasing defect size, biventricular hypertrophy is evident both clinically and on the ECG. With shunt reversal and pulmonary hypertension at systemic levels, right-sided signs are prominent and the murmurs are softer or disappear.

Cardiomegaly and enlargement of the PA conus are not as great as in ASD, except in infants with big shunts.

The second sound in very small VSDs is normal. A_2 is obscured by the pansystolic murmur of larger defects, and with equal ventricular pressures S_2 is single.

Spontaneous closure
This occurs in 30–50% of VSDs. It is common in muscular defects, or defects of the membranous septum. It does not occur in defects adjacent to valves, in infundibular (supracristal) defects, in AV canal type defects or in malalignment defects.

Sites of VSD
Figure 2.1 shows the four common sites simplified;
• *Membranous (infracristal)*. The commonest, just behind the medial papillary muscle of the tricuspid valve, which may oppose it and help to close it spontaneously. On closure, an aneurysm of the membranous septum may occur.
• *Muscular*. Variable in site and may be multiple. Acquired muscular VSD after septal infarction is usually of the Swiss-cheese type.
• *Posterior (AV defect)*. Para-tricuspid defect similar to the site of a VSD in AV canal defect, but this VSD may be present with normal AV valves: 'inlet' VSD.
• *Infundibular ('supracristal')*. A high VSD just beneath the pulmonary valve and below the right coronary cusp of the aortic valve. This may be inadequately supported and prolapses causing aortic regurgitation. This VSD does not close spontaneously.

The infundibular VSD may be associated with malalignment of the infundibular septum, e.g.
VSD + shift of septum to right: Fallot's tetralogy
VSD + shift of septum to left: double-outlet LV with subaortic stenosis

Cardiac catheterization
Confirms a step-up in O_2 saturation in the RV and can quantitate the left-to-right shunt. LV cines in the 45° and 60° LAO views visualize the interventricular septum with head-up tilt. Aortography checks aortic valve competence and excludes PDA or coarctation. RV angiography

Grades of VSD

	Very small	Small	Moderate	Large	Eisenmenger
Thrill	No	Yes	Yes	Yes	No
Murmur and site	Early ejection systolic LSE only	Loud pansystolic. LSE → apex and PA	As in small, but additional mitral diastolic at apex	Pansystolic decrescendo to S_2. Pulmonary ejection systolic + click. Possible pulmonary regurgitation	None at LSE. Ejection systolic. PA (soft) and pulmonary regurgitation
Apex	Normal	Normal or LV+ slight	LV+ RV+ slight	LV+ RV+	RV+ + PA palpable
S_2	Normal. A_2 easily heard	A_2 obscured by mumur, but S_2 split on inspiration	Obscured by murmur	A_2 obscured. P_2 may be loud	Loud single palpable S_2
ECG	Normal	Normal	LV+ LA+ LAD	LV+ LA+ RV+	RV+ RA+ RAD
CXR	Normal	Normal heart size. Mild pulmonary plethora	Slight cardiomegaly PA+. Pulmonary plethora	Cardiomegaly (both ventricles). Large PAs. Pulmonary plethora	Large PAs. No plethora. Peripheral pruning
Differential diagnosis	Mild AS or subAS. Mild PS or infundibular PS	MR. TR. HCM. Pulmonary stenosis	MR. TR. Pulmonary stenosis	Severe MR. Mixed AVD	Eisenmenger ASD. PDA, etc.
Prognosis or treatment	Spontaneous closure	Probable spontaneous closure. Observe	Surgery	Surgery	Medical treatment

Antibiotic prophylaxis (dental procedures, etc.) for all grades

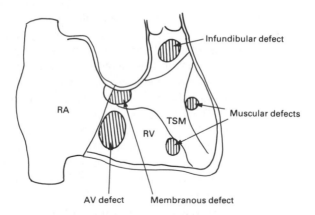

Ventricular septal defects and left ventricular angiography

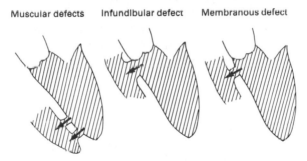

Figure 2.1 Ventricular septal defect. The sites of the four common VSDs are shown, top. TSM = trabecula septomarginalis. The bottom panel shows an LV cineangiogram diagrammatically in the 45° LAO projection with 30° cranial tilt. Muscular VSDs tend to be low in the septum and are often multiple. The infundibular defect is immediately subaortic. The membranous defect tends to be a more discrete jet with a small gap between the jet and the aortic valve.

checks the RVOT. The site of the VSD can be diagnosed at catheter. Muscular VSDs are usually lower in the septum and may be multiple. The infundibular VSD is high, immediately subaortic and there is no gap between the aortic valve and the VSD jet (Figure 2.1). The membranous VSD is usually a discrete jet with a slight gap between the jet and the aortic valve (Figure 2.1).

Complications of VSD

• *Aortic regurgitation*. Occurs in about 5% of VSDs. It may occur with membranous (infracristal) or infundibular (supracristal) defects. The right coronary cusp is unsupported in the infundibular defect and often prolapses into or through the VSD, obscuring it on angiography. With membranous defects the non-coronary cusp may also be involved.

• *Infundibular stenosis.* Muscular infundibular obstruction develops in about 5% of VSDs and is progressive – commoner in older patients and those who have had pulmonary artery banding. Infundibular stenosis improves flooded lungs but causes shunt reversal and cyanosis.

• *Infective endocarditis.* Possible with any VSD with a risk of 0.2% per year. The risk is reduced by VSD closure. All should have antibiotic prophylaxis for dental procedures, etc. Successfully patched VSDs should have antibiotic cover for 3 months after surgery until the patch endothelializes. Infective endocarditis in a VSD with a typical left-to-right shunt presents with pulmonary complications as the infected material is driven into the pulmonary circuit. Patients may present with recurrent atypical pneumonia or pleurisy.

• *Pulmonary hypertension.* VSD is the commonest cause of hyperkinetic pulmonary hypertension (large PAs on the CXR and pulmonary plethora). Calculation of pulmonary vascular resistance at catheter is important because this gradually rises as irreversible intimal hypertrophy develops without causing much change on the chest X-ray.

Associated lesions

• AV canal or simple secundum ASD (see ASDs).
• Aortic regurgitation (see above).
• PDA: a common association (10% of VSDs). The early diastolic murmur heard in the left upper chest may be confused with aortic or pulmonary regurgitation. Aortography is mandatory in VSDs.
• Pulmonary stenosis: valvar (congenital), infundibular (congenital or acquired). The effects depend on the size of the VSD, the severity of the pulmonary stenosis and the systemic vascular resistance. With mild PS, a left-to-right shunt persists. If PS is severe and the VSD small, the condition mimics severe PS alone. If PS is severe and the VSD large, right-to-left shunting occurs (effects similar to Fallot's tetralogy).
• Coarctation.
• TGA, or corrected transposition.
• More complex lesions: DORV, DOLV, truncus arteriosus, tricuspid atresia.
• Gerbode defect. Left ventricular to right atrial shunt. Either direct or through the membranous septum first to RV, then to RA via tricuspid regurgitation.

Management

In infancy, digoxin and diuretics are administered in an attempt to hold the situation. With large defects the baby is catheterized early, with a view to surgery at about 3 months should the child fail to thrive on medical treatment. The VSD is closed, or if multiple, PA banding is performed to reduce pulmonary flow.

If medical treatment is successful, and there are only moderate size defects, the VSD is closed in pre-school years (e.g. age approximately 3 years).

Closure of small defects may be justified on the grounds of infective endocarditis risk, but minute defects are usually left.

The high incidence of spontaneous closure in the first year of life (approximately 50%) must encourage medical management at this age where possible.

Generally surgical closure is indicated for:

• failure to thrive in infancy
• large defects (> 1 cm^2/m^2). Left-to-right shunts ($Q_p : Q_s$) $> 2 : 1$. Increasing heart size on CXR
• RV systolic pressure $> 65\%$ LV systolic pressure if PVR < 8 Wood units (see below)
• increasing aortic regurgitation
• doubly committed VSD (e.g. Fallot's tetralogy)
• previous endocarditis on the VSD.

Management of the child with elevated pulmonary vascular resistance (PVR) is more difficult. If the PVR is < 8 units the VSD is usually closed. If the PVR is > 8 units a lung biopsy may be indicated to assess the severity of intimate proliferation before deciding on surgery. (See table on page 513 for calculation.)

Clamshell closure

The double clamshell device can be used for non-surgical closure of some muscular VSDs which have not closed spontaneously. Unfortunately the device is not suitable for the commoner membranous VSDs as the clamshell can interfere with the aortic or tricuspid valve or cause LVOTO.

2.2 Atrial septal defect (ASD)

From the fifth week of intrauterine life the fetal common atrium starts to be divided by the septum primum. This crescentic ridge grows down from the cranial and dorsal part of the atrium towards the endocardial cushions. The foramen primum develops at the junction of the septum with the endocardial cushions. The foramen secundum develops at the top of the septum primum as the foramen primum closes. The septum secundum develops as a second crescentic ridge to the right of the septum primum, which fuses with the endocardial cushions. The limbic ledge forms the lower part of the septum secundum and the foramen ovale maintains right-to-left atrial flow in fetal life.

Types of ASD (Figure 2.2)
• Patent foramen ovale.
• Primum.
• Secundum.
• Sinus venosus defect.
• IVC defect.
• Coronary sinus anomalies.

Patent foramen ovale (PFO)
Not strictly an ASD. May occur in up to 25% of young children. There is no physiological inter-atrial shunting unless an additional cardiac lesion is present (e.g. pulmonary stenosis when a high RA pressure may cause right-to-left shunting). A PFO does not require closure unless this situation arises. It is useful in catheterization, allowing left atrial catheterization easily. On withdrawal from LA to RA, however, there is a difference in mean pressures. This differentiates a PFO from an ASD, where the mean pressures are the same or virtually so. A PFO does not need prophylactic antibiotics for dental procedures, etc. Rarely, it may allow the passage of a paradoxical embolus. This is increasingly recognized as a cause of stroke following a Valsalva manoeuvre (e.g. straining, heavy lifting, etc.), often in young people. Surgical closure in these patients must be considered.

Pathophysiology and symptoms
Left-to-right shunting at atrial level occurs during the first months of life as the RV becomes more compliant than the LV (which becomes thicker and stiffer in response to systemic pressures). High pulmonary flow results, with flow murmurs audible over pulmonary and tricuspid valves. Pulmonary flow may be five times as great as the systemic.

In young adults the development of pulmonary hypertension is not common but it results in RV pressure approaching systemic levels and the start of shunt reversal (Eisenmenger ASD). It does not occur in infancy.

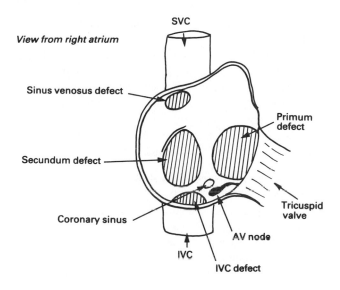

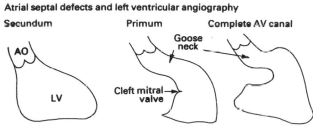

Figure 2.2 The sites of the common ASDs are shown, top. The lower panel shows the LV cineangiogram in the RAO projection diagrammatically. In the secundum ASD this may be normal or show a prolapsing mitral valve. The typical 'goose neck' of primum ASDs or AV canal is shown with a horizontal outflow tract, grossly abnormal AV shape and cleft mitral valve.

Secundum ASD patients are often asymptomatic in childhood and may not be diagnosed until 40–50 years old. Primum ASDs are picked up earlier.

Symptoms or reason for diagnosis:

• The chesty child: resulting from high pulmonary flow.

• Dyspnoea on effort and occasionally orthopnoea (stiff lungs, not LVF).

• Symptomatic. Routine school medical or mass X ray.

• Palpitations. All varieties of atrial dysrhythmias are common especially in the older patient and are not necessarily cured by closing the defect.

- The development of atrial fibrillation and cardiac failure. This is a serious problem in ASDs. RV compliance is reduced, the tricuspid ring dilates further, and tricuspid regurgitation and hepatomegaly occur. Systemic flow falls, the left atrium may enlarge as progressive CCF develops. (In SR the left heart is small in secundum ASD.)
- Paradoxical embolism or cerebral abscess may occur in patients with high RV pressures and shunt reversal.

Infective endocarditis is not a problem with an ASD *per se*, unless there is an associated mitral valve lesion.

Physical signs of secundum ASD
More common in females. May occur as part of the Holt–Oram syndrome (triphalangeal thumbs, ASD or VSD).

Right heart signs are dominant:
- Raised JVP with equal 'a' and 'v' waves.
- RV prominence with precordial bulge in children and large pulmonary conus and flow.
- Pulmonary systolic ejection murmur (flow).
- Fixed split A_2 and P_2 on any phase of respiration is typical although occasionally very slight movement of P_2 can be detected.
- Tricuspid diastolic flow murmur with large left-to-right shunts.
- Systolic thrill in the pulmonary area may occur from high flow and does not necessarily mean additional pulmonary stenosis.
- With AF, signs of tricuspid regurgitation.
- Pulmonary hypertension results in a softer ejection systolic murmur, often an ejection click, the tricuspid flow murmur disappears and P_2 is loud. Pulmonary regurgitation may occur (Graham Steell early diastolic murmur).

Differential diagnosis
In the simple secundum, ASD is with mild pulmonary stenosis (P_2 delayed, softer and moves with respiration).

With larger hearts, pulmonary hypertension and the development of cardiac failure, the conditions confused with an ASD include: mixed mitral valve disease (see Figure 3.2); pulmonary hypertension and/or cor pulmonale; congestive cardiopathy.

Patients with ASDs are usually in SR, with right heart signs most obvious. In AF with low output it is more difficult, but on CXR the pulmonary artery is very large in ASDs and there is pulmonary plethora.

Associated lesions
- *Floppy mitral valve.* (Often overdiagnosed on angiography.)

• *Pulmonary stenosis.* This will cause right-to-left shunting if severe.
• *Anomalous venous drainage.* The sinus venosus defect is almost always associated with anomalous drainage of the right upper pulmonary vein to the right atrium. However, more than one pulmonary vein may be involved. This is checked at cardiac catheter.
• *Mitral stenosis (Lutembacher's syndrome, 1916).* Probably rheumatic mitral stenosis associated with an ASD. Congenital mitral stenosis is a rare possibility.
• As part of more complex congenital heart disease, e.g. TAPVD, TGA, tricuspid atresia, pulmonary atresia with intact ventricular septum.

The sinus venosus defect behaves as a small secundum ASD with its associated right upper lobe anomalous venous drainage.

Chest X-ray
• *Small aortic knuckle.* Large pulmonary artery conus.
• *Pulmonary plethora.* Cardiac enlargement is due to RV dilatation. Right atrial enlargement common.
• Progressive enlargement of both atria once in AF.

ECG
Incomplete or complete RBBB.
Right axis deviation.

Echocardiography
This is all that may be needed in children when PVR is usually normal.

Cardiac catheterization
Cardiac catheterization is performed to document the diagnosis, assess the shunt with a saturation run, check pulmonary and coronary sinus drainage, check RV function and the mitral valve with an LV injection. Thus LV, RV and PA angiograms with follow through are usually required.

Oximetry is performed early in the catheter prior to angiography. If the oxygen step-up is high in the RA there may be a sinus venosus defect. In secundum ASD the step-up is in mid-RA. If the oxygen step-up is very low in the RA near the tricuspid valve and the ASD cannot be crossed with the catheter, consider the possibility of anomalous pulmonary veins draining into the coronary sinus.

In secundum ASD the LV is small and normal. The mitral valve may appear to prolapse. In primum ASD there is the so-called 'goose-neck' appearance with a cleft in the mitral valve (see Figure 2.2) plus some mitral regurgitation which may fill the RA if severe. In complete AV canal the cleft becomes a large gap and the LV has a characteristic appearance in the RAO view. The LAO views visualize the septum. The aorta is small, shifted to the left (large RA).

	Secundum ASD	Primum ASD	AV canal
Presentation	Child or adult	Usually childhood	Infancy
Appearance	Normal	Normal	Down's syndrome
Colour	Normal	Normal	Cyanosis
Signs	2° ASD	As 2° ASD ± MR	As VSD, but S_2 split
Ventricular septum	Intact	Intact	VSD component
Pulmonary hypertension	–	–	+
EGG	RBBB + RAD	RBBB + LAD	RBBB. LAD. long PR or worse
Mitral valve	Occasionally prolapsing usually normal	Cleft anterior leaflet, varying degrees of MR	Severe MR. Grossly abnormal MV and TV

Treatment

Surgical closure is recommended between the ages of 5 and 10 years to avoid late-onset RV failure, tricuspid regurgitation and atrial arrhythmias. Late-onset pulmonary hypertension is uncommon because this is usually established in the first year of life. The calculated left-to-right shunt on saturations should be 2 : 1 or more at atrial level to recommend closure. Small ASDs can be left alone. In the older patient, closure of an ASD is still worthwhile, symptomatic improvement being associated with a reduction in RV size (especially if there is low voltage on RV leads pre-operatively).

Patients with secundum ASDs may have an associated floppy mitral and/or tricuspid valve and regurgitation though this may cause problems years after ASD closure.

Device closure. Recently small- or moderate sized ASDs can be closed percutaneously through the right heart using a variety of different devices. The clam shell device developed in the 1980s was followed by the Sideris buttoned double disc device. Most recently, the Amplatzer device can be inserted through a 7F sheath. Transoesophageal echocardiography during the procedure is helpful. The ASD should be clear of the AV valves and pulmonary veins and have a rim of normal atrial septum to make clam-shell closure possible. Approximately 50% of secundum ASDs may be suitable for device closure. About one-third of patients have small residual leaks, and device embolization occurs in a samll number necessitating catheter removal or surgery. The technique is still in development.

Primum ASD

A more complex and serious lesion than the secundum ASD, it forms part of the spectrum of AV canal defects. It is due to maldevelopment of the septum primum and endocardial cushions. Its most simplified subdivisions are as follows.

• *Primum ASD*. No VSD component. Mitral valve (anterior leaflet) is cleft with associated mitral regurgitation of varying degrees, from none to severe. Sometimes called 'partial AV canal'.

• *Complete AV canal*. Primum type ASD plus VSD component. Mitral and tricuspid valves are abnormal with abnormally short chordae and bridging leaflets stretching across the VSD and joining mitral and tricuspid valves.

It accounts for only 3–5% of congenital heart disease in the first year of life, and less than a tenth of all ASDs.

Associated lesions

• Down's syndrome (very common), Klinefelter's syndrome, Noonan's syndrome, renal and splenic abnormalities.

• Cardiac abnormalities: common atrium; unroofed coronary sinus (left SVC to LA); pulmonary stenosis; coarctation.

Presentation

Primum ASD usually presents in childhood, and the complete AV canal in infancy (heart failure and failure to thrive in infancy with signs of VSD, early childhood with dyspnoea with chest infections and central cyanosis if pulmonary vascular disease develops).

Chest X-ray

• CXR of a simple primum defect resembles a secundum ASD. The AV canal CXR has a large globular heart with pulmonary plethora.

ECG

• RBBB.
• Left axis deviation (cf. right axis in secundum defect).
• Long PR interval.

Conduction defects are common (the AV node is in the inferior portion of the defect), especially junctional rhythms or complete AV

block. If right axis deviation develops it suggests the development of
pulmonary hypertension or additional pulmonary stenosis.

Treatment

Primum ASD. Fifty per cent reach surgery before age 10 years. Early
surgery may help prevent RV dysfunction. The cleft mitral valve is
repaired if there is significant mitral regurgitation and the defect is
closed with a patch.

Complete AV canal. Fifty per cent die within 1 year if untreated.
Options in infancy are banding the pulmonary artery or closure of ASD
and VSD components dividing the bridging leaflets. Subsequent mitral
valve replacement may be necessary, as well as permanent pacing for
AV block. The presence of pulmonary hypertension makes operative
mortality high.

Rarer defects

The IVC defect may be large and allow shunting of IVC blood into LA,
with children becoming slightly cyanosed on effort. It may also occur
following surgical closure of a primum ASD.

Unroofed coronary sinus with a left SVC draining to LA usually
occurs as part of a more complex lesion (e.g. common atrium).

2.3 The patent ductus arteriosus (PDA)

In fetal life the duct allows flow from the pulmonary circuit to the
aorta. It normally closes spontaneously within the first month after
birth. In premature babies it is more likely to remain patent for longer
or permanently. Up to 50% of premature babies have a PDA, especially
those with respiratory distress syndrome. The duct responds less well to
a rise in PO_2 in prematurity and the duct may be silent.
The PDA is more common:
• in children born at high altitudes
• in females
• where there has been history of maternal rubella in the first trimester
of pregnancy (PDA is the commonest congenital heart lesion following
maternal rubella).

Pathophysiology and symptoms

Most children with a PDA are asymptomatic, the condition having been
diagnosed at school medical, etc. With larger ducts a significant left-to-

right shunt occurs causing an increased LV volume load similar to a VSD. Symptoms of LVF are similar. Irreversible pulmonary hypertension may develop in a few cases, causing an Eisenmenger syndrome (approximately 5%).

Differential cyanosis and clubbing may be noticed by the patient who has shunt reversal (blue feet, pink hands), with preferential flow of pulmonary arterial blood down the descending aorta.

In rare instances death is due either to CCF or infective endocarditis.

Physical signs to note
Very small ducts have few signs apart from the continuous machinery murmur in the second left interspace.

Signs to note in a moderate PDA are:
• collapsing pulse with wide pulse pressure (feel the foot pulses in babies)
• thrill, second left interspace, systolic and/or diastolic
• LV+. Hyperdynamic ventricle
• machinery murmur. Loud continuous murmur obscuring second sound in second left interspace and just below the left clavicle, louder in systole. It is not present in the neonate (with the high PVR), but appears as the PVR falls in the first few days
• mitral diastolic flow murmur at apex
• the second sound is usually inaudible.

Pulmonary hypertensive ducts
The diastolic component of the murmur may disappear, and the systolic become shorter with an ejection quality. The second sound is single (loud P_2). Occasionally it is reversed audibly (prolonged LV ejection).

Dilatation of the pulmonary trunk causes an ejection sound and sometimes pulmonary regurgitation.

Associated lesions
• VSD.
• Pulmonary stenosis.
• Coarctation.
• As part of more complex lesions: e.g. pulmonary atresia with intact septum. If collaterals are poor, pulmonary flow is duct dependent. Drug control in this instance is important. In interrupted aortic arch or hypoplastic left heart syndrome, the PDA maintains flow round the body.

Pharmacological control of the PDA

Helping to close the duct in neonatal LVF

Important points are: avoiding fluid overload; normal blood glucose and calcium; diuretics rather than digoxin (AV block in babies). Then use indomethacin 0.2 mg/kg via nasogastric tube given at 6-hourly intervals for a maximum of three doses. An i.v. preparation is not generally available.

There is a risk of renal damage (unlikely with this regime) and the drug should be avoided if there is an elevated serum creatinine (> 150 mmol/l or 1.7 mg/100 ml). Also avoid indomethacin if there is a bleeding disorder.

Helping to keep the duct patent in pulmonary atresia

This is more difficult because sudden deaths have been reported following the use of prostaglandin E_1 (PGE_1), and the cause is unknown.

PGE_1 is infused at 0.1 μg/kg/min via an umbilical artery catheter. The Po_2 rises. Vasodilatation may drop the mean aortic pressure and increase the right-to-left shunt if there is one already. After a few minutes the dose is reduced to 0.05 μg/kg/min or even to 0.025 μg/kg/min.

Other side-effects include fever and irritability. Taken orally, the drug produces troublesome diarrhoea. *It should not be tried except at experienced neonatal centres.*

Differential diagnosis

Includes:
- AP window
- VSD with aortic regurgitation
- coronary AV fistula
- pulmonary AV fistula
- ruptured sinus of Valsalva
- innocent venous hum
- mammary souffle (pregnancy)
- surgical shunts (Waterston, Blalock, etc.).

Cardiac catheterization

This is performed if additional lesions are suspected. The right heart catheter follows a characteristic course from PA down the descending aorta. Associated lesions are excluded by a saturation run (VSD). Aortography indicates duct size and site. LV cine is necessary if a VSD is suspected in addition.

Treatment

Spontaneous closure of the PDA is rare after 6 months of age and a PDA should be closed by the preschool year to avoid the risk of infective endocarditis and the rarer development of LVF or the Eisenmenger reaction. Infective endocarditis on a very small duct is extremely rare and these can be left alone. Infection risk is related to duct size and ducts > 4.0 mm should be occluded. Many of the problems encountered by surgical closure (e.g. haemorrhage, 'recanalization' due to inadequate ligation, phrenic and left recurrent laryngeal nerve palsy) have been obviated by the use of duct occluders implanted in the catheter laboratory.

The first of these was the ivalon plug implanted retrogradely via the femoral artery. The introducing catheter was too big for children. The Rashkind double umbrella device followed in 1979. Femoral arterial and venous sheaths were needed. A pair of miniature back-to-back umbrellas were positioned across the duct under screening, and angiography at the end confirmed correct positioning and successful duct occlusion. This device has now been superseded by a variety of implantable coils which can be positioned in the duct using only a femoral venous sheath. Smaller guiding catheters can be used than with the Rashkind device. The procedure can now be done as a day case.

Problems with the technique are few in skilled hands. The duct may be too large for the occluder or multiple coils resulting in a persistent leak. Usually a single coil is enough to occlude the duct. Embolization of the device down a pulmonary artery is possible in about 1% cases but it can usually be retrieved with a catheter snare. Turbulent flow in the left pulmonary artery may be seen on colour Doppler echocardiography following coil deployment which can cause a degree of LPA obstruction.

2.4 Coarctation of the aorta

A congenital narrowing or shelf like obstruction of the aortic arch. The constriction is usually eccentric, distal to the left subclavian artery, opposite the duct and termed 'juxtaductal'. In extreme form the arch may be interrupted. Recognized types are as follows.

Infantile type

Associated with hypoplasia of the aortic isthmus (a diffuse narrowing of the aorta between left subclavian artery and duct), this was called 'preductal' coarctation. Presentation occurs in the first month of life, with heart failure and associated lesions, which are extremely common.

Adult type

This coarctation is juxtaductal or slightly postductal. The obstruction develops gradually and presentation is commonly between the ages of 15 and 30 years with complications. Associated cardiac lesions are much less common than with the infantile type, apart from a bicuspid aortic valve.

Pseudocoarctation

This is just a tortuosity of the aorta in the region of the duct. There is no stenosis, just a 'kinked' appearance. It is of no haemodynamic significance.

Other severe stenotic lesions may occur in the aorta (e.g. supravalvar aortic stenosis, descending thoracic or abdominal stenoses). The abdominal and descending thoracic aorta stenoses may be due to an aortitis. Classic coarctation may be due to abnormal duct flow *in utero* associated with other anomalies, and the two types are not strictly comparable.

Children with coarctation are usually male. Coarctation in females is suggestive of Turner's syndrome.

Associated lesions

These are very common.
* *Bicuspid aortic valve* (which may become stenotic and/or regurgitant). Approximately 50% of cases, but series vary enormously.
* PDA. The commonest associated shunt.

Postductal coarctation + PDA. Usually left-to-right shunt into the pulmonary artery. If the duct is large, pulmonary hypertension may occur.

Infantile coarctation + PDA. High pulmonary vascular resistance results in right-to-left shunt, with distal aorta, trunk and legs supplied by right ventricular flow through the PDA. Differential cyanosis results (blue legs, pink hands) and heart failure.
* VSD. In isolation or with:

Transposition of the great arteries + VSD + PDA. Complex lesion with differential cyanosis (blue hands, pink feet).

Mitral valve disease. Congenital mitral valve anomalies, stenosis or regurgitation.

Other complex lesions. Primitive ventricle, primum ASD or AV canal.

Aortic arch anomalies. Hypoplastic left heart with hypoplastic aortic root. Aortic atresia. Aortic root aneurysms.

Non-cardiac associations. Berry aneurysms, renal anomalies (especially Turner's syndrome).

Symptoms
• Infantile heart failure is expected in > 50% preductal coarctation. It may also occur with postductal coarctation plus a large PDA (see above).

Postductal coarctation may be missed in childhood presenting in adolescence or early adult life with one or more of the following:

• noticing a vigorous pulsation in the neck or throat
• hypertension, may be symptomless, routine medical
• tired legs or intermittent claudication on running
• subarachnoid haemorrhage from a Berry aneurysm
• infective endocarditis on coarctation or bicuspid aortic valve
• left ventricular failure
• rupture or dissection of the proximal aorta, distal aortic rupture has occurred (e.g. into the oesophagus), aortic rupture is more common in pregnancy
• angina pectoris, premature coronary disease occurs.

Physical signs to note
• Blood pressure in both arms (?left subclavian involved or not). Hypertension with wide pulse pressure in right ± left arm.
• Weak, delayed, anacrotic or even absent femoral pulses compared with right radial. Low blood pressure in legs.
• Prominent carotid and subclavian pulsations.
• Collaterals in older children (not before age 6 years) and adults. Bend the patient forward, with arms hanging down at the sides. Feel round the back with the palm, over and around the scapulae and around the shoulders. Collaterals do not develop in preductal coarctation with PDA because distal aorta supply is from the pulmonary artery.
• Tortuous retinal arteries. Frank retinopathy is not common.
• JVP is usually normal.
• LV hypertrophy.

....

- Murmurs;

Due to bicuspid aortic valve (p. 89).

From the coarctation itself: a continuous murmur with small, tight
coarctation (< 2 mm) heard over the thoracic spine or below the left
clavicle. With larger coarctation the murmur is ejection systolic only.

From collaterals. Ejection systolic, bilateral, front or back of chest. In
interrupted aorta (complete coarctation) the murmurs are due to
collaterals.

From an associated PDA or VSD.

From lower thoracic or abdominal coarctation.

It may be difficult to decide the source of an ejection systolic murmur
in coarctation!

- Second sound. A_2 is usually loud, but not usually delayed beyond P_2.

Chest X-ray

Rib notching occurs from the age of 6–8 years (dilated posterior
intercostal arteries). It does not occur in the first and second ribs. (The
first two intercostals do not arise from the aorta.)

The heart is usually normal in size unless there are associated lesions.

The typical aortic knuckle is absent, and is replaced by a double
knuckle (in postductal coarctations). The upper part is the dilated left
subclavian, the lower the poststenotic dilatation of the descending
aorta.

ECG

Shows left ventricular hypertrophy; RBBB is common.

Echocardiography

May obviate the need for cardiac catheter in the infant with no
associated lesion.

Cardiac catheterization

Is required in children with atypical signs or associated lesions. Babies
can be catheterized from the right heart via a PFO, or from a right
axillary cut-down in older children. Additional lesions are checked
(bicuspid aortic valve, PDA, VSD, etc.) and aortography performed in
the LAO projection to show the coarctation. A coarctation gradient of
40 mmHg is highly significant. The size of the descending aorta is
noted as are site and size of collaterals.

Balloon angioplasty

Some paediatric centres now advocate this as an alternative to surgery as first-line treatment for both infantile and adult-type coarctation but this is controversial as first line treatment. It is not a satisfactory procedure in neonates and infants as there is a high restenosis rate, and patients with a long narrow segment at the isthmus do badly with little or no reduction in coarctation gradient. There is also a risk of a small saccular aneurysm developing at the site of the dilatation (in which case surgical repair is necessary). Surgery itself carries a restenosis risk of 15%.

The technique is much more suitable for restenosis occuring after primary resection than as an initial procedure, and the risk of aneurysm formation is much less for dilatations of restenosis (approximately 7%) than as a primary procedure. A close look around the whole of the circumference of the aorta at the coarctation site is needed after dilatation to check for the small aneurysm.

The major complication is aortic rupture and death occuring within 36 h of the procedure in approximately 2.5% cases.

Surgery

The prognosis without surgery is poor: most patients die before the age of 40 years owing to complications. Severe preductal coarctation in infancy or interrupted aortic arch (usually with PDA + VSD) may require urgent reconstructive surgery.

In postductal coarctation, surgery is performed between 5 and 10 years or at the time of diagnosis, which may be later. Patients with both coarctation and aortic stenosis have the coarctation resected first, and a subsequent aortic valve replacement if necessary.

Recently, extra-anatomical bypass surgery has been developed for coarctation or interrupted aortic arch in older children or adults in which a dacron graft is anastomosed from the ascending aorta to the descending aorta either above or below the diaphragm. This avoids all the problems of surgery at the coarctation site itself such as restenosis or aneurysm formation at the site of the patch aortoplasty.

Follow up

Postoperative hypertension is expected, usually requiring nitroprusside, labetalol, trimetaphan and/or chlorpromazine in the immediate postoperative phase.

Long-term hypertension is also common. All patients should be followed up for life after coarctation resection to check:

- continued hypertension
- the possibility of premature coronary artery disease

• repeat cardiac catheter in infants or early adult life is often performed to check the coarctation site and possible residual gradient, especially if hypertension persists.

2.5 Transposition of the great arteries (TGA; complete transposition, D-transposition)

In its commonest form the aorta arises from the right ventricle and the pulmonary artery from the left ventricle. The aorta lies anterior and to the right of the pulmonary artery (D-loop). There is thus atrioventricular concordance, and ventriculo-arterial discordance. Unless there is an associated shunt (ASD, VSD, PDA), the two circuits are completely separate and life is impossible once the duct closes.

TGA occurs in approximately 1 per 4500 live births (100–200 cases per year in the UK). It is commoner in males. Untreated mortality is high (10% 1-year survival).

Presentation
At birth, with cyanosis that increases in the first week as the PDA closes. Birth weight is normal or high. Progress is poor and progressive cardiac enlargement occurs. As PVR declines in the first weeks of life, high pulmonary flow develops and LVF occurs. Congestive cardiac failure is the commonest cause of death.

When pulmonary vasculature is protected from high flow by pulmonary stenosis, children are often quite active even though very cyanosed. Squatting and cyanotic attacks are uncommon in contrast to the very cyanosed Fallot child.

Physical signs to note
• The commonest cyanotic congenital heart disease causing cyanosis at birth.
• Initially hyperdynamic circulation: bounding pulses in a blue baby.
• Loud (palpable) A_2 retrosternally from anterior aorta. P_2 not heard.
• Murmurs often absent: high pulmonary flow may cause a soft mid-systolic ejection murmur, ejection sound may arise from either aorta or pulmonary artery, right-to-left shunt through VSD may cause a soft early systolic murmur; left-to-right shunt through VSD (high PVR or LVOTO) does not usually cause a murmur.

The signs depend on the level of the PVR, the presence or absence of LVOTO and/or a VSD.

ECG

Is very variable. Usually shows RA + RV + and RAD. Additional LV + and LA + occurs with high pulmonary flow and LV volume overload. It is not so prevalent in patients with additional pulmonary stenosis.

Chest X-ray

Shows pulmonary plethora. Heart has 'egg on its side' appearance and the pedicle is small (aorta in front of PA). The left heart border is convex.

Echocardiography

Is usually diagnostic. The anterior aorta and posterior pulmonary artery are seen. Additional defects such as ASD or VSD, LVOTO, PDA or abnormalities of the AV valves should be looked for.

Differential diagnosis

All causes of cyanosis and pulmonary plethora (see second table, p. 19) but TGA is the commonest.

Also consider Eisenmenger VSD.

If there is LVOTO, lung fields are not plethoric, and the condition may then resemble Fallot's tetralogy or DORV with pulmonary stenosis.

Associated lesions

• PDA may be life saving if there is no VSD. Differential cyanosis occurs.
• VSD.
• VSD + LVOTO (fibrous shelf or fibromuscular tunnel beneath pulmonary valve) = TGA + VSD + LVOTO. These patients have poor pulmonary flow and may have frank cyanotic spells.
• ASD. Usually without PS, and high pulmonary flow occurs.
• Coarctation.
• Juxtaposed atrial appendages.

Prognostically the best situations are TGA + ASD, or TGA + VSD + moderate pulmonary stenosis. The child can survive the early months and does not get the irreversible pulmonary vascular changes (these are usually present by 1 year of age) in children with TGA + large VSD but no protective pulmonary stenosis.

Cardiac catheterization

Confirms normal AV connections, but RV injection fills anterior aorta. The associated shunt is identified. An aortogram shows coronary anatomy plus a possible PDA or coarctation. Injection into the LV shows possible LVOTO. If possible, the PA should be entered to check for PVR (usually easiest via aorta through RV → VSD → LV → PA).

Options for treatment

1 *Prostaglandin infusion.* May be needed for the intensely cyanosed neonate with duct-dependent pulmonary flow until a balloon atrial septostomy can be performed. (See p. 34.)

2 *Rashkind balloon septostomy.* May be life saving in the neonate. Performed at diagnostic catheterization. A PFO is enlarged by inflating the balloon catheter carefully in the left atrium, and sudden traction of the balloon into RA increases atrial mixing. Approximately 70% of babies can be helped through the first year with this technique, and atrial septectomy is not generally needed.

3 *Intra-atrial reconstruction.* Senning or Mustard operation. Usually performed between the age of 6 months and 1 year, these operations separate systemic venous and pulmonary venous return at atrial level.

In the Mustard operation, systemic venous return is diverted through the mitral valve via an intra-atrial baffle into LV thence to PA. Pulmonary venous return is diverted through the tricuspid valve to the right ventricle, thence to the aorta.

Advantages:
- Circuits are separated.
- Cyanosis disappears.
- Child grows with reasonable exercise tolerance.

Disadvantages:
- RV bears load of systemic circulation, both RV muscle and tricuspid valve may not be up to it with RV failure or TR.
- It is not strictly anatomical total correction.
- Postoperative supraventricular dysrhythmias are common (especially with the Mustard procedure).
- Baffle obstruction may occur.

4 *Rastelli procedure for TGA, VSD and LVOTO.* These patients may be shunted early (Blalock). Then at ages 3–4 years the Rastelli procedure is performed. The VSD is enlarged, the pulmonary valve closed and the pulmonary artery ligated just above the pulmonary valve. The LV is connected to the aorta by means of an intracardiac patch. Then an extracardiac valve conduit connects the anterior RV to the pulmonary artery.

This is total correction, with the LV bearing the systemic load.

Problems which can result are a residual VSD, tricuspid regurgitation, conduit compression by the sternum and conduit valve degeneration.

5 *Anatomical correction: the arterial switch.* Switching the great arteries to their correct ventricles is becoming increasingly popular and is anatomical correction. Surgery is performed early in the first few weeks of life while the LV is still capable of generating systemic pressures. LV mass will fall as PVR falls and if the switch is performed too late the LV will fail. Otherwise a two-stage procedure may be needed, with pulmonary artery banding to 'tone-up' the left ventricle. Problems are primarily surgical on account of the delicate surgery of coronary artery relocation. An initial Rashkind balloon septostomy, followed later by a Senning or Mustard procedure, was the standard treatment for TGA but is now being replaced by the arterial switch where possible.

2.6 Corrected transposition (l-transposition)

In its commonest form the aorta lies anterior and to the left of the pulmonary artery (l-loop). It is physiologically corrected in that the circulation proceeds on a normal route although the ventricles are 'switched', i.e.

RA → morphological LV but in RV position → PA
→ LA → morphological RV but in LV position → Ao

There is thus atrio-ventricular discordance and ventriculo-arterial discordance. There is usually situs solitus with the atria normally placed Rarely, the condition presents with situs inversus and dextrocardia. A few cases of corrected transposition have no associated lesions and the individual can live a normal adult life with no symptoms, the RV coping well with systemic load. The presence of associated lesions usually results in presentation in childhood, and the condition is not particularly benign.

Associated lesions: the four most common (Figure 2.3)
- VSD. Shunt from systemic (RV) to venous (LV) ventricle. Occurs in 70–90% of cases depending on series. A 'malalignment' defect: as there is malalignment between the atrial and ventricular septum.
- Pulmonary stenosis in 40%. Often subvalvar due to an aneurysm of the membranous septum bulging out beneath the pulmonary valve.
- AV valve regurgitation. Usually a problem with the tricuspid valve (left-sided) not coping with systemic pressures produced by the RV. Also it is often dysplastic with a typical Ebstein malformation. Mitral (right-sided) prolapse also may occur.

....

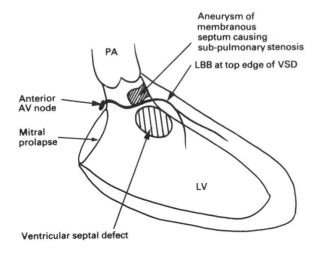

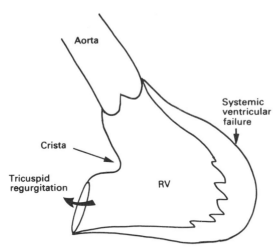

Figure 2.3 Problems in corrected transposition. The upper diagram shows the left (venous) ventricle and the position of the VSD in relation to the bundle. An aneurysm of the membranous septum is shown causing subpulmonary obstruction. The lower diagram shows the right (systemic) ventricle, which is trabeculated. Dysplastic tricuspid valve associated with tricuspid regurgitation. Systemic (RV) ventricular failure is a common cause of death.

• Complete AV block. The AV node is anterior and the bundle runs beneath the pulmonary valve and anterior to the VSD.

Pulmonary valve or VSD surgery runs the risk of inducing AV block (which may occur spontaneously anyway).

....

Presentation
- Systemic ventricular failure (RV) due to tricuspid (left AV valve) regurgitation.
- Congenital complete AV block. Not a benign type of AV block, children may be symptomatic from this alone.
- Cyanotic heart disease mimicking Fallot's tetralogy (subpulmonary stenosis + VSD with venous to systemic ventricular shunting).
- Paroxysmal tachycardia as in Ebstein's anomaly. Anomalies of the conducting system may occur (e.g. additional posterior AV node, WPW, etc.).
- Abnormal EGG in adult life: mimicking anteroseptal infarction.

Physical signs
The best clues to corrected transposition are the clinical findings of second or third degree AV block in a child, e.g.

cannon 'a' waves in the JVP } in third degree block
variable intensity S_1

As in TGA (complete D transposition), A_2 is loud and palpable. In corrected transposition it is heard best in the second left intercostal space – mimicking the loud P_2 of pulmonary hypertension.

There may be signs of left AV valve regurgitation (pansystolic murmur from left sternal edge to apex). There may be an ejection click from the anterior position of the aortic valve.

Chest X-ray
The left-sided aorta produces a 'duck's back' appearance with a straight left heart border, and AV valve regurgitation causes the respective ventricles and atria to enlarge. The left pulmonary artery may be hidden behind the heart and aorta.

ECG
Long PR interval. Higher degrees of AV block. Prominent Q waves in right chest leads (V1–3) but absent Q waves in left precordial leads. Left axis deviation. Q wave in standard lead 3, but no Q wave in lead 1.

Treatment
The commonest early symptom is from complete AV block (20–30%) requiring pacing. Atrial arrhythmias are common (SVT or AF) from about the age of 40 and digoxin and/or amiodarone therapy will be needed. Beware the negative inotropy of other drugs.

Medical treatment for congestive cardiac failure may be needed if the systemic ventricle (RV) fails to cope with systemic workloads. CCF is the commonest cause of death in patients with no associated anomalies. ACE inhibitors should be started early.

Patients may require left AV valve (tricuspid) replacement or repair plus VSD closure. The latter risks the development of complete AV block with the conducting system in the roof of the VSD (see Figure 2.3).

Intracardiac mapping helps identify and avoid bundle damage. Unusual coronary artery anatomy may make ventriculotomy of the venous (LV) ventricle difficult.

Even with the greatest care, permanent pacing may be needed. The establishment of a permanent system is not without problems either. The transvenous wire must grip the endocardial surface of the non-trabeculated (venous) left ventricle.

2.7 Fallot's tetralogy

This is the most common cyanotic congenital heart disease presenting after 1 year of age. It forms part of a spectrum of complex cyanotic congenital heart disease, and is very similar in many respects to double-outlet right ventricle with pulmonary stenosis (DORV + PS), VSD with severe infundibular stenosis, and pulmonary atresia with VSD.

Development of Fallot's tetralogy

In Fallot's tetralogy there is a failure of the bulbus cordis to rotate properly so that the aorta lies more anterior and to the right (dextroposed) than normal. The aorta moves nearer the tricuspid valve and overrides the septum with a 'malalignment' VSD beneath the aortic valve.

Infundibular stenosis develops, with hypertrophy of the septal and parietal bands of infundibular muscle that form part of the crista (Figure 2.4). Obstruction to RV outflow is usually due to a combination of infundibular and valve stenosis, but may be either alone. In addition, RV outflow obstruction may be due to the small size of the pulmonary valve ring or main pulmonary trunk. Peripheral pulmonary stenoses are common. The original tetralogy described by Fallot in 1888 is:

- pulmonary stenosis (Figure 2.4)
- VSD
- overriding of the aorta
- right ventricular hypertrophy

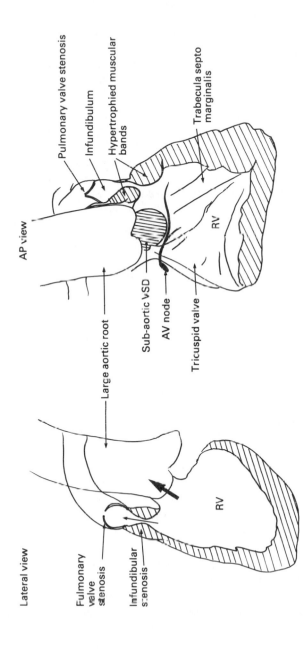

Figure 2.4 Fallot's tetralogy. The left diagram shows a lateral view of the right ventricle with the large aorta overriding the VSD. The severe infundibular stenosis results in the diversion of RV blood straight up into the aorta (heavy arrow). The right panel shows the right ventricle in the AP projection. The VSD is subaortic. Note the hypertrophied bands of the infundiculum. The bundle lies immediately beneath the VSD and is at risk during VSD closure.

Additional anomalies or problems commonly associated are:
- right-sided aortic arch (in 25%)
- absent or hypoplastic left pulmonary artery (more common if arch is right-sided)
- aortic regurgitation due to large aortic ring plus subaortic VSD
- ASD.

Pathophysiology and symptoms

With the large VSD, both ventricles are at the same (systemic) pressure. Pulmonary flow and the degree of right-to-left shunt across the VSD depend on the severity of pulmonary stenosis and the level of systemic vascular resistance (SVR). Increasing SVR will reduce the right-to-left shunt and increase pulmonary flow. Mild pulmonary stenosis may be associated with the 'acyanotic' Fallot child. Pulmonary blood flow may be increased by a patent ductus arteriosus although the association is not that common. Bronchial collaterals develop with increasingly severe pulmonary stenosis.

Infundibular stenosis is a variable obstruction. It increases with time (muscle and fibrous tissue accumulation) and also with hypoxia or acidosis, which may result in cyanotic attacks (infundibular spasm). Infundibular shutdown results in a severe reduction in pulmonary flow and an increased right-to-left shunt of blood from RV straight into the aorta.

Squatting helps cyanosis in two ways, by increasing pulmonary flow and reducing right-to-left shunting:
- increasing systemic vascular resistance
- reduction in venous return – especially of acidotic blood from the legs (acidotic blood promotes infundibular spasm).

Typical clinical presentation

- Patients are not cyanosed at birth (cf. TGA). It usually appears at 3–6 months and increases with time.
- Cyanotic attacks develop. Often with 'stress', crying or feeding. Increasing cyanosis results in syncope and convulsions (see page 492). The pulmonary stenotic murmur may disappear during attacks. Cerebral blood flow may be so severely compromised that permanent neurological damage results.
- Poor growth. Delayed milestones.
- Squatting is common in older children once walking starts. In more

severe cases, children may squat at rest (knees up to chest and buttocks on the ground).
• Symptoms of polycythaemia: arterial or venous thromboses, particularly cerebral, and children must not be allowed to get dehydrated, which can precipitate this. Later in life: gout, acne, kyphoscoliosis, recurrent gingivitis (see Figure 2.10).
• Infective endocarditis.
• Cerebral abscess (absence of lung filter with right-to-left shunt).
• Paradoxical embolism.

Physical signs
• Developing cyanosis, clubbing and polycythaemia.
• JVP: 'a' wave is usually absent (contrast with pulmonary stenosis with intact septum).
• Parasternal heave of RV hypertrophy.
• Palpable A_2 is common (large aorta, too anterior).
• Ejection systolic murmur from left sternal edge, radiating up to pulmonary area, systolic thrill.
• Single second sound (A_2 only).
   The systolic murmur is due to pulmonary stenosis, not the VSD. With cyanotic attacks the murmur becomes quieter or may disappear.
• A diastolic murmur in a Fallot patient may be due to aortic regurgitation (very large aortic root).
• A continuous murmur is due to large aortopulmonary collaterals (heard in the back).

Chest X-ray
The classic heart shape is of coeur en sabot (heart in a boot) appearance with the apex lifted off the left hemidiaphragm by RV hypertrophy. There is a concavity in the usual site of the pulmonary artery. Lung fields are usually oligaemic and pulmonary arteries small. A network of collaterals may be seen around the main bronchi at the hilum. The aortic knuckle is a good size and may be right-sided in about 25% of cases.

ECG
Shows sinus rhythm, right axis deviation and RV hypertrophy with incomplete or complete RBBB. Ventricular ectopics are common, and paroxysmal ventricular tachycardia may be found on 24-hour ECG taping.

Cardiac catheterization (Figure 2.5)

Is needed to assess the anatomy of the RVOT and the main pulmonary artery branches, RV and LV function, site and size of VSD, competence of the aortic valve, coronary anatomy to exclude a PDA or coarctation, and to visualize any previous shunt.

This is best managed with biplane RV cine (and craniocaudal tilt on the AP projection helps visualize the main pulmonary trunk and its bifurcation). An LV cine in the LAO projection will show the VSD and LV function. An aortogram is essential in Fallot's tetralogy.

It is important to visualize the size and anatomy of the pulmonary arteries because this determines the choice of subsequent operation. With severe pulmonary stenosis or pulmonary atresia these may not be seen adequately on RV injection. A retrograde pulmonary vein hand-shot injection (catheter through a PFO or ASD) may show up small true pulmonary arteries.

The most difficult differential diagnosis is from double-outlet right ventricle with subaortic VSD and pulmonary stenosis. In Fallot's tetralogy less than half the aortic valve should straddle the VSD, and in DORV more than half. The final arbiter may be the surgeon. Medical treatment of cyanotic attacks and management of polycythaemia; see **12.4**, p. 492 and **2.10**, p. 60.

Surgery

Initial enthusiasm for complete one-stage repair in the first year of life was tempered by high mortality in many patients, especially those needing a transannular patch on the RV outflow tract.

Total correction under the age of 1 year is usually reserved for those infants who do not need an outflow transannular patch. A Blalock shunt is performed (Figure 2.6) if the anatomy is unfavourable. Under the age of about 3 months a Waterston shunt is preferred, because the subclavian artery is too small for a good Blalock. A second-stage total correction can be performed when the child is larger (age > 2 years). Conditions favouring an initial shunt include: hypoplastic pulmonary arteries, single pulmonary artery, virtual pulmonary atresia and anomalous coronary anatomy.

An alternative to shunting is to try pulmonary valvuloplasty, ballooning the outflow tract and valve, to attempt to improve pulmonary flow and pulmonary artery size as a palliative method before total correction. Recently resection of infundibular muscle, using a modified atherectomy device, has been attempted and percutaneous infundibular resection may become a useful treatment in time.

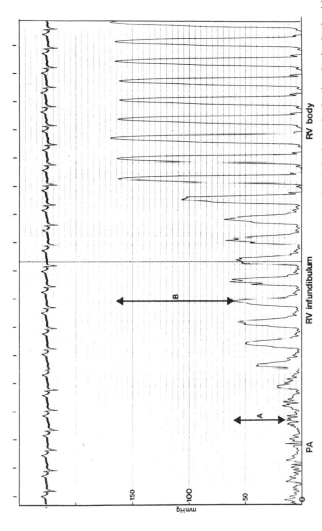

Figure 2.5 Fallot's tetralogy. Right heart withdrawal. PA pressure is normal. The RVOT gradient is both at valve level and subvalve level (infundibular). Valvar gradient (A) = 45 mmHg, and the infundibular gradient (B) = 105 mmHg. Total gradient = 150 mmHg.

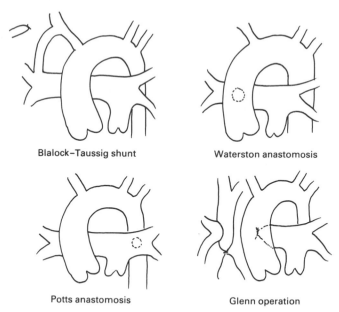

Blalock–Taussig shunt

Waterston anastomosis

Potts anastomosis

Glenn operation

Figure 2.6 Shunt operations for cyanotic congenital heart disease. Blalock–Taussig shunt: either subclavian artery to respective pulmonary artery. Waterston shunt: back of ascending aorta to pulmonary artery. Potts anastomosis: back of pulmonary artery to descending aorta. Glenn operation: SVC to right pulmonary artery only. The Potts operation is rarely used now. The bidirectional Glenn (to both pulmonary arteries) is increasingly popular.

Following total correction there may be further problems:
• RV failure
• tachyarrhythmias
• heart block (see position of bundle just beneath VSD)
• pulmonary regurgitation
• RVOT aneurysm
• problems from initial shunt
• reopened VSD.

RV failure and rhythm problems are the most important. Repeat cardiac catheterization is sometimes necessary in patients following total correction to assess all these factors.

Virtually any arrhythmia may develop in time. Junctional bradycardia or complete AV block requiring permanent pacing, atrial fibrillation requiring anticoagulation and rate control, or paroxysmal VT requiring anti-arrhythmics – usually amiodarone in view of poor RV function.

Pulmonary regurgitation is being recognized as increasingly important in the late development of RV failure. Surgical correction involving a transannular patch often involves late pulmonary regurgitation. Reduction of pulmonary regurgitation using a monocusp valve or a homograft is being attempted to preserve RV function. There is an increasing trend towards transatrial repair for the same reason. Additional peripheral pulmonary artery stenoses can be dealt with by balloon dilatation and stent implantation.

2.8 Total anomalous pulmonary venous drainage (TAPVD)

In TAPVD all four pulmonary veins drain directly or indirectly into the right atrium. There is an associated ASD to allow flow to the left heart. Pulmonary flow is increased and the child is cyanosed. The degree of cyanosis and the severity of symptoms depend on:

• the size of the ASD
• the degree of pulmonary hypertension
• the presence of pulmonary venous obstruction

Cyanosis is more severe if pulmonary flow is reduced (e.g. with irreversible pulmonary hypertension) and if mixing in the atria is poor (e.g. with small ASD or PFO). The child with the least cyanosis is the one with high pulmonary flow, low PVR and good atrial mixing (large ASD). Pulmonary venous obstruction reduces pulmonary flow and increases cyanosis, and is most common with infracardiac TAPVD (see below).

Anatomical possibilities (Figure 2.7)

A variety of venous pathways can conduct pulmonary venous blood to the right atrium. They can be divided into three.

• *Supracardiac.* Venous drainage to the left SVC, which joins the left innominate vein, thence to the right SVC. This vein may occasionally be compressed between the left main bronchus (behind) and the pulmonary trunk (in front).

• *Cardiac.* Venous drainage into a venous confluence (a sort of miniature LA) joining the coronary sinus. Venous drainage directly into RA via one or more ostia.

• *Infracardiac.* The rarest variety. The venous confluence at the back of the heart joins a vertical vein passing down through the diaphragm to join either the IVC or the portal vein. The vein may be obstructed at

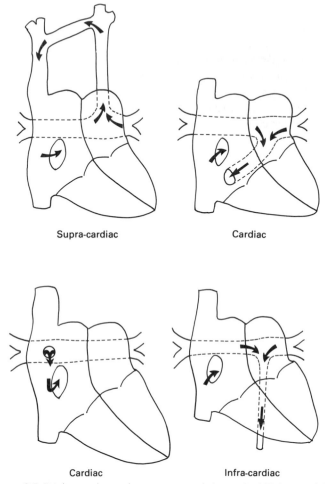

Supra-cardiac   Cardiac

Cardiac   Infra-cardiac

Figure 2.7 Total anomalous pulmonary venous drainage. An ASD is part of the lesion.

the diaphragm, or at the liver if it drains into the portal system. Crying will increase the obstruction and increase cyanosis.

Various combinations of these three are possible (e.g. left lung to vertical vein, right lung direct to RA).

Pathophysiology and symptoms

In many ways the condition is similar to an ASD (left-to-right shunt into RA, pulmonary plethora, RV hypertrophy) but the patients are cyanosed. As in ASD, the LV is usually small, the RV doing the extra shunt work. Most infants also have a PDA. High pulmonary flow in a child causes cardiac failure, recurrent chest infections and poor growth development.

Additional pulmonary venous obstruction causes cyanosis at birth, dyspnoea and early death in pulmonary oedema.

Patients with high pulmonary flow plus a large ASD may be only slightly cyanosed, tolerate the lesion well and survive into adult life.

Physical signs
In patients with no venous obstruction (usually supra-cardiac TAPVD), similar to those in ASD (page 28) with additional:
• cyanosis (mild to moderate, depending on pulmonary flow)
• a continuous murmur (hum) either high up the LSE or in the aortic area; this is the venous hum of high flow in the SVC with TAPVD to the left innominate vein (supracardiac).

In patients with venous obstruction (usually infracardiac TAPVD) look for:
• prominent 'a' wave in JVP with pulmonary hypertension, but difficult to see in babies
• sick infant, vomiting, deeply cyanosed, tachypnoea, CCF
• no murmurs, loud P_2, gallop rhythm.

Chest X-ray
The supracardiac type shows the 'cottage loaf' heart, or the 'snowman in a snowstorm'. The wide upper mediastinal shadow is caused by the dilated SVC and anomalous vein (left SVC) to the left innominate. The pulmonary plethora and pulmonary venous congestion cause the snowstorm appearance. Pulmonary plethora may not be obvious in the neonate. With additional pulmonary venous obstruction there are additional signs of pulmonary oedema. The left ventricle and left atrium are small, thus marked cardiomegaly is uncommon.

ECG
Similar to a secundum ASD in mild cases. With pulmonary hypertension marked RAD and RV hypertrophy occur with P pulmonale and RV strain pattern (T-wave inversion V1–4).

Echocardiography
May be useful in defining cases with pulmonary venous obstruction. Septal motion is paradoxical in patients with high pulmonary flow and

unobstructed pulmonary veins (RV volume overload). In children with pulmonary hypertension and pulmonary venous obstruction, septal motion is usually normal. Two-dimensional echocardiography is useful in defining pulmonary venous anatomy, the venous confluence and the site of drainage.

Differential diagnosis
The sick neonate: consider other pulmonary causes for cyanosis and tachypnoea: (respiratory infection, aspiration of meconium, etc.). Arterial Po_2 should improve by these patients breathing 100% O_2 for 5 min. Echocardiography is helpful.

In cyanosed children with pulmonary plethora on the CXR consider: TGA, primitive ventricle, truncus arteriosus, single atrium.

In patients with gross pulmonary venous obstruction, other causes have to be considered, e.g. cor triatriatum, congenital mitral stenosis.

Cardiac catheterization
Pulmonary angiography with follow through is necessary in order to detect the pulmonary venous anatomy. A saturation run is needed with sampling also in low IVC and left innominate vein. All pulmonary veins must be identified.

If infants are < 2 months old, Rashkind balloon septostomy may help by increasing ASD size and allowing better mixing, with reduction in cyanosis and an increased Po_2.

Surgery
Total correction is necessary for all cases of TAPVD, as there is no long-term palliative operation and medical treatment alone carries about a 90% 1-year mortality. Most of the infracardiac type have some form of venous obstruction and a low cardiac output. This means surgery on a sick infant with a high operative risk (15–20%). Children with a supracardiac or cardiac type with a large ASD and good mixing initially fare better but develop established pulmonary vascular disease unless totally corrected early. Deep hypothermia and total circulatory arrest may be needed for the operation.

Supracardiac type. The common pulmonary vein is anastomosed to the back of LA. ASD is closed and left SVC ligated.

Cardiac type. The inter-atrial septum is refashioned, depending on the exact anatomy, to include the drainage site of the pulmonary veins into the LA. The coronary sinus may be included in the LA.

Infracardiac type. The common pulmonary vein is anastomosed to the back of the LA. The ASD is closed and the descending anomalous vein ligated.

Recurrence of pulmonary venous obstruction post-operatively is uncommon but carries a very poor prognosis.

2.9 Tricuspid atresia

Anatomy (Figure 2.8)

A rare cause of cyanotic heart disease. The tricuspid valve is completely imperforate or more commonly non-existent, being replaced by muscle and/or fibrous tissue. Systemic venous blood crosses an essential ASD into a large LA and LV. The mitral valve is usually normal. The circuit is usually completed by a VSD. Blood flows from left to right through this VSD into a small RV into the pulmonary arteries. Pulmonary flow may be limited by pulmonary stenosis or too small a VSD. There may in addition be a coarctation or a PDA.

Pathophysiology and symptoms

There are two main types of tricuspid atresia which dictate the early symptoms:

• *Common type*: normal great vessel position (normal ventriculo-arterial connections). Usually have pulmonary stenosis, with poor pulmonary flow, small pulmonary arteries or a small VSD.

The poor pulmonary flow in infancy results in intense cyanosis from birth. Cyanosis may deteriorate after the first year, with the additional development of infundibular stenosis resulting in cyanotic attacks.

CXR shows small heart, straight right heart border and oligaemic lung fields. ECG shows RA strain, left axis deviation and LV hypertrophy. This pattern is uncommon in cyanotic congenital heart disease (see second table on page 19).

• *Less common type*: transposed great vessels (discordant ventriculo-arterial connections). PA arises from LV and is of good size with no pulmonary stenosis. As the PVR falls in the first few weeks of life, pulmonary flow increases (unrestricted by pulmonary stenosis), the circulation becomes hyperdynamic with pulmonary congestion and possible additional mitral regurgitation (functional from a dilated LV and mitral annulus). If uncorrected, patients develop congestive cardiac failure (mostly LV) and pulmonary vascular disease.

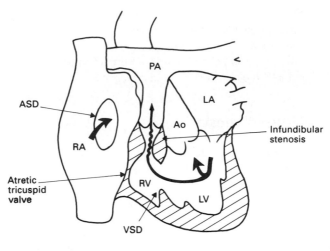

Fontan Operation

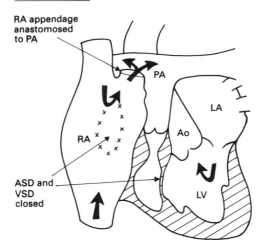

Figure 2.8 Tricuspid atresia.

CXR shows a large heart with pulmonary plethora and congestion. ECG shows normal or even right axis.

Echocardiography

This is vital. It shows one large AV valve (mitral). Large RA with bulging septum into LA. Connections of the great vessels and size of VSD should be seen. Doppler studies will quantify degree of mitral regurgitation and presence of a possible PDA.

Cardiac catheterization

The most important pieces of information that cannot be established with the two-dimensional echo are the PA pressure and anatomy (and ? subpulmonary stenosis). Unfortunately it is commonly impossible to reach PA with a catheter if the great vessels are not transposed. The surgeon may have to be content with pictures of the pulmonary arteries from the LV cine. Aortography to check for PDA or coarctation.

Options for surgical treatment

Pulmonary flow too small:

1 Rashkind balloon septostomy if ASD too small.

2 Consider shunt (e.g. bidirectional Glenn, or Blalock) to enlarge pulmonary arteries.

Pulmonary flow too great:

3 PA banding in first year of life.

All with a view to:

4 Fontan operation, 'total correction' from about age 2 years onwards.

The Fontan operation

The systemic and venous circulations are separated using the LV as the systemic pumping chamber, dispensing with the small RV and connecting the right atrial appendage directly to the right or divided main pulmonary artery. The ASD and VSD are closed. Blood from the venae cavae thus flows to RA → PA → PV → LA → LV → aorta. There are a variety of modifications of the Fontan procedure depending on the exact great vessel anatomy. Caval valves are unnecessary. The best results occur if:

• child still in sinus rhythm with minimal atrial dysrhythmias
• normal or low PA pressures with low PVR
• good LV function
• minimal or no mitral regurgitation.

With the best haemodynamics to start with, operative mortality is now < 10%, but late complications do occur and atrial arrhythmias can prove a major problem. Cardiac output falls sharply if the child develops atrial fibrillation with signs and symptoms of right heart failure. Long-term anti-arrhythmics may be needed to attempt to maintain sinus rhythm.

2.10 Cyanotic congenital heart disease in the adult

In adults, inoperable cyanotic congenital heart disease is usually due to the Eisenmenger situation with PA pressure at systemic level and bidirectional shunting through an ASD, VSD or patent ductus arteriosus. It may also be caused by incompletely corrected Fallot's tetralogy, or more rarely Ebstein's anomaly, pulmonary atresia or truncus.

In a few young patients, heart–lung transplantation has offered the only hope of a cure for the Eisenmenger syndrome. Early results are good and at least one woman has had a child following heart–lung transplantation.

Careful follow up of these patients is essential because there are also a great number of non-cardiac problems which must be considered.

Polycythaemia

This is due to erythropoietin production secondary to chronic hypoxaemia. Although theoretically physiological, it is counterproductive as it results in hyperviscosity and hypervolaemia. This results in headaches, blurred vision and a 'muzzy' head. Patients appear plethoric with suffused conjunctivae. Retinal veins are engorged and tortuous. Pruritus may be a nuisance particularly after getting out of a hot bath. More serious complications include venous (and less often arterial) thrombosis, gout and peptic ulceration.

Regular venesection is usually necessary and should aim to keep the packed cell volume (PCV) between 0.5 and 0.55 (50–55%). Two drip lines are required for simultaneous venesection and the administration of the same volume of a plasma expander/colloid. It is important to avoid any fall in circulating volume. A strict aseptic technique is required as these patients often have acne and are vulnerable to infection. Generally it is sensible just to remove one unit of blood (450–500 ml) over 1–2 h and to measure the PCV the following day once equilibration has occurred.

Following venesection, the patient should feel improved with a clearer head, better exercise tolerance, less dyspnoea and a better appetite.

It is better to decide on venesection on the basis of the PCV rather than the haemoglobin level. Iron deficiency may develop with repeated venesection. If iron therapy is administered the patient may rapidly become polycythaemic again. There is a fine balance between excessive

venesecting causing dyspnoea from anaemia and inadequate
venesection causing it from hyperviscosity.

Bleeding disorders
Paradoxically in a condition where thrombosis is common, bleeding
abnormalities also occur. Platelet function may be abnormal and
clotting factors may be deficient. Occult gastrointestinal bleeding
(peptic ulceration) and haemoptysis may in part be due to this. Fresh
frozen plasma and/or platelet transfusions may be needed especially
pre- and postcardiac catheterization or surgery.

Dental hygiene
Frequent visits to the dentist are often necessary, since adults may
contract periodontal disease and gingivitis. A dental brace is a
particular hazard for this group, with the risks of infected gums
seeding the circulation and causing a cerebral abscess.

Skin
Acne is a common problem and septic foci must be treated early.
Long-term tetracycline therapy may be indicated.

Cerebral abscess
This is a recognized hazard of dental or skin sepsis, the passage of
bacteria across a septal defect being due to the bidirectional shunt. The
development of neurological symptoms or signs, drowsiness or a
pyrexia of unknown origin (PUO) requires urgent investigation, a
cerebral CT scan and a neurological expert.

Gout
A common complaint that can usually be managed with long-term
allopurinol 100–300 mg od. Renal function must be checked in these
patients.

Pregnancy and contraception
This is contraindicated as it carries a very high maternal mortality
(> 60% with Eisenmenger VSDs). Spontaneous abortion is very
common. It is very important to give early and clear contraceptive
advice to all women with cyanotic congenital heart disease. The pill is
best avoided (thrombosis risk). The intrauterine contraceptive device is
best avoided (bleeding and endocarditis risk). The best advice is

sterilization by tubal ligation. This is probably achieved most safely by a mini-laparotomy rather than by a laparascopic technique.

In the very unlikely event of a woman refusing all this advice and coming to term the outlook is grim. Caesarian section should be considered electively at 36–38 weeks with great care paid to volume replacement and oxygenation. Epidural anaesthesia has been recommended rather than a general anaesthetic (see below) but the systemic vascular resistance must not fall.

High altitudes
Heights of > 1000 m should be avoided unless inhaled oxygen is available. Patients should receive inhaled oxygen throughout commercial flights and should avoid flights in light aircraft without oxygen.

Vigorous exercise
Should be avoided. Right-to-left shunting may increase as systemic vascular resistance falls with muscle bed dilatation. Arrhythmias and sudden death have been provoked by effort.

Antibiotic prophylaxis
Routinely given prior to any dental or surgical procedure.

General anaesthesia
Is not contraindicated but may be hazardous. Dehydration and hypotension must be avoided, with the risk of increasing the right-to-left shunt. Ketamine 1–2 mg/kg is a good drug for induction, having little effect on systemic or pulmonary vascular resistance. Volume replacement and small doses of phenylephrine (2 µg/kg) may be needed to keep up the arterial pressure. Postoperative heparinization will help prevent venous thrombosis.

Heart–lung transplantation (see also page 259)
With a very limited donor supply it is sensible to refer patients who may be suitable for this early rather than to wait for a crisis. Patients generally should be < 50 years old. Results are not as good as for heart transplantation alone. The main indication for this is a rapid deterioration in symptoms, e.g.
- end-stage pulmonary vascular disease
- frequent haemoptysis
- syncope at rest

- refractory arrhythmias
- severe hypoxaemia causing angina
- refractory right heart failure.

Single-lung transplantation with correction of the intracardiac defect may be a possibility in the younger patient who is deteriorating. The results of this operation are not yet quite as good as combined heart and lung transplantation. Problems with with the single lung transplant include postoperative early pulmonary oedema in the transplanted lung, breakdown of the bronchial anastomosis and late obliterative bronchiolitis.

Relative contraindications to transplantation include:
- malignant disease
- moderate or severe renal or hepatic dysfunction (creatinine clearance < 50 ml/min)
- severe chest deformity
- previous lung resection or pleurectomy
- positive serology (HIV, hepatitis B or C)
- pulmonary aspergillosis
- active infection
- on high-dose steroids
- multisystem disease, e.g. diabetes, collagen vascular disease, etc.
- active peptic ulceration
- peripheral vascular disease
- psychiatric condition, drug or alcohol abuser.

The final decision is team based and also involves assessment of the patient's social circumstances, family support, etc. Both the patient and his/her family need to know both the risks of the operation, and the subsequent management which places considerable demands on them.

3 Valve Disease

3.1) Acute rheumatic fever

Although there has been a sharp reduction in the incidence of rheumatic fever this century in the western world, it is still the cause of nearly half of the cardiac disease in the Third world, especially in the younger age groups. The decline of the disease in the UK has been ascribed partly to a reduction in virulence of the *Streptococcus*, partly to the reduction in overcrowding and improved living conditions, and partly to the early use of antibiotics for tonsillitis by general practitioners. We should not get complacent about rheumatic fever and think of it as a disease of the past: new cases still occur in the UK and recently there have been several outbreaks in the USA, not necessarily confined to the poorer areas. Peak age is 5–15 years. The disease is rare under the age of 5 years. It tends to be a recurrent illness unless prevented, with patients often having three or more attacks by the age of 20 years.

Aetiology
Pharyngeal infection with Lancefield Group A streptococci triggers a subsequent attack of rheumatic fever about 2 to 3 weeks later in > 3% of children.

Antigenic mimicry is thought to be the most likely explanation. A carbohydrate in the cell wall of the Group A *Streptococcus* is similar to a glycoprotein in the human cardiac valve. It is thought an autoimmune reaction occurs. Antibodies to the streptococcal cell wall cross-react with valve tissue: hence the latent period after the initial pharyngeal infection while the antibody response is mounted. Other cross-reacting antibodies have been found: one cross-reacting with the myocardial sarcolemma could account for the myocarditis, and another to the caudate nucleus for Sydenham's chorea. Anti-heart antibodies found during an acute attack may be cause or effect.

Diagnosis
This is purely clinical. The Jones criteria (1944) have been revised several times and are shown below. For diagnosis there must be:
- evidence of a preceding beta-haemolytic *Streptococcus* infection
- two major criteria, or
- one major and two minor criteria.

Revised Jones criteria for rheumatic fever diagnosis are listed in the table.

Major	Minor	In addition
Carditis	Fever	Recent streptococcal infection
Arthritis	Previous rheumatic fever	History of scarlet fever
Sydenham's chorea	Raised ESR or CRP	Positive throat swab
Erythema marginatum	Arthralgia	Raised ASO titre
Subcutaneous nodules	Long PR interval	Raised anti-DNase B titre

The differential diagnosis includes acute juvenile arthritis (Still's disease), a connective tissue disease, infective endocarditis serum sickness, drug hypersensitivity and many viral illnesses causing pericarditis. Children frequently present with a fever and joint pains and have a soft innocent mid-systolic flow murmur and a third heart sound. These alone are very non-specific.

Rheumatic fever can affect any of the cardiac tissues. It causes a pancarditis: pericardium, myocardium (including the conduction tissue) and endocardium (including the valves). The histological marker is the Aschoff node (1904), which may persist in the myocardium long after the disease is over. They were found in the atrial appendage of patients who had a closed mitral valvotomy.

Clinical features

Carditis and arthritis are the only common features.

• *Carditis*. Usually causes no symptoms in first attack. The commonest evidence is a soft pericardial rub or a soft apical pansystolic murmur of mitral regurgitation. An early diastolic murmur is very unusual in a first attack. Valve stenosis does not occur at this stage. There may be a soft mid-diastolic murmur (Carey Coombes) but this does not necessarily indicate subsequent mitral stenosis. There may be a small pericardial effusion but tamponade or constriction does not occur. A prolonged PR interval on the ECG is non-specific.

• *Arthritis*. A migrating polyarthritis usually of larger joints: flitting from one joint to another. It does not cause chronic arthritis. If arthritis is used as a major criterion for the diagnosis, arthralgia cannot be used as a minor one.

• *Nodules*. Small (often smaller than a pea), mobile and painless on extensor surfaces of elbows, wrists, ankles and spine. They are rare (probably < 5% of cases).

• *Erythema marginatum*. Also unusual. This occurs mainly on the trunk

but not on the face. It is an evanescent geographical-type rash with slightly raised red edges and a clear centre. The patches change shape with time. It does not itch and is not indurated.
• *Sydenham's chorea (St Vitus' dance)*. Does not occur for several months after rheumatic fever. Unilateral or bilateral involuntary quasi-purposeful movements sometimes associated with facial grimacing. Since the initial illness is easily missed this may be the first manifestation of the disease.

Investigations
There are no specific tests. ESR, and C-reactive protein, anti-streptolysin O and anti-deoxyribonuclease B titres are measured and should be raised, or be rising on the second estimate. Anti-hyaluronidase antibody also serves as a measure of previous streptococcal infection. The echo is used to detect the very early changes of stretching of the anterior mitral chordae.

Treatment
Treatment with salicylates or steroids does not prevent the development of subsequent rheumatic heart disease. It is important to establish the diagnosis, which may mean waiting until arthritis or carditis is definite.
• Salicylates rapidly reduce fever and arthritis. Dose is 100 mg/kg/day in children. Serum salicylate levels should be 15–20 mg/100 ml. Toxicity produces tinnitus and hyperventilation.
• Steroids are used rather than salicylates for patients with definite carditis. Prednisolone approximately 3 mg/kg/day in divided doses for 2 weeks tapering off quickly. If symptoms recur the course is restarted.
• Diazepam is used for Sydenham's chorea. Neither salicylates nor steroids have any effect on this.
• Penicillin. Immediate treatment with benzathine penicillin 1.2 million units i.m. Eliminates any remaining streptococci. Prevention of further attacks by using penicillin V (phenoxymethyl penicillin) 250 mg bd on a regular basis until the patient is considered beyond risk (e.g. up to the age of 30 years). For penicillin hypersensitivity use sulphadiazine 500 mg bd.

Most cases settle within 4–6 weeks. Occasional cases need longer courses of therapy plus treatment for congestive cardiac failure. Long term myocardial damage is often forgotten in the concentration on valve lesions.

Mitral stenosis

This is almost always secondary to rheumatic fever, although only half the patients have a positive history. The incidence is declining although many cases from the third world are severe. Two-thirds of patients are female.

Aetiology

Valvar

1 Rheumatic. Almost all cases. All the rest are rare.
2 Congenital: isolated lesion or associated with ASD (Lutembacher's syndrome). Some of these cases may be rheumatic mitral stenosis plus a patent foramen ovale.
3 Mucopolysaccharidoses. Hurler's syndrome. Glycoprotein deposition on the mitral leaflets.
4 Endocardial fibroelastosis spreading on to the valve.
5 Prosthetic valve. Usually only in mechanical valves (e.g. Starr–Edwards, Björk–Shiley).
6 Malignant carcinoid.

Inflow obstruction
Conditions which mimic mitral stenosis, e.g.
• left atrial myxoma
• left atrial ball valve thrombus
• hypertrophic obstructive cardiomyopathy (page 127)
• cor triatriatum (stenosis of a common pulmonary vein).

Pathogenesis
Group A (usually Type 12) streptococci have cell wall antigens which cross-react with structural glycoproteins of the heart valves. Very small nodules (macrophages and fibroblasts) develop on the valve edge and the cusp gradually thickens. Stenosis occurs at three levels:
• commissures: these fuse with the valve cusps still mobile
• cusps: the valve leaflets become thick and eventually calcified
• chordae: these fuse, shorten and thicken.
    A combination of all three results in a 'fish-mouth' buttonhole orifice.

Pathophysiology and symptoms
1 Dyspnoea on effort: orthopnoea and PND. A rising left atrial pressure is transmitted to pulmonary veins. Secondary pulmonary

arterial hypertension results. Pulmonary oedema may be precipitated by:
- development of uncontrolled AF
- pregnancy
- exercise
- chest infection
- emotional stress
- anaesthesia.

2 Fatigue: due to low cardiac output in moderate-to-severe stenosis. A doubling of cardiac output quadruples the mitral valve gradient. The loss of atrial transport when AF develops results in a fall in cardiac output. Exercise tolerance on the basis of four classes is based on the New York Heart Association criteria (see page 4).

3 Haemoptysis. May be due to:
- bronchial vein rupture: 'pulmonary apoplexy', large haemorrhage but not usually life threatening
- alveolar capillary rupture: pink frothy sputum in pulmonary oedema
- pulmonary infarction: in low output states and immobile patients
- blood-stained sputum: in chronic bronchitis associated with attacks of dyspnoea.

4 Systemic emboli: in 20–30%.

Thrombus develops in large 'stagnant' left atrium and atrial appendage, mainly in patients with AF, low output and large atria. It may be the presenting symptom. Mesenteric, saddle and iliofemoral emboli are common. Ball valve thrombus may occur in LA.

5 Chronic bronchitis: common in MS. Due to oedematous bronchial mucosa.

6 Chest pain: like angina. In patients with RV hypertrophy secondary to pulmonary hypertension – even with normal coronaries. Coronary embolism may occur.

7 Palpitations: paroxysmal AF with fast ventricular response.

8 Symptoms of right heart failure: pulmonary hypertension and possible functional tricuspid regurgitation: hepatic pain on effort (hepatic angina), ascites, ankle and leg oedema.

9 Symptoms of left atrial enlargement compressing other structures:
- left recurrent laryngeal nerve, hoarseness (Ortner's syndrome)
- oesophagus, dysphagia (beware potassium replacement tablets causing oesophageal ulceration)
- left main bronchus, very rarely causing left lung collapse.

10 Infective endocarditis (page 373): rare in pure mitral stenosis.

Physical signs (Figure 3.1)

1 S_1 loud, as mitral valve is open throughout diastole and is suddenly slammed shut by ventricular systole. It indicates mobile leaflets.

2 A_2–OS interval shortens with increasing severity of stenosis. LA pressure 'climbs' up LV pressure curve approaching in time aortic valve closure. (See cardiac catheterization, page 496.)

3 The length of the diastolic murmur is an indication of the severity of stenosis.

Differential diagnosis

1 Causes of inflow obstruction (HCM, LA myxoma, ball-valve thrombus).

2 Causes of rumbling mitral or tricuspid diastolic murmur:
  • aortic regurgitation (page 99; Austin–Flint)

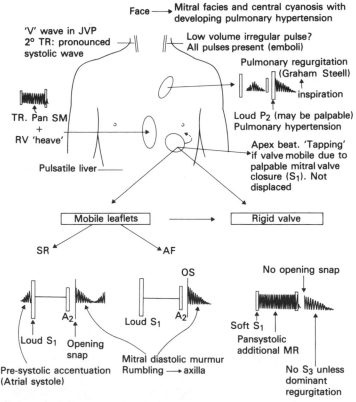

Figure 3.1 Physical signs of mitral stenosis.

- flow murmur in ASD, this may be confusing (see Figure 3.2)
- tricuspid stenosis, diastolic murmur accentuated by inspiration, best sign is slow 'y' descent on JVP.

3 Causes of early diastolic sound resembling opening snap:
- constrictive pericarditis } sudden cessation of early
- restrictive myopathy   } rapid ventricular filling.

4 Causes of loud S_1: tachycardia and hyperdynamic states (valve still open at end diastole, and forceful closure by hypercontractile LV).

ECG
Atrial fibrillation (in sinus rhythm P mitrale). RV hypertrophy. Small voltage in lead V1. Progressive right axis deviation.

Echocardiography (see **12.3**)
In pure mitral stenosis with mobile leaflets this obviates the need for cardiac catheterization. It may show:
- thickened mitral leaflets with the posterior leaflet moving anteriorly in diastole. Mitral opening coincides with snap on phonocardiogram.
- reduced diastolic closure rate (E–F) slope of mitral anterior leaflet
- small LV (unless additional MR present). Slow diastolic filling
- pulmonary valve may be flat with absent 'a' wave opening (in pulmonary hypertension)
- calcification of mitral leaflets or mitral annulus.

Echocardiography is also very useful in distinguishing the 'mimics' of mitral stenosis. It will diagnose a left atrial myxoma, HCM and aortic regurgitation. It is very useful as a guide to the severity of mitral stenosis and to document the results of mitral valvotomy. The mobility of the mitral leaflets is easily seen with this technique.

Cardiac catheterization
Should be unnecessary in young patient with a mobile valve and no signs of mitral regurgitation. It is contraindicated in pregnancy when echocardiography is essential. A patient with atrial myxoma diagnosed

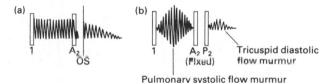

Figure 3.2 Similarity on auscultation between: (a) mixed mitral valve disease, and (b) ASD.

by echo should not be catheterized. (The LV catheter may knock fragments off a prolapsing myxoma.) A myxoma requires urgent surgery.

Cardiac catheterization is advisable in patients who have had a previous valvotomy in order to assess the mitral valve and the degree of regurgitation. It is necessary in patients with signs of mitral regurgitation. Doppler echocardiography can be diagnostic. See **12.3**.

Catheterization is also required in patients with signs of other valve disease, symptoms of angina (coronary angiography), signs of severe pulmonary hypertension and when the mitral valve is calcified on CXR (Figure 3.3). If mitral valve replacement is envisaged, coronary angiography is usually performed (especially in the elderly).

The mean mitral gradient is calculated at rest and, if this is low, also on exercise (straight-leg raising). The mitral valve area can be calculated if the cardiac output is measured (page 496).

Medical treatment

1 Digoxin: in atrial fibrillation only. If fast AF is not slowed by standard doses, either a small dose of verapamil or beta-blocking agent should be added. There is no evidence that digoxin prevents the development of AF in patients who are still in sinus rhythm.

2 Diuretics are necessary to reduce preload and pulmonary venous congestion. They may help delay the need for surgery.

3 Anticoagulants are still controversial. They should be used in patients who:

- have had a previous systemic/pulmonary embolism
- have a mitral prosthesis (tissue or mechanical)
- have low-output states with right heart failure

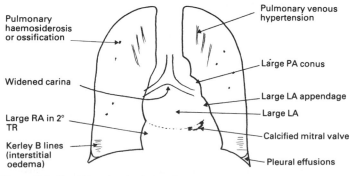

Figure 3.3 Chest X-ray in mitral stenosis.

- are in AF with moderate mitral stenosis and who have not had an atrial appendicectomy.

Anticoagulants are not of proven benefit in sinus rhythm. They should be avoided in pregnancy if possible (see page 112). Patients who have had a mitral valvotomy and atrial appendicectomy can probably be managed without anticoagulants provided they do not fall into the above categories.

Cardioversion (pages 318–320)

May be attempted if the development of AF is recent and the patient is anticoagulated. If not, there is a risk of systemic emboli.

Heparinization for 24 hours prior to cardioversion is not adequate. There is nothing to be gained by repeated cardioversions. AF should be accepted and the ventricular rate slowed. Amiodarone or flecainide may help prevent the development of AF in patients who have been successfully cardioverted.

Infective endocarditis (page 373)

Is rare in pure mitral stenosis.

Acute rheumatic fever

Should be thought of in any young patient presenting for the first time with mitral stenosis. Histology of the atrial appendage will help in diagnosis. Prevent further attacks with penicillin 250 mg bd or sulphadiazine 500 mg bd. It should be continued in young women to age 40 years.

Intervention

Symptomatic decline in mitral stenosis is gradual but the development of atrial fibrillation usually causes a sharp deterioration in symptoms. Some form of intervention is needed in those patients with Class 3 or 4 NYHA effort tolerance and some patients with Class 2 who find it difficult to work or to manage the housework. Mitral valve area of < 1 cm^2 is an indication for intervention. This now consists of mitral valvuloplasty, open mitral valvotomy or mitral valve replacement. There is still no perfect mitral prosthesis, and intervention aims to preserve where possible the native mitral valve, especially in the younger patient.

Mitral valvuloplasty

The development of the Inoue balloon is a great advance from the original double-balloon and two-wire technique, and mitral valvuloplasty has now replaced the operation of closed mitral valvotomy. It is the technique of choice for patients with pure mitral stenosis but no regurgitation or mitral valve calcification. It can be performed in any age group, however, the results are best in the younger age group where the subvalve mitral chordae have not become thickened and fused. It can be performed in the mid-trimester of pregnancy.

Prior to mitral valvuloplasty it is important to establish with trans-oesophageal echocardiography that there is no thrombus in the left atrial appendage. Transthoracic echocardiography cannot be relied on for this information. Valvuloplasty is avoided with:
- left atrial or left ventricular thrombus
- history of systemic emboli
- more than Grade 1 mitral regurgitation
- thickened rigid mitral leaflets
- thickened fused mitral chordae
- moderate or severe mitral calcification.

Figure 3.4 shows the technique. The procedure only requires light sedation, as with a routine cardiac catheter. The choice of balloon size (26, 28 or 30 mm) is dictated by the patient's height (see table).

Patient height (cm)	Maximum balloon diameter (mm)
≤ 147	24
> 147	26
> 160	28
> 180	30

Following trans-septal puncture via the right femoral vein, the Inoue balloon is advanced into the left atrium over a curly guide wire (Figure 3.4a). The distal portion of the balloon is inflated slightly and the balloon advanced to the apex of the left ventricle (Figure 3.4b). The balloon is then gradually withdrawn until it is positioned across the mitral valve and free of the subvalve apparatus (Figure 3.4c). On balloon inflation the distal portion inflates first, then the proximal portion to form an hourglass shape with the waist across the mitral valve (Figure 3.4d). Finally, with continuing inflation the waist disappears and the commissures are split. The residual mitral valve gradient is measured directly and the degree of mitral regurgitation, if any, assessed by left ventriculography or Doppler echocardiography. In correctly selected patients the results are startlingly good with at least a doubling of the valve area. A tiny ASD is left but this is of no

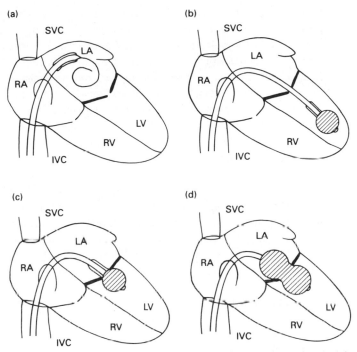

(a) (b)

(c) (d)

Figure 3.4 Stages in mitral valvuloplasty (a) The balloon is advanced to the left atrium via a trans-septal puncture and curly guide wire through the fossa ovalis. (b) The guide wire is withdrawn, the distal portion of the balloon is inflated and advanced to the left ventricle. (c) The balloon is drawn back to the mitral valve. (d) The balloon is fully inflated. The proximal portion of the balloon now inflates forming an hourglass shape, and this waist finally disappears with maximum inflation.

significance and the shunt is trivial if any. Long-term results cannot be quoted yet but the procedure is considered as good as a closed valvotomy with benefit expected for 10–15 years.

An echocardiographc score has been devised which is useful prognostically. Valve leaflet mobility, thickening, calcification and subvalve chordal thickening are graded 0–4 and added together (worst possible score 16). High scores (> 8) fare badly. A low LVEDP is also important as a good prognostic indicator.

Surgery

1 *Closed mitral valvotomy (closed commissurotomy).* Performed through a left thoracotomy without bypass. Rarely performed now due to the development of mitral valvuloplasty. The contraindications to a closed valvotomy are the same as for valvuloplasty (see above), but include also patients with severe lung disease or chest deformity and the elderly frail patient in whom a valvuloplasty may still be possible.

2 *Open mitral valvotomy (open commissurotomy).* Performed on cardiopulmonary bypass through a median sternotomy. It is used in patients who have already had a mitral procedure (previous closed valvotomy or valvuloplasty) or in whom there are other features: e.g. mild mitral regurgitation or calcification, a history of emboli, demonstrable thrombus in the left atrium, or in whom there is concern about the subvalve chordae.

3 *Mitral valve replacement.* Needed for heavily calcified and rigid mitral valves, those with unacceptable mitral regurgitation, severe chordal thickening and fusion or two previous valvotomies or valvuloplasties.

Mitral restenosis occurs over a period of years following valvuloplasty or valvotomy. It is due to turbulent flow across thickened valve leaflets resulting in platelet and fibrin deposition. It is least likely to occur where a good valvuloplasty or valvotomy with pliable leaflets results in good mitral flow. Early restenosis (within 5 years) usually means an inadequate valvuloplasty or valvotomy. Patients may do well with an open valvotomy. Late restenosis may need valve replacement due to degenerative change and calcification in the valve.

3.3 Mitral regurgitation

This may be due to abnormalities of the mitral annulus, the mitral leaflets, the chordae or the papillary muscles. Chordal or papillary muscle dysfunction is subvalvar mitral regurgitation. Many disease processes affect the valve at more than one level.

Aetiology (see table on page 80)

Functional mitral regurgitation
Is probably a combination of mitral annulus dilatation and papillary muscle malalignment. It occurs in LV dilatation from any cause, commonly in dilated cardiomyopathy (DCM) and ischaemic heart disease.

Annulus calcification
Occurs in the elderly and is more common in females, diabetics and patients with Paget's disease. It commonly affects the posterior part of

the mitral annulus and is often visible as a calcified band at the back of the heart on the lateral chest X-ray with calcium in the posterior AV groove. The calcium may involve the mitral leaflets, causing mitral regurgitation, and eventually the conducting system. Very severe ring calcification may make mitral valve replacement impossible. In its milder form it causes no mitral valve problem and may be a chance finding on CXR or echocardiography.

Mitral annular calcification is an independent risk factor for stroke with a relative risk twice that of controls. This is independent of other risk factors such as AF, or congestive cardiac failure.

Valvar regurgitation
Is commonly due either to rheumatic fever, infective endocarditis or the floppy valve. In rheumatic causes the cusps are thickened, with fused commissures and often a 'fish-mouth' orifice. Patients commonly have combined MS and MR.

Chordal rupture
Is often idiopathic. Myxomatous degeneration in the floppy valve syndrome may also involve the chordae, which stretch and eventually rupture. Ischaemia may cause chordal rupture.

Papillary muscle dysfunction
Inferior infarction commonly causes posterior papillary muscle dysfunction with characteristic signs (see below). Anterior papillary muscle dysfunction is much rarer and signifies a large anterior infarct with probable additional right coronary artery disease.

The floppy valve
This forms a spectrum of conditions from an asymptomatic patient with a mid-systolic click, to one with severe mitral regurgitation from chordal rupture. (It has also been called: mitral leaflet prolapse, mitral click systolic murmur syndrome, Barlow's syndrome, myxomatous degeneration of the mitral valve, billowing mitral valve syndrome.) It occurs as the following:
• an isolated lesion often in asymptomatic patients
• associated with other conditions, e.g. secundum ASD, Turner's syndrome, PDA, Marfan's syndrome, osteogenesis imperfecta, pseudoxanthoma elasticum, cardiomyopathy, WPW syndrome

It occurs in approximately 4% of the normal asymptomatic population It has been grossly overdiagnosed echocardiographically and is a cause of cardiac neurosis. It is due to progressive stretching of

Aetiology of mitral regurgitation

Mitral annulus	Mitral leaflets	Chordae	Papillary muscles
Senile calcification	*Infective*	*Elongation/rupture*	*Dysfunction/rupture*
Degeneration	Endocarditis	Marfan	Ischaemia
Functional dilatation	Rheumatic	Ischaemia	Infarction
Ring abscesses		Endocarditis	Abscess
Marfan		Trauma	Infiltrations
	Congenital	Rheumatic	Sarcoid
	1° ASD	Idiopathic	Amyloid
	AV canal	Ehlers–Danlos	Myocarditis
	Clefts	Parachute MV	Hurler's
	Perforations		
	Absence		*Malalignment*
	(2° ASD)		LV dilatation}
			LV aneurysm
	Connective tissues disorders		HCM
	Marfan		Endocardial
	PXE		fibroelastosis
	Osteogenesis imperfecta		Corrected TGA
	Ehlers–Danlos		

Floppy valve

the mitral leaflets, with weakening due to acid mucopolysaccharide deposition in the zona spongiosa. The chordae are also involved. Tricuspid prolapse may coexist.

- Some patients have non-specific atypical chest pain (non-anginal) and palpitations.
- Infective endocarditis prophylaxis is necessary for those patients with a murmur. An isolated mid-systolic click does not merit them.
- Rarely, complications develop, for example: progressive mitral regurgitation requiring MVR, cerebral emboli, dysrhythmias may be ventricular with associated re-entry and pre-excitation pathways, sudden death.

Pathophysiology and symptoms

Mild cases of MR may be asymptomatic for many years. Most patients fall into one of two groups depending on the time course of events, and the size/compliance of the left atrium.

In acute MR the small LA cannot absorb the regurgitant fraction and the systolic wave is transmitted to the pulmonary veins, with resulting acute pulmonary oedema. In long-standing MR the LA is large, it can absorb the regurgitant fraction and the 'v' wave transmitted to the pulmonary veins is small. See table below.

Symptoms are similar to mitral stenosis in the chronic state. Haemoptysis and systemic emboli are less frequent.

Generally, pulmonary hypertension and right heart symptoms are not as frequent in MR as in pure MS. Infective endocarditis is more common in MR, however.

Acute	Chronic
Sudden onset dyspnoea and pulmonary oedema	Chronic dyspnoea and fatigue
Small LA. 'Non-compliant'	Large LA. 'Compliant'
Usually still in SR	Usually in AF
? Apical thrill if chordal rupture	? Associated mitral stenosis
Often ejection quality systolic murmur	Pansystolic murmur
Pulmonary hypertension	Pulmonary hypertension less severe
Large 'v' wave in wedge trace	Lower 'v' wave on wedge trace except on effort

Common causes	
Chordal rupture	Rheumatic valve
Acute inferior infarction with posterior papillary muscle dysfunction (rupture is rarer)	Floppy valve
	Functional MR
Infective endocarditis	

Physical signs in the floppy valve syndrome

These vary with the degree of mitral regurgitation. With mild or moderate degrees of mitral regurgitation, signs peculiar to the floppy valve syndrome are shown below. With severe regurgitation physical signs are less specific.

Apex beat

A double apex may be noted in some patients with a floppy valve Tensing of the chordae in mid systole may cause this mid-systolic dip. It is best felt when the patient is lying on his or her left side.

Murmurs

As LV volume diminishes in mid systole the floppy valve starts to prolapse and a mid-systolic click (tensing of chordae) often precedes the murmur of mitral regurgitation (there may be more than one click). In very mild cases a mid-systolic click with no murmur is common.

The smaller the ventricle the earlier the systolic click and the longer the murmur, which gets louder up to S_2. The signs may be altered by various manoeuvres in a similar way to HCM (page 130) (Figure 3.5).

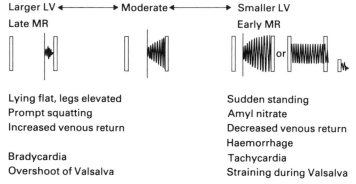

Larger LV ←————→ Moderate ←————→ Smaller LV
Late MR   Early MR

Lying flat, legs elevated   Sudden standing
Prompt squatting   Amyl nitrate
Increased venous return   Decreased venous return
                                                  Haemorrhage
Bradycardia   Tachycardia
Overshoot of Valsalva   Straining during Valsalva

Figure 3.5 Mitral regurgitation in the floppy valve syndrome.

Differential diagnosis

1 *Aortic valve stenosis:* the floppy valve has a normal or slightly collapsing pulse. The mid-systolic click occurs after the carotid upstroke.

2 *HCM:* this is more difficult because both may have similar pulses, double apex beats and murmurs getting louder on amyl nitrate inhalation. HCM does not have a mid-systolic click and more LV+.

3 *VSD:* here the murmur is usually pansystolic with a thrill both maximum at the left sternal edge. Differentiation from subvalvar regurgitation with posterior chordal rupture may be impossible clinically, especially if associated with myocardial infarction.

4 *Papillary muscle dysfunction:* classically postinferior infarct. The murmur may be late systolic but without a click. In more the severe cases the murmur is pansystolic.

5 *Tricuspid regurgitation:* an 'inspiratory' murmur loudest at the left sternal edge. Best sign is prominent systolic waves in the JVP.

Physical signs in chronic valvar mitral regurgitation (Figure 3.6)

1 Sudden premature ventricular emptying due to MR results in early aortic valve closure. The murmur may continue through A_2. S_2 is thus more than normally split and P_2 may be loud if additional pulmonary hypertension is present.

2 Features to suggest chordal rupture as opposed to valvar regurgitation:
- sinus rhythm
- apical thrill in systole

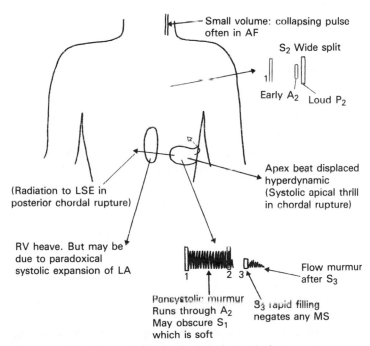

Figure 3.6 Physical signs in chronic valvar mitral regurgitation.

• murmur is more ejection in quality and sometimes mid- to late systolic.

3 In posterior chordal rupture the jet is directed to the anterior wall of the left atrium. The murmur is often loudest at the left sternal edge. In anterior chordal rupture the jet is directed posteriorly and the murmur may be loudest in the back.

Important points in mitral regurgitation clinically

• The intensity of the systolic murmur is absolutely no guide to the severity of the regurgitation. Prosthetic valve regurgitation may be inaudible.

• A murmur maximal at the left sternal edge may be mitral regurgitation.

• Mitral regurgitant murmurs may be pansystolic, late-crescendo systolic or ejection systolic in quality.

• Check P_2 moves on inspiration to exclude ASD.

ECG

1 AF in chronic disease. If in SR: LA+.

2 Left ventricular hypertrophy.

3 A few cases show right ventricular hypertrophy in addition.

Echocardiography

1 To show left atrial size with systolic expansion.

2 May show a flail mitral leaflet with chaotic movement.

3 May show posterior mitral leaflet prolapse – late or pansystolic: vegetations on mitral valve, mitral annulus calcification.

4 Dilated LV with rapid filling. Dimensions relate to prognosis.

5 Rapid diastolic mitral closure rate (steep E–F slope) due to rapid filling.

6 Mean VCF (circumferential fibre shortening) often increased with good LV function.

7 Possibly additional floppy tricuspid or aortic valves.

8 Doppler will establish size and site of regurgitation jet.

Chest X-ray

• Left ventricular dilatation enlarging the ventricular mass and left heart border.

• LA dilatation in chronic cases. Rarely, giant left atrium may occur with calcified wall.

....

• Mitral valve calcification, signs of pulmonary venous congestion, Kerley B lines as in mitral stenosis.

Cardiac catheterization

Is necessary to confirm the diagnosis and exclude other valve and coronary disease. Left ventricular function is assessed. Coronary angiography is also performed.

The size of the 'v wave in the pulmonary wedge or left atrial pressure trace depends on the severity of mitral regurgitation and the size of the left atrium. In severe cases of acute mitral regurgitation the 'v' wave may reach 50 mmHg or more (Figure 3.7). The height of the 'v' wave increases sharply with effort.

Left ventricular angiography in the 30° right anterior oblique projection will show the severity of the regurgitation. In severe cases the regurgitant jet fills the pulmonary veins in one systole. The angiogram will also help identify the cause. In rheumatic mitral regurgitation there are usually one or more discrete jets through an immobile valve with associated stenosis.

In the floppy valve or chordal rupture the regurgitant jet is over a broad front, and the prolapsing leaflet can usually be seen. Posterior papillary muscle dysfunction is usually associated with inferior

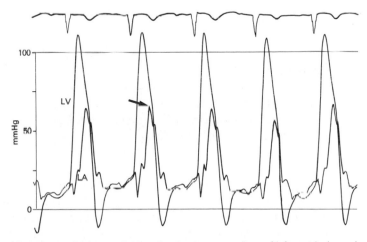

Figure 3.7 Mitral regurgitation. Simultaneous recordings of left ventricular and left atrial pressures (recorded from PA wedge position) in a patient with acute mitral regurgitation from ruptured chordae. The 'v' wave reaches 60 mmHg due to the severe regurgitation and the small left atrium. The patient is still in sinus rhythm. The peak of the 'v' wave is arrowed.

hypokinesia. Spurious mitral regurgitation may be produced by ectopic beats or by a catheter too near the mitral valve or subvalve apparatus.

Medical treatment (page 225; heart failure)
• As in mitral stenosis fast AF is treated with digoxin.
• Anticoagulants are not indicated unless there is: a history of systemic embolism; a prosthetic mitral valve, either xenograft or mechanical; additional mitral stenosis with a low output.
• Diuretics are needed to reduce pulmonary venous congestion and left ventricular preload.
• Afterload reduction has been shown to reduce the regurgitant fraction and may even abolish it altogether. Acute cases can be treated with i.v. nitroprusside, chronic ones with oral ACE inhibitors.
• In acute mitral regurgitation with chordal rupture and pulmonary oedema, artificial ventilation and full monitoring as in cardiogenic shock may be necessary (page 252).
• Infective endocarditis should be considered (page 371).

Prognosis
As in chronic aortic regurgitation, chronic mitral regurgitation is a relatively well-tolerated lesion if left ventricular function is preserved. Approximately 60% of patients with chronic MR are alive 10 years later. Prognosis depends on LV function.

Poorer prognostic features are:
• symptomatic history > 1 year
• atrial fibrillation
• patients aged > 60 years
• angiographic ejection fraction < 50%
• angiographic LVEDV > 100 ml/m^2
• echocardiographic dimensions of left ventricle: end-systolic dimension > 5 cm; end-diastolic dimension > 7 cm.

Surgery
Mitral valve replacement (MVR) for pure MR has been less successful than for pure mitral stenosis, possibly because MVR has been delayed until LV function is irreversibly impaired. Overall operative mortality is 5% for elective surgery.
1 *Acute mitral regurgitation with chordal rupture:* surgery is necessary because medical treatment alone carries a poor prognosis. Mitral valve repair may be possible in some cases (e.g. plication of mitral cleft or commissure, advancement of posterior cusp in floppy valve).

Annuloplasty is not usually satisfactory. Recurrent mitral regurgitation may occur following mitral repair. Most patients need MVR.

2 *Chronic mitral regurgitation:* MVR should be performed before LV function deteriorates irreversibly. Surgery is indicated for symptoms of increasing fatigue and dyspnoea (NYHA Grades 3 and 4). Also in patients with Grade 2 symptoms who have enlarging heart on CXR and increasing dyspnoea.

3 *Postinfarct mitral regurgitation:* papillary muscle infarction or rupture usually requires urgent MVR without delay. Intensive vasodilator therapy or IABP may hold the situation for a few hours but is no substitute for surgery.

Aortic stenosis

Levels of aortic stenosis

Aortic stenosis may occur at three levels and the three are not mutually exclusive.

1 Valvar aortic stenosis.

2 Supravalvar aortic stenosis.

3 Subvalvar aortic stenosis. This may be due to:
- discrete fibromuscular ring
- hypertrophic obstructive cardiomyopathy (HCM)
- tunnel subaortic stenosis
- anomalous attachment of anterior mitral leaflet: e.g. in AV canal, or parachute deformity of mitral valve with fused papillary muscles.

Various anatomical combinations may occur: a discrete fibromuscular ring with supravalvar stenosis and/or a grossly hypertrophic upper septum. In severe cases in childhood the term 'higgledy-piggledy' left heart has been used to describe pathology in the subvalve region, the valve and aorta occurring together.

The term 'fixed subaortic' stenosis has been used to describe a group of conditions: discrete fibromuscular ring and tunnel subaortic stenosis as opposed to variable obstruction due to muscular hypertrophy in HCM. The division is artificial because the conditions may coexist, and 'fixed' obstruction may be gradually acquired.

Valvar aortic stenosis

The commonest cause of aortic stenosis. It does not have a single aetiology (Figure 3.8).

1 *Congenital valvar abnormality.* The commonest cause of isolated aortic stenosis, 72% in one series. More frequent in males (4 : 1).

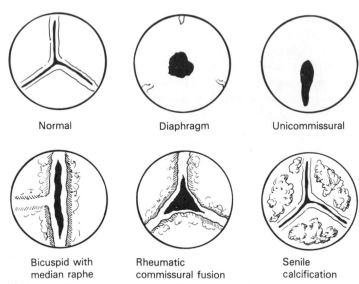

Normal   Diaphragm   Unicommissural

Bicuspid with
median raphe

Rheumatic
commissural fusion

Senile
calcification

Figure 3.8 Diagrammatic summary with valve viewed from above.

- Bicuspid valve (approximately 1% of the population). The commonest form of congenital heart disease. Both types become increasingly fibrotic and calcified with age, the bicuspid valve being the commonest cause of aortic valve stenosis in the age group 40 to ≥ 60 years.
- Other degrees of commissural fusion: unicommissural with eccentric hole, or even diaphragm (three fused cusps) with central orifice. Unicuspid aortic valve is the commonest cause of aortic stenosis presenting under the age of 1 year. It often presents as part of the hypoplastic left heart syndrome.

2 *Senile calcification of a normal valve.* Occurs in the age group > 60 years. The valve is tricuspid. The commissures are not fused, but the cusps are immobilized by heavy calcification. This often causes an ejection systolic murmur, but frank aortic valve stenosis is not so common.

3 *Inflammatory valvulitis.* Rheumatic fever results in commissural fusion of a tricuspid valve. The valve is usually regurgitant also (Figure 3.9). Rheumatoid arthritis may cause nodular thickening of aortic valve leaflets and, rarely, a degree of aortic stenosis usually with regurgitation.

4 *Atherosclerosis.* Severe hypercholesterolaemia in homozygous Type II

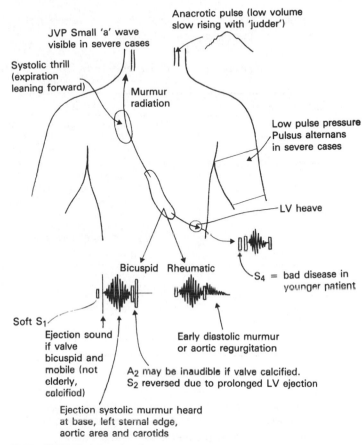

Figure 3.9 Typical signs in valvar aortic stenosis.

hyperlipoproteinaemia. Gross atheroma involves aortic wall, major arteries, aortic valve and coronary arteries.

Disease progression
Valvar obstruction gradually increases even in children who may be asymptomatic. Progressive valve calcification occurs, and may be visible on the chest X-ray from about the age of 40 years onwards. The severity of the calcification correlates roughly with the degree of stenosis.

Pathophysiology and symptoms
1 *Compensated:* good LV function with valve area > 1 cm². May be

asymptomatic. Children may be asymptomatic with severe disease. Adults may not present until age > 60 years.

2 *Angina:* occurs with normal coronary arteries. Due to imbalance of myocardial oxygen supply/demand. See table below.

Increased demand	Decreased supply
↑ Cardiac work ↑ Muscle mass from hypertrophy ↑ Wall stress from high intracavity pressure: both in systole and diastole	Prolonged systole with shorter diastole Reversed coronary flow in systole from venturi effect of narrow valve orifice High intramural pressure in systole preventing systolic coronary flow Low aortic perfusion pressure in diastole with high LVEDP Rarely calcification extending to coronary ostia

3 *Dyspnoea:* occurs due to high diastolic pressures in the left ventricle increasing with exercise. As LV function deteriorates (or AF occurs) orthopnoea or PND supervene.

4 *Giddiness or syncope on effort:* possible reasons are:
- high intramural pressure on exercise, firing baroreceptors to produce reflex bradycardia and vasodilatation
- skeletal muscle vasodilatation on exercise with no increase in cardiac output or additional rhythm disturbance
- development of complete AV block with aortic ring calcium extending into the upper ventricular septum

5 *Systemic emboli:* often retinal or cerebral. Amaurosis fugax may be the presenting symptom especially when the valve is calcified. Small flecks of calcium and/or platelet emboli may be seen wedged in retinal arterioles on ophthalmoscopy.

6 *Sudden death:* may occur in 7.5% of cases, even before severe ECG changes develop, e.g. in children.

7 *Infective endocarditis:* page 371.

8 *Congestive cardiac failure:* severe aortic stenosis may present for the first time as CCF with a large heart, very low pulse volume and soft murmurs, or no audible murmurs at all.

Physical signs
See Figure 3.9, page 89.

Coexisting lesions

In addition to the fact that an aortic valve abnormality may coexist with subvalvar stenosis, both lesions may occur with certain other congenital cardiovascular defects, e.g.

- aortic valve stenosis (bicuspid valve) + coarctation of the aorta (e.g. Turner's syndrome)
- aortic valve stenosis + coarctation + PDA
- VSD ± pulmonary stenosis
- as part of the hypoplastic left heart syndrome
- corrected TGA
- supravalvar stenosis with pulmonary artery branch stenosis.

ECG in aortic valve stenosis

1 Should be in sinus rhythm. If in AF, suspect additional mitral valve disease or ischaemic heart disease.

2 P mitrale with prominent negative P-wave component in V_1 (due to high LVEDP).

3 LV hypertrophy.

4 'Strain pattern' in lateral chest leads. In children T-wave inversion in inferior leads often occurs first. Severe aortic stenosis may occur with a normal ECG in children.

5 Left axis deviation (due to left anterior hemiblock).

6 Poor R wave progression in anterior chest leads.

7 LBBB or complete heart block with calcified ring (in approximately 5% of cases).

Following aortic valve replacement there is often a reversion of the P- and T-wave changes gradually over the years, and a reduction in LV voltage as the LV mass is reduced.

Chest X-ray

May show:

- left ventricular hypertrophy
- calcified aortic valve (in age > 40 years), calcium on lateral view will be above and anterior to oblique fissure
- post-stenotic dilatation of ascending aorta (not specific for valvar stenosis, e.g. may occur with fibromuscular ring in subvalvar stenosis)
- pulmonary venous congestion and signs of LVF
- *Note:* check for rib notching and small or 'double' aortic knuckle in coarctation.

Echocardiography

May show:
- bicuspid valve (eccentric 'closure' line) with reduced valve opening
- calcified valve (multiple echo-bands)
- LV hypertrophy, assess LV function
- diastolic fluttering of anterior mitral leaflet if additional aortic regurgitation is present
- assessment of aortic valve gradient from Doppler echocardiography may be a substitute for cardiac catheterization in the younger patient (see page 478). Two-dimensional echocardiography gives more information about the valve and LV function, but cannot provide coronary artery anatomy.

Cardiac catheterization

May be performed to:

1 Document the aortic valve gradient (Figure 3.10) or calculate the valve area (see Figure 12.32). Peak systolic gradient of > 100 mmHg and valve area < 0.5 cm^2 = severe aortic stenosis.

2 Assess LV function.

3 Perform coronary angiography to document possible CAD and check the coronary ostial anatomy. Bicuspid aortic valve is associated with a dominant left coronary artery and short main stem.

4 Check the aortic root.

Indications for surgery

1 In children, aortic valvotomy or valvuloplasty is performed in symptomatic patients or asymptomatic with severe stenosis.

2 In adults, aortic valve replacement is recommended once symptoms develop. The natural history of medically treated patients who are symptomatic is poor. (Average survival is 2–3 years with angina or syncope, 1–2 years with cardiac failure.)

In patients who are asymptomatic but have documented severe stenosis and a deteriorating ECG, valve replacement is also recommended.

3 The decision to operate on the elderly patient must depend on:
- adequate hepatic and renal function
- adequate lung function (forced expiratory volume in 1 second, FEV$_1$ preferably > 0.8–1 l)
- reasonable adult weight (> 40 kg)
- the severity of additional coronary disease or LV dysfunction.

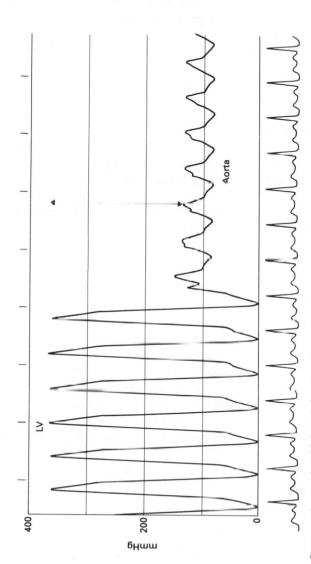

Figure 3.10 Severe aortic stenosis. Withdrawal of catheter from left ventricle to aorta in a man with severe aortic stenosis due to a calcified bicuspid aortic valve. LV pressure is 360/0–40 and aortic pressure is 130/80. Peak-to-peak gradient is 230 mmHg (arrowed).

Average operative mortality for isolated aortic valve replacement is now < 5%. The need for additional coronary revascularization or the presence of poor LV function increases the risk (10–20%). Long-term survival post-AVR depends on presence of:

- additional CAD and history of infarction
- heart size increasing pre-operatively
- low cardiac output
- pulmonary hypertension.

Aortic valvuloplasty

This technique has proved of some value in a very small group of elderly patients with severe aortic stenosis who are considered inoperable (very poor lung function, renal failure, etc.). It is of more value to the paediatric cardiologist in a child with aortic stenosis who is too small for an aortic valve replacement. It is performed percutaneously in the catheter laboratory. The technique involves insertion of one or two balloons across the aortic valve via guide wire(s). The balloon can usually be advanced across the valve retrogradely but the distal end of the balloon may damage the left ventricular septum and cause arrhythmias. The balloon is usually inflated to 4–9 atm for up to 1 min. The procedure usually causes an abrupt reduction in cardiac output during inflation and the patient should be well atropinized and not hypovolaemic.

Following valvuloplasty there is a gradient reduction, and usually an increase in aortic valve area. Long-term results vary, and some workers have found only a temporary improvement in aortic valve area. Complications include profound bradycardia, hypotension, tamponade, systemic emboli and death in a few cases. In addition there is a significant problem with entry site complications, some patients needing femoral artery repair. This problem is receding with use of a long arterial sheath.

Aortic valvuloplasty cannot be considered an alternative to aortic valve replacement. It is of some value to a very small group of infirm patients, or a group of children with congenital aortic stenosis. Its benefits may only be temporary but in children it may gain time until the child has grown enough for an aortic valve replacement. It has even been performed on the fetus *in utero* with success.

Supravalvar aortic stenosis (Figure 3.11)

This is caused by a constricting ridge of fibrous tissue at the upper margin of the sinuses of Valsalva. The coronary ostia are below the

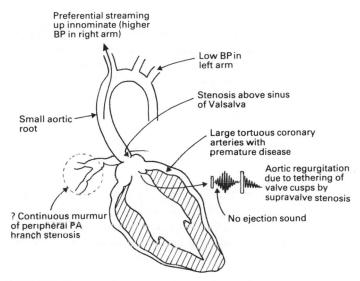

Preferential streaming
up innominate (higher
BP in right arm)

Low BP in
left arm

Stenosis above sinus
of Valsalva

Small aortic
root

Large tortuous coronary
arteries with
premature disease

Aortic regurgitation
due to tethering of
valve cusps by
supravalve stenosis

? Continuous murmur
of peripheral PA
branch stenosis

No ejection sound

Figure 3.11 Diagrammatic summary of supravalvar aortic stenosis.

stenosis. Rarely, the obstruction is a more generalized hypoplasia of ascending aorta.

Associated conditions

Williams' syndrome (autosomal dominant with variable penetration). Children with:
- elfin facies (large mouth with protruding upper lip, high forehead, epicanthic folds, recessed nasal bridge, mental retardation, strabismus, low-set ears)
- hypervitaminosis D and hypercalcaemia
- other cardiac lesions: peripheral pulmonary artery stenoses, valvar pulmonary stenosis, aortic valve regurgitation
- mesenteric artery stenoses, thoracic aortic aneurysms
- rubella syndrome.

Cardiac lesion and signs

Supravalvar aortic stenosis should also be considered in a child who has additional aortic regurgitation, no ejection sound and blood pressure in the left arm lower than the right. The CXR does not show post-stenotic dilatation of the ascending aorta.

Symptoms are those of valvar stenosis. Coronary arteries are characteristically large but tend to have premature arterial disease due to the high pressure below the supravalvar stenosis.

....

The supravalvar shelf and the adherent aortic cusps may rarely isolate the coronary artery orifice ('house-martin's nest' appearance on angiogram) and acute myocardial infarction or sudden death occur.

The pulmonary arterial stenoses may improve with time and the RV pressure then falls. The left-sided lesions often gradually get worse. In patients initially managed medically, repeat catheterization is often needed to check on possible deterioration of the supravalvar aortic lesion. An example of a catheter withdrawal tracing from LV to aorta in this condition is shown in Figure 4.3 (page 134).

Surgery
Is less satisfactory than for aortic valve stenosis. It may only be possible if the ascending aorta is of reasonable size. A gradient from LV to ascending aorta of > 70 mmHg would be an indication for operation. The narrowed segment may be enlarged by inserting an ellipse- or diamond-shaped patch of woven dacron or pericardium.

Discrete fibromuscular subaortic stenosis
Approximately 10% of congenital aortic stenosis. The fibromuscular ring obstructs the left ventricular outflow tract immediately beneath the aortic valve. It never presents under the age of 1 year and is probably an acquired lesion associated with congenital abnormality of the ventricular muscle. About half the affected patients have additional cardiovascular lesions.

Distinction from valvar aortic stenosis
This may be very difficult. Discrete fibromuscular subaortic stenosis is a possibility if:
- there is aortic regurgitation (thickening of valve due to high-velocity jet through obstruction or even attachment to the right coronary cusp)
- absent ejection sound (Figure 3.12)
- no valve calcification.

Post-stenotic dilatation of ascending aorta may or may not occur and is not reliable diagnostically.

Echocardiography
Is invaluable in establishing the diagnosis. On M-mode it may show the following:
- very early systolic closure of aortic valve (right coronary cusp especially), and systolic fluttering of aortic leaflets
- cluster of subaortic echoes above anterior mitral leaflet.

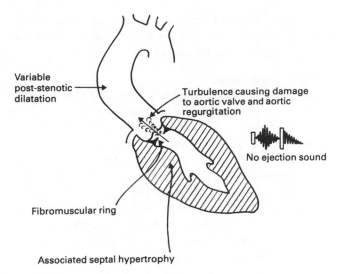

Variable post-stenotic dilatation

Turbulence causing damage to aortic valve and aortic regurgitation

No ejection sound

Fibromuscular ring

Associated septal hypertrophy

Figure 3.12 Diagrammatic summary of discrete fibromuscular subaortic stenosis.

Two-dimensional echocardiography may show the subaortic shelf clearly in the long-axis view in older children. The differentiation of the echoes from the aortic valve itself in younger children may be difficult.

Cardiac catheterization
Confirms subaortic obstruction. The ring is visualized on LV angiography. The degree of the obstruction can be measured and additional aortic regurgitation assessed.

Surgery
Excision of the fibromuscular ring is possible, but often residual abnormal LV muscle remains (very similar to HCM). The ring is excised through the aortic valve. There is usually a small residual gradient and sometimes mild aortic regurgitation. Follow up with repeat cardiac catheterization is necessary to exclude recurrent obstruction. Occasionally, aortic valve replacement is required later for aortic regurgitation.

3.5 Aortic regurgitation

This may be due to primary disease of the aortic valve or to aortic root disease with dilatation and stretching of the valve ring. The

97

regurgitation may be through the valve or, rarely, down a channel adjacent to the valve ring (e.g. ruptured sinus of Valsalva aneurysm aorto–left ventricular tunnel).

Pathophysiology

Often moderate aortic regurgitation is tolerated with no symptoms:
- aortic regurgitation results in an increase in left ventricular end-diastolic volume (LVEDV) and end-systolic volume (LVESV)
- the stroke volume (SV) is high in compensated cases
- left ventricular mass is raised with LV hypertrophy
- compensatory tachycardia reduces the regurgitant flow per beat by shortening diastole, and allows an increase in cardiac output.

As the regurgitation increases and LV function deteriorates:
- LVEDP rises and may eventually equal aortic diastolic pressure
- premature mitral valve closure occurs, preventing diastolic forward flow through the mitral valve
- LVEDV rises further but stroke volume falls.

Aetiology

Congenital	Acquired
Valve disease	
Bicuspid valve	Rheumatic fever
Supravalvar stenosis	Infective endocarditis
Discrete subvalvar fibromuscular ring	Rheumatoid arthritis (valve nodules)
Supracristal VSD with prolapse	SLE
of right coronary cusp	Pseudoxanthoma elasticum
	Hurler's syndrome and other
	mucopolysaccharidoses
Aortic root disease	
Ruptured sinus of Valsalva aneurysm	Dissection (Type A)
	Hypertension
	Cystic medial necrosis, e.g. Marfan's
	syndrome
	Osteogenesis imperfecta
	Giant cell aortitis
	Arthritides with aortitis, e.g. ankylosing
	spondylitis, Reiter's syndrome,
	psoriasis
	Syphilis
	Trauma

Symptoms

As in aortic stenosis, but angina and syncope are much less common. Unlike aortic stenosis, aortic regurgitation is a well-tolerated lesion if gradual compensatory mechanisms can occur. Even moderate aortic regurgitation may be tolerated for years. However, acute valvar aortic regurgitation or ruptured sinus of Valsalva is poorly tolerated and quickly produces LVF or congestive cardiac failure. Intensive medical therapy followed by investigation and surgery is often necessary.

Eponyms associated with aortic regurgitation (Figure 3.13)
1 Austin–Flint murmur. Due to vibrations in diastole of anterior mitral leaflet: oscillating between regurgitant jet and antegrade blood flow from left atrium. Very similar to mitral stenosis, but S_1 is quiet and there is no opening snap.
2 Duroziez's sign: to-and-fro murmur audible over femoral arteries.
3 Quincke's pulse: capillary pulsation in fingertips or mucous membranes.
4 Traube's sign. 'pistol-shot' sound audible over femoral arteries. Presence of additional aortic stenosis is detected by the bisferiens carotid pulse.
5 De Musset's sign: head bobbing due to collapsing pulses.

Differential diagnosis
• Pulmonary valve regurgitation, e.g. in patients who have had total correction of Fallot's tetralogy or postpulmonary valvotomy. Patients with pulmonary hypertension secondary to mitral valve disease (Graham Steell murmur).
• Patent ductus arteriosus. Machinery murmur usually loudest in second left interspace.
• VSD with aortic regurgitation. Usually right coronary cusp prolapses into or through a supracristal VSD. The prolapsing cusp may cause right ventricular outflow tract obstruction. (Retrosternal thrill, harsh pansystolic murmur, early diastolic murmur.)
• Ruptured sinus of Valsalva aneurysm. Usually right coronary sinus ruptures into RV outflow tract or RA. Sudden onset chest pain and CCF with high JVP. Consider this in patients with aortic regurgitation and signs of right heart failure as it is unusual in aortic regurgitation.
    More rarely:
• Coronary AV fistula. This presents during adult life with LVF due to left-to-right shunt (into RA, RV or coronary sinus).
• Pulmonary AV fistula, e.g. in patients with Osler–Rendu–Weber syndrome + bronchiectasis, cyanosis and $2°$ polycythaemia.
• Aorto-pulmonary window. Usually large communication with resultant pulmonary hypertension. Rarely survive to adult life.

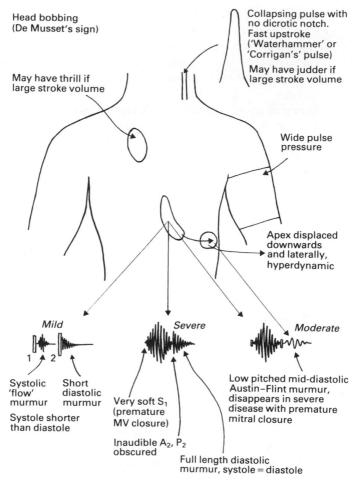

Head bobbing
(De Musset's sign)

Collapsing pulse with
no dicrotic notch.
Fast upstroke
('Waterhammer' or
'Corrigan's' pulse)

May have judder if
large stroke volume

May have thrill if
large stroke volume

Wide pulse
pressure

Apex displaced
downwards
and laterally,
hyperdynamic

Mild

Severe

Moderate

1 2

Systolic
'flow'
murmur

Systole shorter
than diastole

Short
diastolic
murmur

Very soft S_1
(premature
MV closure)

Inaudible A_2, P_2
obscured

Full length diastolic
murmur, systole = diastole

Low pitched mid-diastolic
Austin–Flint murmur,
disappears in severe
disease with premature
mitral closure

Figure 3.13 Typical signs of aortic regurgitation. Left sternal edge: use stethoscope diaphragm with patient sitting forward and breath held in expiration. Apex (to hear S_3 and Austin–Flint murmurs): use bell with patient lying on left side.

- Aorto–left ventricular tunnel.
- Persistent truncus arteriosus. Again patients rarely survive to adult life (early pulmonary hypertension, cyanosis, VSD + truncal valve regurgitation).

ECG

Left ventricular hypertrophy with diastolic overload pattern (prominent

Q waves in anterolateral leads). ST depression and T-wave inversion occur as the condition deteriorates.

Echocardiography
May show:
- LV function and dimensions. Exercise may help detect early LV dysfunction.
- Aortic valve thickening. Possible 'vegetations' on aortic valve.
- Diastolic fluttering of anterior mitral leaflet (may be audible as the Austin–Flint murmur).
- Premature mitral valve closure. Occasionally only the 'a' wave opens the mitral valve at all in severe cases.

More rarely:
- aortic root dimensions and possible 'double' wall in aortic dissection
- flail aortic leaflet prolapsing into LV outflow tract.

Chest X-ray
May show:
- aortic valve calcification uncommon in pure AR
- large LV
- ascending aorta may be very prominent (e.g. dissection) or aneurysmal (e.g. Marfan's syndrome, syphilis)
- calcification of ascending aorta (syphilitic AR)
- signs of pulmonary venous congestion or pulmonary oedema.

Cardiac catheterization
It is necessary to document:
1 The severity of the aortic regurgitation.
- Grade I – dye just regurgitant, not filling the ventricle
- Grade II – dye gradually accumulating to fill the whole ventricle
- Grade III – dye filling the whole ventricle, but cleared each systole
- Grade IV – dye filling the ventricle in one diastole, never cleared.

2 The anatomy of the aortic root, and to check the regurgitation is valvar and not ruptured sinus of Valsalva, to exclude dissection, to check for rarer congenital defects mimicking aortic regurgitation.
3 To assess LV function. With severe aortic regurgitation the LVEDP equals the aortic end-diastolic pressure.
4 To check coronary arteries and coronary ostia.
5 Additional valve disease.

Indications for surgery
1 Symptoms of increasing dyspnoea and LVF.

2 Consider AVR if:
- enlarging heart on CXR (> 17 cm on PA film)
- pulse pressure > 100 mmHg (especially if diastolic < 40 mmHg)
- ECG deterioration with T-wave inversion in lateral chest leads.

Sixty-five per cent of patients with all three of these criteria will either die or develop CCF within 3 years.

3 Ruptured sinus of Valsalva aneurysm.

4 Postinfective endocarditis if not responding to medical treatment.

3.6 Pulmonary stenosis

Obstruction to RV outflow may be at several levels, as in aortic stenosis.

Peripheral pulmonary artery stenosis. Stenoses of main trunk of pulmonary artery or more distal stenoses. These stenoses may be localized or diffuse. Commonly associated with supravalvar aortic stenosis and infantile hypercalcaemia. Also part of the rubella syndrome associated with PDA.

Pulmonary valve stenosis. A common isolated lesion (7% of congenital heart lesions). Also occurs as part of Noonan's syndrome, Fallot's tetralogy, rubella syndrome. It is rarely acquired, e.g. carcinoid syndrome.

Pulmonary infundibular stenosis. Rare as an isolated lesion. Usually associated with a VSD, or as part of Fallot's tetralogy or just in association with pulmonary valve stenosis.

Subinfundibular stenosis. This rarest form has been described. It may occur as part of right-sided HCM.

Pathophysiology and symptoms
The effects of pulmonary stenosis depend on its severity and the structure and function of the rest of the right heart, i.e. RV function (systolic and diastolic), competence of the tricuspid valve, presence or absence of a VSD, presence or absence of an ASD/PFO, maintenance of sinus rhythm.

With good RV function and a competent tricuspid valve plus sinus rhythm, moderate pulmonary stenosis can be tolerated with no symptoms.

Very severe 'pinhole' pulmonary stenosis is virtual pulmonary atresia and may lead to early infant death, especially if the duct closes.

The additional presence of an ASD or PFO may lead to right-to-left shunting (e.g. on effort), with cyanosis.

RV failure is the commonest cause of death, with gross cardiac enlargement. Common symptoms are thus:

- dyspnoea and fatigue (low cardiac output), not orthopnoea or PND
- cyanosis (if ASD or PFO)
- RV failure with ascites, leg oedema, jaundice, etc.
- retarded growth in children.

Symptoms which are uncommon (unlike aortic stenosis) are angina, syncope on effort and symptoms from infective endocarditis. Patients may be aware of pulsation in the neck from the giant 'a' wave in the JVP.

Physical signs to note

Characteristic facies may be:

- rounded plump face with isolated pulmonary valve stenosis
- Noonan's syndrome ('male Turner')
- Williams' syndrome (hypercalcaemia + supravalvar aortic stenosis + pulmonary artery stenoses), elf-like facies, JVP: prominent or giant 'a' wave, RV hypertrophy, palpable RVOT thrill.

Valve stenosis (Figure 3.14)

With mild valve stenosis there is an ejection sound, ejection systolic murmur, and A_2 and P_2 clearly heard and widely split. As the stenosis becomes more severe, the murmur is longer and obscures A_2. P_2 is delayed still further and is softer. With severe stenosis P_2 becomes inaudible and the ejection sound disappears as the valve calcifies. The murmur radiates towards the left shoulder and over the left lung posteriorly.

With infundibular stenosis there is no ejection sound and the murmur may be more prominent at the left sternal edge.

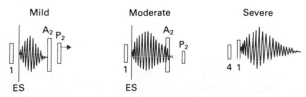

Figure 3.14 Grades of pulmonary stenosis.

Differential diagnosis

Differential diagnosis is from aortic valve or subvalvar stenosis, VSD, Ebstein's anomaly, ASD and innocent RVOT murmurs in children.

ECG

Shows right axis deviation, right atrial hypertrophy, 'P pulmonale', right ventricular hypertrophy, incomplete or complete RBBB.

Chest X-ray

There is poststenotic dilatation of the pulmonary artery, but lung fields are oligaemic, in contrast to ASD. RV hypertrophy causes some cardiac enlargement with the apex lifted off the left hemidiaphragm.

With severe long-standing pulmonary stenosis the heart may be very large with an enormous right atrium. (The wall-to-wall heart.) This appearance is seen in:

• severe pulmonary stenosis in the adult
• Ebstein's anomaly
• large pericardial effusion (chronic)
• mitral stenosis with giant atria
• dilated cardiomyopathy
• Uhl's anomaly (RV hypoplasia).

Cardiac catheterization

Is necessary to document the gradient and site of the stenosis.

The size of the pulmonary arteries and possible additional stenoses in them. Additional lesions must be excluded – especially PDA, VSD, ASD and left-sided obstructive lesions. RV functions are important. The position and comparative size of the great vessels are important in more complex lesions (e.g. Fallot's tetralogy, DORV with PS, TGA with VSD and PS).

Pulmonary valvuloplasty

Pulmonary valvuloplasty is now an acceptable alternative to surgery. Good reduction of pulmonary valve gradient is obtained, long-term results are good and RV hypertrophy on the ECG regresses.

Surgery

Pulmonary valvotomy and/or infundibular resection should be considered if there is RV failure, or if peak systolic gradient at valve/subvalve level is > 70 mmHg. Emergency surgery may be needed in infants. An additional PFO/ASD or VSD is usually closed. With severe valve stenosis a transannular patch may be needed.

3.7 Tricuspid valve disease

The commonest tricuspid valve disease is functional regurgitation secondary to pulmonary hypertension. Tricuspid valve destruction from infective endocarditis is increasingly seen in drug addicts. Other forms of tricuspid valve disease are uncommon (see table).

Congenital lesions	Acquired lesions
Tricuspid atresia	Functional regurgitation
Tricuspid hypoplasia	Destruction from infective endocarditis
Ebstein's anomaly (page 106)	(page 371)
Cleft tricuspid valve (AV canal)	Rheumatic involvement
	Floppy valve
	Endocarditis due to hepatic carcinoid
	Fenfluramine, Phentermine

Tricuspid regurgitation (TR)

Dilatation of the tricuspid valve ring with deteriorating right ventricular function is common in patients with pulmonary hypertension from any cause. It often occurs in patients with rheumatic mitral valve disease and pulmonary hypertension. The development of atrial fibrillation in ASDs is associated with tricuspid regurgitation. AF is expected with any significant degree of TR, both RA and RV dilate with the change to AF and the regurgitation worsens.

Symptoms

If any, there may be fatigue, hepatic pain on effort, pulsation in the throat and fullness in the face on effort, ascites and ankle oedema.

Signs

Systolic 's' wave in the JVP with rapid 'y' descent, if still in sinus rhythm (rare) prominent 'a' wave also, RV heave, soft inspiratory pansystolic murmur at LSE, pulsatile liver, ankle oedema and possible ascites and jaundice, peripheral cyanosis.

Treatment

Some degree of TR can be tolerated in the ambulant patient by conventional diuretic therapy and digoxin. Spironolactone, amiloride or an ACE inhibitor should be part of the regime. Support stockings may help prevent troublesome ankle oedema and venous ulceration.

In more severe and symptomatic patients a period of bed rest and i.v. diuretic therapy is needed. The symptoms quickly recur usually, once the patient is mobilized. In these cases tricuspid valve replacement must be considered. Tricuspid annuloplasty does not often result in any lasting benefit.

Tricuspid stenosis (TS)

This is rare, almost always rheumatic, and associated with additional mitral or aortic valve disease. Symptoms are as in TR.

Signs

Slow 'y' descent in JVP, Prominent 'a' wave if in SR, RV heave absent, tricuspid diastolic murmur at LSE best heard on inspiration and after effort. At cardiac catheterization even a gradient of 3–4 mmHg across the tricuspid valve is highly significant. RV angiography usually shows additional TR. The only treatment is valvuloplasty or valve replacement.

Ebstein's anomaly

A tricuspid valve dysplasia with downward displacement of the valve into the body of the ventricle. The tricuspid leaflets are abnormal; they may be fused, perforated or even absent and their chordae are abnormal. The clinical picture depends on:
- severity of tricuspid regurgitation
- RV function. The atrialized portion of the RV is thin walled and functions poorly
- rhythm disturbances. These are frequent. Both SVT and VT. There is often an abnormal conducting system with Type B (right-sided) WPW syndrome.
- associated lesions, commonly ASD or PFO; pulmonary stenosis; corrected transposition. Less commonly mitral stenosis, Fallot's tetralogy.

Presentation

Infancy. Heart failure from severe tricuspid regurgitation with chronic low output. Cyanosis from right-to-left shunting at atrial level (PFO or ASD). This may increase when a PDA closes as pulmonary flow is reduced still further. Prognosis at this age is poor.

Older child or young adult. This may be with a murmur noticed at school medical, or paroxysmal SVT. Mild forms may be asymptomatic.

Physical signs

Depend on above lesions. Usually the child is cyanosed, with elevated JVP and hepatomegaly.

At LSE listen for pansystolic murmur (TR), S_3 (RV), tricuspid diastolic murmur.

Chest X-ray

Shows very large right atrium in symptomatic cases often with oligaemic lung fields. With large globular hearts consider: pericardial effusion pulmonary stenosis, dilated cardiomyopathy as alternatives.

ECG

Shows RBBB. RAD. RA + (P pulmonale). Sometimes Type B WPW. Echocardiography is diagnostic, see page 474.

Treatment

Is medical initially to control symptoms of right heart failure and arrhythmias if present.

RV angiography is diagnostic, but frequently produces rhythm disturbances which may be difficult to control. Simultaneous measurement of intracardiac electrogram and pressure shows at one point an RA pressure, but an RV cavity electrogram.

Tricuspid valve replacement plus closure of an ASD is possible but results are generally not good.

Alternatively a tricuspid annuloplasty can be performed with plication of the atrialized portion of the right ventricle.

3.8 Prosthetic cardiac valves

Types

There is no perfect valve prosthesis. A knowledge of possible valve problems and complications is necessary for long-term management of these patients and regular follow up by experienced physicians essential. Currently there are three main types of prosthesis. (See Figure 3.15.)

Mechanical valves

These may be of the ball-in-the-cage type (Starr–Edwards, introduced in 1960), single-tilting disc (Björk–Shiley, introduced in 1969, Medtronic Hall) or double-tilting disc (St Jude, CarboMedics). All patients with mechanical valves require anticoagulation for life. The valves are very

(a)

(b)

(c)

(d)

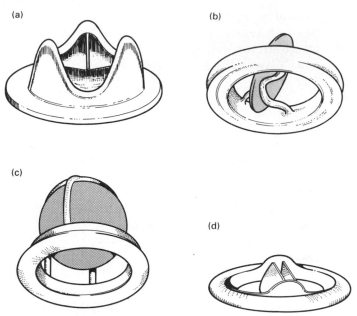

Figure 3.15 Examples of prosthetic valves. (a) Carpentier–Edwards porcine xenograft. Only the three wire stents (cloth-covered) are radio-opaque. (b) Björk–Shiley disc valve. The single disc is pyrolite carbon and is not radio-opaque. (c) Starr–Edwards ball valve. The mitral valve shown has four struts, and the aortic prosthesis has three. The silastic ball is not seen on the CXR. (d) St Jude medical bileaflet valve shown in this picture in the open position. This is a low-profile valve with two pyrolite carbon discs. The CarboMedics valve is similar.

durable, but have a higher thromboembolism rate than xenografts. Very occasionally a patient or their partner may be disturbed by the audible valve clicks.

Biological valves

Xenografts. These are manufactured from porcine valves (Carpentier–Edwards, Hancock, Wessex) or from pericardium (Ionescu–Shiley, Hancock) mounted on a frame. Aortic xenografts can be managed without anticoagulants, but most patients with mitral xenografts are in AF and should also be anticoagulated. Biological valves do not have good long-term durability and may need replacing at about 8–10 years. Unfortunately they have poorer durability in young patients. However, they are better in elderly patients.

Homografts. These are cadaveric aortic or pulmonary valves. They are either be transferred into a nutrient antibiotic medium and be stored for up to 4 weeks, or frozen for long-term storage. Availability is limited. A homograft should be considered the valve of first choice in a young patient requiring an aortic valve replacement. The use of an inverted homograft in the mitral position is not successful. Anticoagulation is not needed. Durability is better than xenografts, but deterioration in valve function is possible in time. They are also useful in replacing infected aortic valves being more resistant to reinfection than other valves.

Outpatient follow-up problems

Systemic embolism

This may occur with any valve prosthesis, but is commonest with mechanical valves: approx. 1% per year even with the best anticoagulant control. Absolutely rigorous anticoagulant control is necessary: aim to keep the INR between 2.5 and 3.5 for a Starr–Edwards valve and between 3.0–4.0 for a disc valve. If a patient with good warfarin control has a small (e.g. retinal) systemic embolism, and the valve prosthesis sounds normal then:
- check for infective endocarditis, blood cultures, FBC, ESR, CRP
- echocardiography for possible visible vegetations or intracardiac thrombi, transoesophageal echocardiography is superior to transthoracic for mitral prosthetic vegetations or left atrial thrombus
- consider transient rhythm changes (e.g. paroxysmal AF), check 24-hour tape
- consider non-cardiac source, e.g. innominate or carotid bruit.

If all tests are negative and valve function is normal then dipyridamole 100 mg tds is added to the warfarin. If a further event occurs add soluble aspirin 75 mg od after the biggest meal of the day. Aspirin is a more effective anti-platelet agent than dipyridamole in this situation but carries a greater risk of bleeding from the gut. Dipyridamole itself can cause dyspepsia.

If further emboli occur on this triple regime, a redo valve replacement must be considered. The risks of redo valve surgery are higher with a mitral (10%) than an aortic (5%) prosthesis. In the absence of infection and a functionally otherwise normal valve it may be preferable to 'ride out' the episodes, especially in the elderly.

Dental care

Meticulous dental care is absolutely vital for patients with prosthetic cardiac valves, and physicians should check that 6-monthly dental visits are made. Much dental work may need to be done prior to valve surgery, such as extraction of infected roots, but more complex restorative work usually has to wait until several months following valve replacement. Close liaison with the dentist is essential. Extractions are usually easier to manage with a short hospital admission. There are two big problems: the need to stop the warfarin and for parenteral antibiotic cover.

• Warfarin can be stopped for about 4–5 days prior to dental work, provided it is restarted immediately afterwards. Attempts to reverse the INR with vitamin K should be avoided as it makes subsequent anticoagulation difficult. If bleeding is a problem fresh frozen plasma is needed but its effects are only temporary and repeated doses are usually necessary. If vitamin K has to be given, use small incremental doses, e.g. 1–3 mg only.

• Antibiotic cover must be intravenous and is also detailed in Chapter 9. Ampicillin 1 g plus gentamicin 120 mg i.v. prior to the procedure with amoxycillin 0.5 g orally at 6 hours. For patients who are sensitive to penicillin: vancomycin 1 g slowly i.v. over at least an hour plus gentamicin 120 mg i.v.

These regimes are irksome but unavoidable and substituting oral amoxycillin alone is inadequate cover.

Infection (see also Chapter 9)

Prosthetic valve endocarditis (PVE) carries a mortality of up to 60% and it is a condition requiring urgent referral to a cardiothoracic centre. Patients should be reminded in the clinic to report any unexplained malaise, fever, weight loss, dyspnoea, etc. and should avoid antibiotics until seen by a cardiologist.

Endocarditis developing within the first 4–6 months of valve replacement is usually due to *Staphylococcus epidermidis*, which colonizes the valve at the time of operation. Patients with a history of a perioperative wound infection need particularly careful follow up. Prosthetic valve endocarditis occurring 6 months or more after surgery may be due to a wide variety of organisms, as in native valve endocarditis. A high index of suspicion is needed, particularly if patients have:

• had dental treatment in the last 6 months, uncovered by parenteral antibiotics

- noticed a change in their valve sounds
- a new symptom, however vague: dyspnoea, night sweats, myalgia, anorexia, etc.
- had a recent course of antibiotics.
  Clinically the search for signs of PVE is as for native valve infection. Additional points to note are as follows.
- In mechanical valves the opening and closing sounds of either ball or disc should be clear and sharp, not muffled. Vegetations may restrict ball or disc movement and muffle the relevant prosthetic sounds.
- A mitral xenograft should have no murmurs. An aortic xenograft may have a soft ejection systolic murmur only.
- Very significant PVE may have developed without the presence of an audible regurgitant murmur. A new murmur is a vital clue, but unchanged sounds cannot be relied on. New murmurs in PVE occur late.
- Splinter haemorrhages are common.
- Check for mild haemolysis even in the absence of a new murmur. ?Urinary urobilinogen.
- Check ECG for PR interval prolongation (septal abscess).
- Echocardiography is vital, to look for vegetations and abscess formation. Doppler echo is needed to establish valve regurgitation or a paraprosthetic leak. Transoesophageal echocardiography is particularly valuable if available.
- Radiological screening may show rocking of the prosthetic valve ring due to dehiscence. This usually occurs in the presence of obvious valve regurgitation and is a late and ominous sign.

  If there is any doubt, the patient should be admitted and fully investigated. (See Chapter 9.) Most cases of prosthetic valve endocarditis need a redo valve replacement, and this should be performed early.

  A knowledge of normal prosthetic valve sounds is important. Figure 3.16 shows normal Starr–Edwards aortic and mitral prosthetic sounds.

Pregnancy

In a woman of childbearing age the choice of valve prosthesis is difficult. A xenograft involves a further valve operation at 8–10 years but avoids the problems of anticoagulation. A mechanical valve may avoid the need for a further operation but anticoagulation is mandatory. In young women who want to have children a homograft is the valve of choice in the aortic position, accepting the need for a redo valve replacement at about ≥ 10 years. In the mitral position a

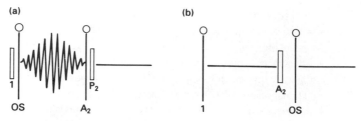

Figure 3.16 Normal Starr–Edwards prosthetic valve sounds. (a) *Aortic valve*. A normal first sound is followed by a prosthetic opening sound. There should be a soft aortic systolic ejection murmur. The ball closing sound is equivalent to A_2. The pulmonary component (P_2) is only heard in patients with wide RBBB. Diastole should be silent. (b) *Mitral valve*. The first heart sound is the mitral ball valve closing. There should be no systolic murmur. A_2 is soft but should be heard distinct from the ball opening sound (OS) which follows. The A_2–OS interval gives an indication of left atrial pressure as in mitral stenosis, a short interval indicating high LA pressure. Diastole should be silent.

mitral valve repair may be possible in patients with a floppy valve. If a valve replacement is unavoidable it is better to opt for a mechanical valve and its long-term durability. A redo mitral valve replacement carries twice the risk of an aortic redo and a mitral xenograft deteriorates faster in younger patients. Xenografts may deteriorate particularly rapidly during pregnancy.

Problems with warfarin in pregnancy
• *Fetal haemorrhage*. Warfarin crosses the placenta but vitamin K-dependent clotting factors do not: the immature fetal liver cannot manufacture them. Good maternal anticoagulant control unfortunately does not prevent fetal haemorrhage.
• *Teratogenicity*. Fetal malformation occurs in 5–30% of reported cases. Chondrodysplasia punctata and stippled epiphyses may occur with abnormal development of the brain (mental retardation, corpus callosum agenesis, ventral midline dysplasia with optic atrophy) and face (nasal hypoplasia). The typical embryopathy occurs with exposure to warfarin at 6–12 weeks gestation. CNS abnormalities may occur due to exposure in the second trimester.
• *Spontaneous abortion*. The risks of this are increased partly due to fetal and placental haemorrhage.
• *Delivery*. The patient must be switched from warfarin to heparin at about 36 weeks. This is a good time to admit the patient, administer the heparin i.v. (1000 units/hour initially).

• *Breast feeding.* Is not a problem with warfarin. Mothers can be restarted on warfarin and continue to breast feed.

Problems with heparin in pregnancy. Heparin does not cross the placenta and hence does not cause fetal malformation or fetal haemorrhage. Retroplacental bleeds and spontaneous abortion can still occur. There are, however, additional major problems with heparin.

• *Administration and compliance.* This has to be by subcutaneous self-injection throughout pregnancy from 6–36 weeks. Low-dose heparin (5000 units bd) is ineffective. The recommended dose is 7000 units s.c. tds or 10 000–12 500 units bd s.c. This is a major undertaking for any patient and often unacceptable. It has to be started very early to avoid the teratogenic effect of warfarin in the first trimester. The switch from warfarin to heparin has to be immediately on obtaining a positive pregnancy test. However, a patient may not realise she is pregnant for several weeks, by which time warfarin may have had its effect.

• *Osteoporosis.* This may occur after > 5 months of heparin therapy, with demonstrable reduction in bone density. The cause is unknown. There is a little evidence that it may be reversible on stopping the heparin.

• *Alopecia.* May occur in some patients.

• *Thrombocytopenia.* This is common but usually asymptomatic. It is more common with heparin derived from bovine lung than with porcine gut (an IgG–heparin immune complex is formed). It usually occurs 3–15 days after starting the heparin and returns to normal if the drug is stopped within 4 days.

• *Lipodystrophy and bruising.* May occur at injection sites.

Recommendations for anticoagulant regime during pregnancy. There is no ideal regime. Earlier enthusiasm for subcutaneous heparin has waned because of the major logistical problems and the dangers of ineffective anticoagulation.

It is safer from the mother's point of view to stick to effective warfarin control throughout the pregnancy and then to switch to i.v. heparin with a hospital admission at 36 weeks. These patients often require a short labour with a low threshold for Caesarean section, and heparin is stopped about 6 hours prior to delivery. It is restarted as soon as possible after delivery with the warfarin being restarted at 2 days postpartum.

With this regime the mother must appreciate the fetal malformation risk, which is realistically < 10%.

Haemolysis

This may occur with either mechanical or tissue valves. Although unusual it is more common in patients who have mechanical valves. It may develop severely acutely, usually associated with acute valve regurgitation (e.g. a flail mitral leaflet), or on a milder more chronic basis. Mild haemolysis may easily be missed. Additional intercurrent infections will exacerbate the anaemia. Prosthetic valve endocarditis must be considered in any patient with haemolysis.

Starr valves with cloth-covered struts were introduced in 1967 in an attempt to reduce systemic emboli. Unfortunately, cloth disruption and haemolysis tended to develop and these valves have been replaced by metal-tracked valves.

Patients are anaemic and possibly mildly jaundiced. There is urobilinogen and haemosiderin in the urine. Serum LDH levels are raised and haptoglobins lowered. The blood film shows fragmented cells (schistocytes), microcytosis and polychromasia. The Coombs test is negative.

Mild haemolysis in the absence of infection may be managed with iron and folic acid supplements and occasional transfusion. Usually redo valve surgery is required.

Structural valve failure

Mechanical valves. Failure is fortunately rare with mechanical valves. Ball variance with early Starr–Edwards valves was due to absorption of lipid by the silastic ball: the ball altered shape or even split.

The Björk–Shiley 60° Convexo–Concave single-disc valve (C–C valve) has had problems, with minor strut fracture allowing the disc to escape. All Björk–Shiley valves manufactured after 1975 have a radio-opaque ring marker in the edge of the tilting disc. In a patient presenting in acute LVF, where valve sounds are inaudible, screening the valve will show this ring is missing if the strut is fractured. The disc may be spotted in the peripheral circulation wedged in an artery. About 4000 patients are alive in the UK with C–C valves and the risk of strut fracture is about 7 per 10 000/year of whom two-thirds die acutely. The risk of a mitral redo valve replacement far exceeds this. Some patients may request a redo operation but most will just require close follow up. The greatest risk seems to be in patients with a large-size mitral prosthesis (31 and 33 mm) and a weld date between 1.1.81 and 30.7.82.

Duramedics bileaflet valves (withdrawn in 1988) also rarely had a problem with fracture of the valve housing mechanism. Most will have been explanted now.

Tissue valves. Gradual deterioration in all tissue valve function is to be expected, particularly in the young patient. Usually there is a gradual increase in valve regurgitation, but the valve may calcify and stenose. Most tissue valves will require a redo replacement at 7–10 years.

Acute tissue valve deterioration is due to a cusp tear. It is a difficulty with any tissue valve, and has been a problem with pericardial valves. The patient presents in acute pulmonary oedema. In patients with a mitral xenograft there is often a characteristic apical whooping systolic murmur and apical systolic thrill. The diagnosis is confirmed by Doppler echocardiography. Urgent redo valve replacement is needed. The torn cusp is not suitable for repair.

Valve dehiscence

This occurs when sutures cut out, causing paraprosthetic valve regurgitation. It may occur in patients requiring valve replacement for uncontrolled infective endocarditis because the surrounding tissue is so oedematous and friable. It is common in patients with aortic valve endocarditis who have a mycotic aortic root aneurysm and need an aortic valve replacement. Patients with Marfan's syndrome are at risk, with the surrounding tissue friable from cystic medial necrosis. It may also occur following a mitral valve replacement where the annulus is heavily calcified. As a sign of prosthetic valve endocarditis it usually occurs at a late stage.

A mild paraprosthetic leak may be tolerated well and treated medically, provided it is not infected. Haemolysis is common. Echocardiography with colour flow mapping is diagnostic. Transoesophageal echocardiography is superior for mitral leaks.

Valve thrombosis

This is usually due to inadequate anticoagulant control and is fortunately rare. Patients present with symptoms from valve obstruction and valve sounds are muffled or absent. Large infected vegetations (especially fungal) may also cause valve obstruction. Echocardiography is again diagnostic. Acute tricuspid valve thrombosis may be rescued temporarily by thrombolysis but this should not be considered for aortic or mitral valve thrombosis with the risk of systemic embolism. Urgent redo valve replacement is needed for all cases.

A chronic non-infected pannus of tissue may rarely encroach on the valve (usually mitral) from the annulus and gradually cause valve obstruction. Redo surgery again is essential.

Myocardial failure

This will cause deterioration in a patient's condition in spite of a perfectly functioning prosthetic valve. It may be due to:
- muscle disease due to previous rheumatic fever
- ventricular hypertrophy and fibrosis due to previous valve disease (e.g. aortic stenosis)
- coronary artery disease
- infective endocarditis directly affecting ventricular muscle (see Chapter 9)
- long cardiopulmonary bypass, especially in patients with ventricular hypertrophy
- systemic or pulmonary hypertension
- coronary emboli
- pre-operative poor ventricular function with severe mitral regurgitation. Mitral valve replacement once involved removal of the papillary muscles and it also increases afterload: this may provoke left ventricular failure
- additional uncorrected valve disease
- rarely unrelated myocarditis or muscle infiltration.

Treatment will depend on the cause. Most patients will improve with the addition of diuretics and an ACE inhibitor (**6.1**, page 230).

Rhythm problems

The three commonest are the development of complete heart block following an aortic valve replacement, atrial fibrillation following a mitral valve replacement and ventricular arrhythmias in patients with myocardial disease.

Complete heart block (CHB). This is common following aortic valve replacement for severely calcified aortic valves and usually occurs during or very soon after surgery. Dual-chamber pacing is needed with the presence of left ventricular hypertrophy. VVI pacing alone in this situation usually produces the pacemaker syndrome (**7.7**, page 302).

CHB may also result from a septal abscess in infective endocarditis. In patients with native endocarditis it is an indication for urgent temporary pacing, followed by valve surgery with epicardial pacing for a day or two followed by the implantation of a permanent pacemaker before the warfarin is started.

Atrial fibrillation and atrial flutter. These are common following cardiopulmonary bypass, and particularly so in patients in sinus rhythm undergoing a mitral valve replacement. Pre-operative treatment with amiodarone (**7.16**, page 348) may help prevent this. Treatment when it occurs is along standard lines (**7.12** page 315). If sinus rhythm was present pre-operatively DC cardioversion should be considered before the patient goes home.

Malignant ventricular arrhythmias. These may occur in patients with severe ventricular hypertrophy, or in patients who have very poor ventricular function. They may cause sudden death in patients who have apparently made a good recovery from surgery. Diuretic-induced hypokalaemia and hypomagnesaemia must be avoided as must digoxin toxicity. The pro-arrhythmic effects of anti-arrhythmic drugs must be remembered.

4 The Cardiomyopathies

These heart muscle diseases of unknown cause are divided into three functional categories:

1 dilated cardiomyopathy (DCM)
2 hypertrophic cardiomyopathy (HCM)
3 restrictive cardiomyopathy.

The restrictive group now includes patients with endomyocardial fibrosis and/or eosinophilic heart disease. These were once known as a fourth group of obliterative cardiomyopathies in which the apex of either or both ventricles is obliterated by fibrous tissue. However, the functional result is a small stiff ventricle and they are now classified with the restrictive group.

These three groups do not include rare specific heart muscle diseases (e.g. connective tissue diseases, haemochromatosis, metabolic and endocrine disease) in which cardiac involvement occurs as part of a systemic disease (see Chapter 11).

4.1 Dilated cardiomyopathy

A dilated flabby heart with normal coronary arteries. The definite diagnosis can only be made following cardiac catheterization, as ischaemic heart disease may sometimes present as heart failure in patients who have never had angina.

Factors incriminated as a possible cause include: alcohol, undiagnosed hypertension, viral infection, autoimmune disease and puerperal heart failure. Thyrotoxicosis may rarely present as a dilated cardiomyopathy. There is a rare form of X-linked dilated cardiomyopathy. Studies of first degree relatives of patients with DCM have shown that about 20% of first-degree relatives have a degree of ventricular enlargement and 3% have definite DCM.

Pathophysiology and symptoms

Progressive dilatation of both ventricles (usually LV > RV) with a low cardiac output and tachycardia produces fatigue, dyspnoea, and later oedema and ascites typical of congestive cardiac failure.

Additional problems result from the following:

- Functional valvar regurgitation. Dilated mitral and tricuspid valve rings plus poor papillary muscle function.
- Systemic or pulmonary emboli. Mural thrombus is common in either ventricle.
- Atrial fibrillation: especially in DCM secondary to alcohol. A further reduction in cardiac output occurs with the development of AF.

121

- Paroxysmal ventricular tachycardia.
- Secondary renal failure or hepatic failure. Further salt and water retention, secondary hyperaldosteronism and hypoalbuminaemia all contributing to the oedema.

Typical signs

A cool, peripherally cyanosed patient with very poor exercise tolerance or a bedridden patient.

- Blood pressure: low. Small pulse pressure (e.g. 90/75).
- Pulse: small volume. Thready. May be in AF. If in sinus rhythm may have pulsus alternans. Usually rapid (> 100/min).
- JVP: raised to the angle of the jaw. May have prominent 'v' wave of tricuspid regurgitation.
- Apex: displaced to anterior or mid-axillary line. Diffuse.
- Auscultation. Gallop rhythm (summation if in SR) with functional mitral regurgitation and/or tricuspid regurgitation.
- Pleural effusions and possible crepitations.
- Hepatomegaly. Mild jaundice. Ascites. Oedema of legs and sacrum.

Check also for signs of hypercholesterolaemia, excessive alcohol intake, previous hypertension (fundi) or collagen disease. Check thyroid for bruit.

Investigations

Chest X-ray shows moderate-to-gross cardiac enlargement with signs of left ventricular failure, pleural effusions or pulmonary oedema.

ECG shows sinus tachycardia usually with non-specific T-wave changes. Poor R-wave progression in anterior chest leads may be mistaken for old anterior infarction.

Echocardiography shows large left and right ventricles with very poor septal and posterior wall movement. Two-dimensional echo may show mural thrombus. There is often a small pericardial effusion. Ejection fraction is very low. Doppler studies may quantitate the degree of mitral regurgitation.

Cardiac catheterization can be dangerous in patients with very poor LV function and precipitate acute pulmonary oedema, systemic emboli or arterial occlusion. It may be necessary once a patient has been 'dried out' to:

- confirm the diagnosis and document normal coronaries
- exclude LV aneurysm
- check on the severity of associated mitral regurgitation.

Ventricular biopsy is no longer indicated for the diagnosis but will still be needed for research. Histological confirmation of acute myocarditis with infiltration of the interstitial tissue by T lymphocytes (confirmed on immunohistochemistry) is only found in 10% of patients. There are many non-specific and non-diagnostic changes. Early excitement with the use of DNA probes with *in situ* hybridization to find viral RNA within the biopsy fragments has proved unfounded as this has now been found as frequently in control specimens. The viral genome may persist within the myocardium long after the acute phase of the disease.

Blood tests: viral titres (especially for the Coxsackie and enterovirus group) and an auto-immune screen as a routine. Blood grouping and HLA typing if transplantation is considered. Measure thyroid function if in AF. Routine serum iron and iron binding capacity (see **11.6**, page 425).

Autoantibodies to alpha- and beta-myosin heavy chains are found in ≤ 25% of patients with DCM at the time of diagnosis. The titre may gradually fall after an initial episode of acute myocarditis. They are thought to be a marker of disease rather than pathogenetic: in fact the presence of antibody is associated with a milder disease course and better functional capacity 1 year later.

Management

Complete prolonged bed rest with careful fluid balance monitoring, daily weight and some fluid restriction are required. Intravenous diuretics are usually needed. Digoxin is indicated in AF or if a loud S_3 persists in spite of diuretics and bed rest. Beta-blockers are not used even with an inappropriate tachycardia. An ACE inhibitor is usually necessary but starting with very low doses (see **6.1**, page 231). Anticoagulation is very important in all patients with DCM even if in sinus rhythm. Only small doses of warfarin may be needed (hepatic congestion); 24-hour ECG monitoring is performed to check for AF or VT.

There is no indication to use steroids and immunosuppression, for these have no influence on prognosis even in confirmed myocarditis.

Prognosis

About 50% of patients with DCM will die in 2 years from initial diagnosis and then mortality is about 4%/year thereafter. Transplantation offers the only hope of long-term survival for patients not responding to medical therapy.

Cardiac transplantation (see also page 257)

Conventional cardiac surgery has little to contribute. Mitral valve replacement is considered when mitral regurgitation is severe but carries an increased risk if the ejection fraction is very low, and even if the patient survives there may be little improvement in a ventricular function. Left ventricular volume reduction (wedge resection of a segment of the ventricle avoiding the papillary muscles) is an operation of interest but as yet unproven long-term benefit. Cardiac transplantation in the younger patient carries the only hope of long-term survival and good life style. Transplantation centres vary in their top age limit for accepting cases. This is usually between 50 and 60. It is important that the patient is referred early before the development of renal failure, recurrent chest infections and cardiac cachexia, which greatly influence operative risks and post-operative survival.

Patients with systemic disease may not necessarily be refused. Insulin-dependent diabetics have been transplanted successfully. Specific conditions must be discussed in advance with the transplant centre.

Future trends

A small number of patients with DCM have been treated with recombinant human growth hormone 14 IU/week. Over 3 months there was a reduction in LV dimensions, an increase in LV wall thickness and myocardial mass and an improvement in exercise capacity. The study was uncontrolled but this is an exciting possible alternative to transplantation which needs further study.

Exclusions

In patients with suspected DCM it is important to exclude conditions that resemble it and may respond to surgery:
• pericardial constriction
• severe aortic stenosis with LVF
• severe mitral regurgitation
• LV aneurysm
• severe pulmonary stenosis
• severe Ebstein's anomaly.

In low-output states these conditions may produce few or no murmurs. Echocardiography is important in these exclusions.

4.2 Hypertrophic cardiomyopathy (HCM)

First described 1958 by Teare, who noted asymmetric septal

hypertrophy in nine adults, eight of whom died suddenly. It is known by other terms, such as IHSS (idiopathic hypertrophic subaortic stenosis), familial hypertrophic subaortic stenosis, ASH (asymmetric septal hypertrophy) and DUST (disproportionate upper septal thickening), although the last two are really just echocardiographic terms.

Although the pathology, haemodynamics and natural history of the condition are well described we are ignorant of the causes of sudden death and have made little difference to the progression of the disease with medical treatment.

Inheritance

About 70% cases are inherited as an autosomal dominant with a high degree of penetrance and equal sex distribution. In the rest genetic defects cannot yet be identified. Spontaneous mutations occur accounting for sporadic cases. More than 30 missense mutations (a single amino acid mutation) have been found in the B myosin heavy chain gene on chromosome 14 alone. This genetic heterogeneity may account for the different clinical spectrum in HCM. The mutation type may be important prognostically and allows preclinical diagnosis. Mutations recognized so far include the following.

Chromosome	Mutation on gene coding for:	Cases (%)	Associations
1q3	Troponin-T	15	Worst prognosis
7q3			WPW syndrome
11p13	Myosin binding protein C	10–15	
14q11	Beta-myosin	30	
15q2	Alpha-tropomyosin	3	

Pathogenesis

Unknown. It has been suggested that the abnormal arrangement of myocardial cells in the septum may be the result of excessive catecholamine stimulation due to a genetic abnormality of neural crest tissue (cf. association of HCM with hypertension, with lentiginosis and phaeochromocytoma). A very similar lesion occurs in Friedreich's ataxia.

Pathology

Hypertrophy of the ventricular septum compared with the LV free wall. The abnormal muscle fibres are short, thick, and fragmented. There is fibrosis. The nuclei are large and the fibres are arranged in whorls. These findings may be patchy but are concentrated in the septum. The pathological changes have been found in the RV outflow tract in patients with a VSD, and in the RV of infants with pulmonary atresia. The subvalve obstruction occurs between the thickened interventricular septum and the anterior leaflet of the mitral valve and its apparatus (Figure 4.1).

The mitral apparatus is either sucked forward in systole (venturi effect of high-velocity jet), or pulled by malaligned papillary muscles. The mitral value becomes thickened and may be regurgitant.

It is possible to have ASH without obstruction. Hypercontractile ventricles may look like HCM on LV angiography but have no gradient at rest or on provocation (may be seen in first degree relatives of patients with HCM). Occasionally the obstruction seems more apical in site. The condition is similar to true HCM.

Pathophysiology and symptoms (Figure 4.2)

The symptoms may be identical to aortic valve stenosis. It may present at any age.

1 Angina, even with normal coronaries.

  • Possibly due to excessive muscle mass exceeding coronary supply. High diastolic pressures producing high wall tension preventing diastolic coronary flow. High systolic stress increasing myocardial oxygen demand. Excessive internal work for any level of external work due to increased frictional and viscous drag. The disarrayed

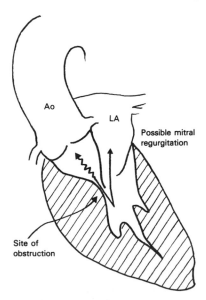

Figure 4.1 Site of obstruction in HCM.

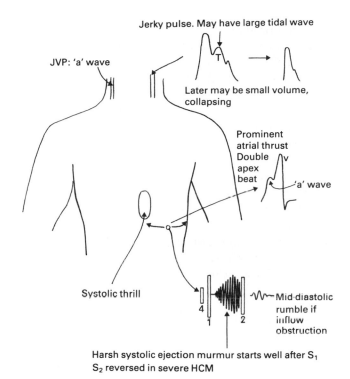

Figure 4.2 Clinical signs of HCM.

hypertrophy results in inefficient transfer of rising muscle tension to muscle shortening
- Abnormal narrowing of small coronary vessels.
2 Dyspnoea.
- Due to poor LV compliance, resulting in a stiff ventricle in diastole. LVEDP is high. Atrial transport is vital. Symptoms become rapidly worse if AF supervenes. Thick papillary muscles may result in 'inflow obstruction'.
- Due to associated mitral regurgitation.
3 Syncope and sudden death: as in aortic valve stenosis. But also:
- Extreme outflow obstruction due to catecholamine stimulation (effort or excitement).
- Known association with Wolff–Parkinson–White syndrome; rapid AV conduction down accessory pathway leading to VF in patients who develop AF or sinus tachycardia.
- Massive myocardial infarction.

Risk stratification

Determining which patients are at risk of sudden death remains a great problem. The search for a marker with high predictive accuracy continues. Poor prognostic features are as follows.

History
- Young age at diagnosis (< 14 years).
- Syncope as a presenting symptom.
- Family history of HCM with sudden death.

Holter monitoring

Non-sustained VT in adults. Occurs in about 25% of adults with HCM. The attacks are usually asymptomatic and often occur at night when vagal tone is high. However non-sustained VT remains the best non-invasive marker for sudden death with a sensitivity of 69% and specificity of 80%. However predictive accuracy is low at 22%, as the incidence is low in children.

Invasive electrophysiology

Increased ECG fractionation. This is still experimental. Preliminary studies involving paced RV electrograms at various RV sites have shown increased fractionation in survivors of VF.

Ventricular provocation (page 335) is a procedure not without risk in HCM. VT can rapidly degenerate into VF and the prognostic value of inducing VF is uncertain.

Peripheral vascular responses

Fall in systolic pressure on exercise, or failing to increase systolic pressure by > 20 mmHg. About one-third of patients with HCM fail to increase their blood pressure normally on effort. The reason for this vasodepressor response is unknown (possibly mediated by LV baroreceptors firing off under very high pressure causing peripheral vasodilatation). It tends to occur in the younger patient, those with the smaller LV cavity and those with a family history of sudden death.

Prognostic genotyping

See section on inheritance (above). Identification of the mutation type appears to carry prognostic significance, e.g. the troponin-T mutation is the worst, patients often dying in the 18–24 age range after the puberty growth spurt.

Other features

Features which have not proved of prognostic benefit in HCM include the following.

Non-invasive electrophysiology. Unfortunately theoretically useful markers such as QT dispersion, heart rate variability and late potentials on the signal averaged ECG, have not proved of prognostic value.

Invasive haemodynamics. The severity of the resting subvalve gradient is of no prognostic value. The severity of the LV hypertrophy is not related to sudden death risk.

Identification of myocardial ischaemia. The presence of ST segment depression is common in baseline ECGs with such marked LV hypertrophy. Neither thallium-201 scanning nor positron emission tomography have proved of value yet in documenting ischaemia. Thallium-201 perfusion defects are common in HCM. Coronary sinus metabolic studies with atrial pacing may prove helpful.

Natural history

Annual mortality in children (< 14 years) is 5.9%. Generally children are less symptomatic (apart from syncope). Annual mortality rate in those aged 15–45 years is 2.5%.

Symptom severity is not closely related to haemodynamic estimates of LVOTO. Some patients may develop endstage congestive cardiac failure with rapidly enlarging heart and reduction in LVOT gradient (postmyotomy patients are said to do this more frequently).

Differentiation from aortic valve stenosis

The three conditions most likely to be confused with HCM are:
1 Aortic valve stenosis.
2 'Subvalve' mitral regurgitation (e.g. chordal rupture).
3 VSD.

	Valve stenosis	HCM
Carotid pulse	Anacrotic	Jerky
Thrill	Second right interspace	Lower sternum to left
Ejection sound	May be present	Absent
Aortic EDM	Often present	Rare (postsurgery)
Manoeuvres to vary obstruction	Fixed	Variable

'Subvalve' mitral regurgitation, VSD and HCM may have small volume 'jerky' pulses, a harsh ejection systolic murmur and a systolic thrill. The thrill in mitral regurgitation is usually apical in chordal rupture (but may be more anterior in posterior chordal rupture).

Therefore the demonstration of variable obstruction is very important.

Some of these manoeuvres can be performed at the bedside and are therefore useful in the differentiation from aortic valve stenosis.

Relevance to medical therapy

1 Patients with angina due to HCM should not receive nitrates.

2 Digoxin should only be prescribed when atrial fibrillation is established and irreversible, or if considerable cardiac enlargement occurs when left ventricular outflow tract obstruction has already fallen.

Variation in LV outflow obstruction

Increased	Decreased
(Murmur louder and longer)	(Murmur softer and shorter)
Reducing ventricular volume	Increasing ventricular volume
Sudden standing	Squatting
Valsalva (during)	Valsalva (after release)
Amyl nitrate inhalation	Mueller manoeuvre (deep inspiration against a closed glottis)
Nitroglycerine	
Hypovolaemia	Handgrip
Excessive diuresis	Passive leg elevation
Increasing contractility	Decreasing contractility
Beta-agonists, e.g. isoprenaline	Beta-blockade (acute i.v.)
Post-extrasystolic potentiation	

? CALCIUM ANTAGONISTS

Decreased afterload	Increased afterload
Alpha-blockade	Alpha-agonists
	Phenylephrine
	Handgrip

3 Diuretics must be used carefully.

4 The role of beta-blockade:

- Acute i.v. beta-blockade is well documented to reduce the sub valve gradient and lower LVEDP. It may increase left ventricular end-diastolic volume (LVEDV). Beta-blockade is thus the mainstay of therapy for symptoms of angina, dyspnoea, giddiness and syncope.

Long-term studies of its efficacy are awaited. There is still no evidence to suggest that it alters long-term prognosis or reduces the incidence of sudden death.

• Large doses of beta-blocking agents are sometimes used (e.g. propranolol ≥ 160 mg tds).

5 The role of calcium antagonists.

• This is still debatable. It depends on the balance between the negative inotropic effect and the vasodilating action of the various drugs.

• Nifedipine has a more pronounced vasodilating action than a negative inotropic action and should be avoided.

• Verapamil has a less vigorous vasodilating effect and more pronounced negative inotropic effect. The claims that it reduces septal thickness have not been substantiated. It should be avoided in patients on beta-blockade. It not as effective an anti-arrhythmic drug as amiodarone in HCM. It can be used as an alternative to beta-blockade. As with beta-blockers, large doses are needed (240–480 mg/day) but the dose should be increased gradually.

Verapamil should be avoided in patients if there is a substantial outflow tract gradient as it may precipitate hypotension and pulmonary oedema.

6 Disopyramide.

A small trial of i.v. disopyramide has shown it can substantially reduce the LVOT gradient. Oral disopyramide is an alternative to beta-blockade and patients may find a better exercise capacity on this.

7 Dysrhythmias.

AF: should be cardioverted as soon as possible even in large hearts. Patients who will not revert should be digitalized. Amiodarone taken orally may induce version to sinus rhythm.

Non-sustained ventricular tachycardia is common occurring in 25% patients on Holter monitoring and the likeliest cause of sudden death (see Risk stratification, above). Propranolol and verapamil are not effective at abolishing this and have no effect on prognosis. Low-dose amiodarone should be tried (plasma levels 0.5–1.5 mg/l) which helps avoid long-term side effects (pages 348–350) and has been shown to be effective. Alternatives are flecainide, mexiletine or disopyramide.

Patients with refractory VT on drug therapy should be considered for an implantable cardioverter defibrillator (ICD)

8 Pregnancy with HCM is generally well tolerated. Beta-blocking agents should be withdrawn if possible (small-for-dates babies and fetal bradycardia may occur as side-effects of beta-blockade). Vaginal

delivery is possible but excessive maternal effort should be avoided. Haemorrhage may increase the resting gradient and volume replacement should be available. Ergometrine may be used. Epidural anaesthesia is probably best avoided as it may cause vasodilatation and hence an increased gradient. Antibiotic prophylaxis for delivery is advised. There is a strong chance the child will be affected.

9 Infective endocarditis may occur in HCM. Routine antibiotic prophylaxis should be given for dental and surgical procedures (page 392).

10 Systemic emboli may occur and require anticoagulation.

Echocardiography (page 472)

Several features in association are diagnostic.

1 Mid-systolic aortic valve closure (occurring later than discrete fibromuscular ring obstruction). Mid-systolic fluttering of aortic valve.

2 ASH. Grossly thickened septum compared with posterior LV wall, with reduced motion of the septum. Angulation of the echo beam may produce false positives on M-mode.

3 Small LV cavity with hypercontractile posterior wall.

4 SAM. Systolic anterior movement of the mitral apparatus. This may demonstrate contact between the anterior mitral leaflet and septal wall in systole. This contact has been used to quantitate the severity of the obstruction.

5 Reduced diastolic closure rate of anterior mitral leaflet. This is due to slow LV filling in diastole with low LV compliance. Echocardiography is useful in assessment of the results of drug treatment.

6 Continuous-wave Doppler studies using the apical four-chamber view with the sample volume in the left ventricular outflow tract show a characteristic dynamic envelope with a concave leading edge.

Electrocardiography (Figure 12.1)

Usually abnormal even in asymptomatic patients (only about 25% have no symptoms plus a normal ECG).

Commonest abnormalities:

• LV hypertrophy plus ST- and T-wave changes, progressive and steeper T-wave inversion with time

• deep Q waves in inferior and lateral leads (septal hypertrophy and fibrosis)

• pre-excitation and WPW syndrome.

• ventricular ectopics.

• ventricular tachycardia on ambulatory monitoring.

Cardiac catheterization

M-mode and two-dimensional echocardiography have reduced the need for diagnostic catheterization. The LV is very irritable, and entering the LV with a catheter often provokes ventricular tachycardia. The procedure should document:

- the severity of the resting gradient, or provocation of a gradient if none at rest, a typical withdrawal gradient is seen in Figure 4.3.
- the presence of mitral regurgitation
- the possibility of an additional fibromuscular ring
- the state of the coronary arteries
- electrophysiological investigation may be needed in patients with WPW syndrome
- postoperative assessment.

Dual chamber pacing

This is an encouraging alternative to surgery, performed in the absence of the usual conduction indications. Depolarization from the RV apex alters septal motion and reduces the subaortic gradient. Initial results show the gradient may be halved with considerable improvement in symptoms. Long-term results and the effects on mitral regurgitation are unknown. The pacemaker should be programmed with a short AV delay to ensure that every ventricular complex is paced. Some patients will in addition have chronotropic incompetence (failure of heart rate to increase on effort) and benefit from DDDR pacing rather than just DDD pacing (see pages 306–308).

Dual chamber pacing is cheaper and probably safer than surgery and should be considered as the initial procedure in patients with symptoms resistant to drug therapy, particularly in the older and more frail patient and those with mitral regurgitation.

Septal infarction

The injection of alcohol down the first septal artery at cardiac catheterization has been shown in a very few cases to reduce the outflow tract gradient. This is still an experimental technique and controversial.

Surgery

Reserved for severely symptomatic patients (angina, dyspnoea and syncope) in spite of vigorous medical treatment.

A myotomy/myomectomy is performed (through the aortic valve). This reduces the LVOT gradient more substantially than DDD pacing.

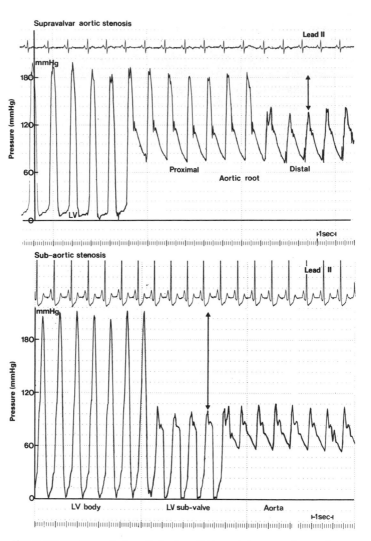

Figure 4.3 Withdrawal of a catheter from LV to aorta in supravalvar aortic stenosis (top panel) and in subaortic stenosis (lower panel) in this case hypertrophic obstructive cardiomyopathy. Both recorded on slow sweep speed. The gradients are represented by vertical arrowed bars. In supravalvar AS the gradient is within the aortic root itself (see page 95). In HCM the gradient is between the LV body and the subaortic chamber. See also Figure 4.1.

The development of LBBB postoperatively may help reduce the obstruction. A mitral valve replacement is sometimes needed in addition for mitral regurgitation (using a low-profile valve).

Surgery in early series carried some risk (10–27%), usually due to malignant postoperative ventricular dysrhythmias. The risks are lower now (< 10%) with the use of amiodarone for documented VT and patient's symptoms can be dramatically improved with surgery. Complete AV block may occur as a result of myomectomy and, if it does, dual-chamber pacing is essential as the LV muscle is stiff and atrial transport vital to maintaining the cardiac output.

4.3 Restrictive cardiomyopathy

Clinically this may be identical to constrictive pericarditis. Whereas surgery is necessary for pericardial constriction, it is of no benefit to and possibly harmful to patients with restriction (see pages 366–369).

Causes
- Iron-storage diseases (see **11.6**).
- Scleroderma (see **11.11**).
- Amyloidosis (see **11.3**).
- Loeffler's eosinophilic endocarditis and endomyocardial fibrosis (EMF), both known as 'eosinophilic heart disease'.
- Sarcoidosis (see **11.10**).

Patients with amyloid heart disease or sarcoidosis may have additional mitral or tricuspid regurgitation. Q waves on chest leads of the ECG are common and may be confused with old infarction. Atrial systolic failure (due to amyloid infiltration) increases the symptoms of congestion. Stagnation of blood in an inert atrium or atrial fibrillation increases the risk of systemic emboli and anticoagulation may be needed. Digoxin has an evil reputation in amyloid heart disease.

Differentiation of constrictive pericarditis from amyloid heart disease
This is difficult. Both restrictive myopathy and constrictive pericarditis may have:
- raised JVP with prominent 'x' and 'y' descents (Figure 8.3)
- normal systolic function
- LVEDV < 110 ml/m^2
- absence of LV hypertrophy

....

• rapid early diastolic filling with diastolic dip and plateau waveform (Figure 8.4).

The best technique to differentiate the two conditions is at cardiac catheter.

• LVEDP and RVEDP are different especially at end expiration in restriction usually by > 7 mmHg (identical in constriction).

• Cardiac biopsy is usually diagnostic.

• The search for amyloid elsewhere, e.g. urinary light chains; gum or rectal biopsy may help but cannot prove cardiac amyloid.

• Technetium pertechnetate scanning is positive in amyloid heart disease, with uptake in the infiltrated muscle.

• SAP scan. [123]I labelled serum amyloid protein is an alternative to technetium. It is valuable for identifying amyloid in other organs, but unfortunately not particularly good for cardiac amyloid.

5 Coronary Artery Disease

Contents

5.1 Pathophysiology of angina

Relevance to medical therapy

Ischaemia develops if myocardial oxygen (O_2) demand exceeds supply. Cellular acidosis and lactate release occur before ST segment depression on the ECG, which in turn precedes angina. ST depression occurring in the absence of pain is called silent ischaemia (see below). Oxygen supply is increased by increasing coronary flow (autoregulation) rather than by increasing oxygen extraction from coronary artery blood. Coronary AV O_2 difference remains constant at approximately 11 ml/100 ml blood. Coronary dilatation in response to ischaemia is probably mediated via adenosine, which is the ideal messenger because it has a very short half-life. Adenosine may be the cause of anginal pain when released from the ischaemic cell, acting as a self-protecting mechanism. Determinants of the O_2 supply/demand ratio are shown in the table below. Angina therapy works by improving this ratio.

Mechanisms of angina therapy

↑ O_2 supply	↓ O_2 demand
Length of diastole ↑ : beta-blockade	Heart rate ↓ : beta-blockade
Coronary tone ↓ : nitrates, calcium antagonists	Contractility ↓ : beta-blockade
LV diastolic pressure ↓ : nitrates	Wall tension ↓ :
O_2 capacity of blood ↑ : transfusion if anaemic	LV pressure ⎫ nitrates
	LV cavity radius^2 ⎭
Aortic perfusion pressure: improve if hypotensive or hypovolaemic	
Coronary atheromatous stenoses: angioplasty or surgery	

Coronary tone

Coronary tone is under neurogenic and humoral control. Coronary arterial smooth muscle contains alpha-, beta-1, dopamine and parasympathetic receptors. Beta-blockade is avoided in patients with proven coronary spasm (unopposed alpha-receptor activity). Cardioselective agents are used with care in patients with angina plus possible vasospasm (Raynaud's phenomenon or migraine).

The coronary endothelium is now known to be very important in the release of vasoactive substances, some causing constriction and others dilatation (see table). Many vasodilators act by releasing endothelial-derived relaxant factor (EDRF) from the endothelial cell, which in turn increases intra-cellular cyclic guanylate cyclase (cGMP), which results in muscle relaxation. EDRF is nitric oxide. Some vasodilators only work in

Regulators of coronary tone

Vasoconstrictors	
Mechanical	Systolic compression (intramural arteries), muscle bridge (epicardial artery)
Alpha-adrenoceptor agonists	Noradrenaline Adrenaline High-dose dopamine (> 15 µg/kg/min) via noradrenaline, Ergotamine, ergonovine (partial alpha-agonist and $5\text{-}HT_2$ agonist)
Endothelium produced	Thromboxane A_2 (and from platelets) Endothelin Prostaglandin F series
Adventitial nerve plexus	Neuropeptide Y
Other hormones	Vasopressin, angiotensin II
Vasodilators	
Mechanical	Diastolic relaxation
Metabolites from ischaemic myocardium	Adenosine, bradykinin, CO_2, H^+
Alpha-receptor antagonists	e.g. Prazosin, phenoxybenzamine
Angiotensin II antagonists	Captopril, enalapril
Beta-receptor agonists	($\beta_1 > \beta_2$) e.g. dobutamine, isoprenaline
Dopamine receptor agonist	Low-dose dopamine (< 5 µg/kg/min)
Phosphodiesterase inhibitors	Papaverine, methylxanthines (aminophylline)
Voltage-dependent calcium channel blockers	Nifedipine, diltiazem, verapamil
Potassium channel openers	Minoxidil, nicorandil, diazoxide
Purine receptor agonist	Adenosine (A_2 receptor), peripheral > coronary vessels
Direct stimulator of intracellular cGMP	Nitrates, atrial natriuretic peptide
Endothelium produced	Endothelial-derived relaxant factor (EDRF): nitric oxide, prostacyclin (PGI_2), Calcitonin gene-related peptide (CGRP), substance P, vasoactive intestinal peptide (VIP), prostaglandin E series

the presence of an intact endothelium (e.g. acetylcholine) but others are independent of an intact endothelium (e.g. nitrates and isoprenaline). If the endothelium is denuded, acetylcholine may even cause coronary constriction.

The role of prostaglandins in coronary tone is still poorly understood. Prostacyclin (PGI_2) is derived from intact endothelium and acts locally to cause dilatation, by increasing intracellular cyclic AMP (Figure 5.1). It acts in opposition to platelet-derived thromboxane A_2 (TXA_2), a potent vasoconstrictor.

Nitrates probably work by forming nitric oxide which stimulates guanylate cyclase, increasing intracellular cGMP. The action of some vasodilators on the vascular smooth muscle cell is shown in Figure 5.1. The physiological effects of beta-blocking agents are shown in Figure 5.3, and of nitrates in Figure 5.4.

In spite of our increasing knowledge of vasoactive substances released by the coronary endothelium, a few patients still present with absolutely typical angina but angiographically normal coronary arteries (see table below).

Chest pain with normal coronary arteries

There are many causes of chest pain which may mimic angina in patients with angiographically normal coronary arteries. There are also a large number of cardiac causes some of which are ischaemic

Chest pain with normal coronary arteries

Non-cardiac	Cardiac–ischaemic	Cardiac–non-ischaemic
Poor history	Angiogram misinterptretation	Pericarditis
Musculoskeletal pain	e.g. ostial stenosis,	Mitral valve prolapse
Cervical root pain	coronary arteritis,	Aortic dissection
Thoracic root pain	wrong projection	
Anaemia	Coronary spasm	
Thyrotoxicosis	Microvascular angina	
Hyperventilation	Syndrome X	
Pneumothorax	Linked angina	
Asthma	Coronary emboli,	
Oesophagitis	e.g. atrial myxoma,	
Oesophageal spasm	mural thrombus,	
Gastritis	vegetation	
Peptic ulcer	Aortic valve stenosis	
	Severe LV hyertrophy	
	e.g. HCM,	
	hypertension	

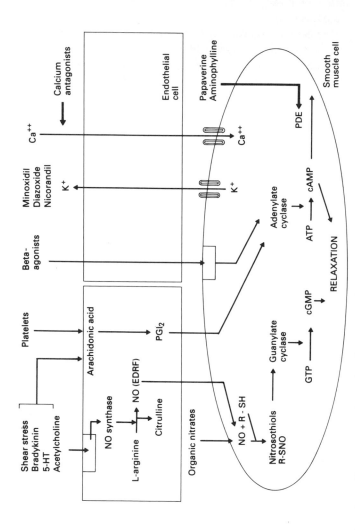

Figure 5.1 Action of vasodilators on smooth muscle cells. From Weatherall, D.J., Ledingham, J.G.G. & Warrell, D.A. (eds). Oxford *Textbook of Medicine*, 3rd edn. (Oxford University Press, 1994.)

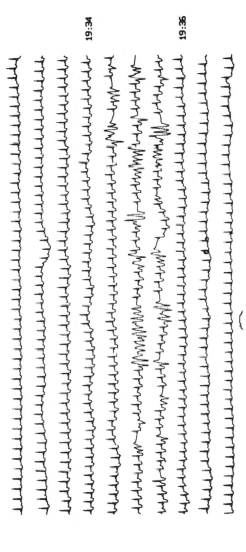

19:34

19:36

Figure 5.2 Sample from a continuous 24-hour ECG recording, showing the development of silent ST segment depression followed by a burst of non-sustained ventricular tachycardia. The silent ischaemia gradually resolves.

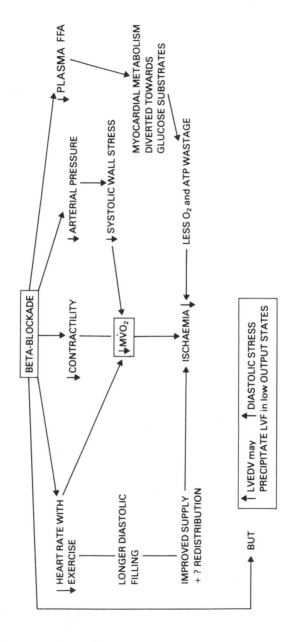

Figure 5.3 Mode of action of beta-blockade in reducing myocardial oxygen consumption.

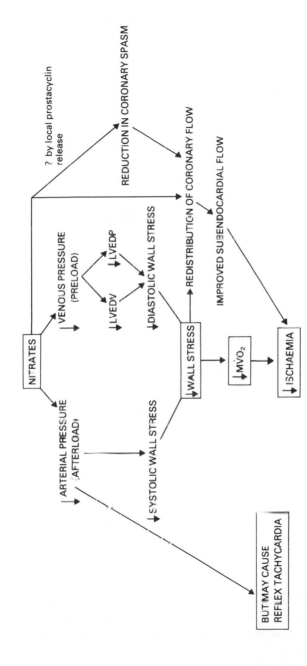

Figure 5.4 Mode of action of nitrates in reducing myocardial oxygen consumption

Coronary spasm

This is thought to be the cause of variant angina described by Prinzmetal in 1958. Angina is typical in site but comes on unpredictably at rest, sometimes provoked by cold or hyperventilation, and associated with ST elevation on the ECG. The spasm is usually localized to a segment of an epicardial coronary artery and in about half the cases there is an associated atheromatous lesion at the site of the spasm but in the rest the vessels look normal once the spasm has relaxed. Myocardial infarction may occur if the spasm cannot be reversed. Earlier studies provoked spasm at angiography with intracoronary ergonovine but this has not always proved to be reversible with intracoronary nitrates. Patients treated with nitrates and calcium antagonists but not beta-blockade (unopposed α effects). Coronary angioplasty in patients with coexisting atheroma may provoke spasm postdilatation.

Cardiac syndrome X

This term has been applied since 1981 to a group of patients who have:
- typical angina pectoris
- a positive treadmill stress test
- angiographically normal coronary arteries.

These patients probably represent a heterogeneous group including some with normal hearts. They are often middle aged women and in some their chest pain is not always typical: e.g. prolonged, or sharp in quality or in the left chest. There is evidence that their angina is ischaemic. Several studies have shown that these patients have abnormal coronary flow reserve: they do not increase coronary flow normally on response to adenosine, dipyridamole or papaverine. This is thought to be due to inappropriate vasomotor tone of the small resistance vessels (< 100 μm diameter – invisible on angiography). There is documented failure of endothelial-dependant dilatation. Slow coronary flow is often seen in the larger epicardial vessels on coronary angiography in patients with syndrome X. Other cardiac abnormalities found in some patients with syndrome X include:
- perfusion abnormalities on stress thallium scanning
- abnormal intramural arteries (< 100 μm) on cardiac biopsy
- abnormal systolic and diastolic function (high LVEDP, abnormal filling rates)
- ischaemia proven on coronary sinus lactate studies with atrial pacing
- myocardial damage: conduction abnormalities, e.g. LBBB, mitochondrial swelling, etc.

In such a heterogeneous group, these findings are not always consistent in every patient. Other studies suggest a more generalized smooth muscle abnormality with oesophageal dysmotility and abnormal forearm hyperaemic responses. Oestrogen deficiency in female patients has been suggested as an aetiological factor as oestrogen causes both endothelial-dependent and -independent vasodilatation.

Whatever the cause of syndrome X, patients angina responds well to nitrates and calcium antagonists. Beta-blockade should be avoided unless there is a resting tachycardia or systemic hypertension. H_2 receptor antagonists are tried for patients with poor symptom relief or any suggestion of acid reflux (see linked angina, below). Low-dose imipramine (25–50 mg at night) may help. Patients can be reassured that their prognosis is good. Their angina should not be dismissed as of no consequence. Follow up is often needed to help with recurrent symptoms.

Linked angina

This is the generation of angina in patients with syndrome X by oesophageal reflux. Instillation of acid into the oesophagus of patients with syndrome X has been shown to reduce coronary flow reserve, not occurring in the denervated heart of transplanted patients. A neurogenic cardio-oesophageal reflex has been incriminated affecting the coronary microvasculature. This compounds an already confusing diagnostic problem. Oesophageal pain may mimic cardiac pain in many respects. Exertion can cause oesophageal reflux anyway, and patients with syndrome X often have gastro-oesophageal problems (e.g. small hiatus hernia in the middle-aged female).

Metabolic syndrome X (Reaven, 1988)

Unlike cardiac syndrome X with which, unfortunately, it is easily confused, there is a high incidence of occlusive coronary disease in this condition. It consists of patients with insulin resistance, low HDL levels, hypertriglyceridaemia, systemic hypertension and upper-body obesity. They also have raised levels of plasminogen activator inhibitor (PAI-1) There is an interesting overlap, however, as insulin resistance has been found in some patients with cardiac syndrome X.

Silent myocardial ischaemia

Episodes of ST depression occurring without chest pain are termed silent ischaemia. This may be documented on an exercise test or during 24-hour Holter monitoring using FM recording equipment (Figure 5.2). Silent asymptomatic ST depression has been found to occur in 2.5% of the male population.

It is now appreciated that silent ischaemia represents impaired myocardial perfusion. It occurs in patients with chronic stable angina and ≤ 75% of episodes of ST depression on 24-hour Holter monitoring may be silent. Generally the more severe the ST depression the more likely it is to be felt by the patient as angina. The frequency of silent ischaemia on the 24-hour tape parallels the exercise test result: the more positive the exercise test and the worse the exercise tolerance, the greater the incidence of silent ischaemia.

Silent ischaemia on Holter monitoring occurs more commonly in the morning. This circadian rhythm is mirrored by the increased incidence of myocardial infarction in the morning. It occurs in about 10% of patients following myocardial infarction.

Patients with frequent episodes of silent ischaemia should be investigated along conventional lines, with exercise testing and subsequent coronary angiography if indicated. Conventional medical treatment for stable angina reduces episodes of silent ischaemia. Beta-blockade will reduce the episodes of silent ischaemia and will abolish the early morning peak of silent ST depression.

Prognostic importance

Silent ischaemia is perhaps surprisingly of no prognostic importance in patients with chronic stable angina as shown in the TIBET study. Exercise testing is more sensitive at detecting ischaemia and there is no need to perform continuous ambulatory ST-segment monitoring in this group. However, it is of considerable prognostic value in patients with unstable angina probably representing a ruptured unstable plaque. Patients with unstable angina who have silent ischaemia on ECG monitoring need urgent coronary angiography.

Ischaemic preconditioning

Brief periods of ischaemia (2–15 mins) can protect the myocardium from possible subsequent lethal ischaemia. This protection is probably mediated via the adenosine A_1 receptor activating intracellular protein kinase C. The subsequent target is uncertain. This self-protecting mechanism may explain why patients who have a history of angina prior to infarction have a better prognosis than those who have a sudden infarct with no preceding angina. It is a phenomenon also noticed during PTCA, with second and subsequent inflations being less painful and with less ST segment shift.

Hibernating myocardium

This is chronic reversible LV dysfunction due to prolonged reduction in coronary flow. Oxygen supply is enough to keep myocytes alive and metabolizing, but insufficient to allow them to contract. This is important as inert myocardium on angiography may be assumed to be dead, infarcted tissue, but will recover function following bypass grafting.

Hibernating myocardium can be diagnosed by the following.

• Infusing low-dose dobutamine during echocardiography. Hibernating muscle will be induced to contract

• Positron emission tomography (PET) scanning. Perfusion is studied using ^{13}N ammonia, and metabolism with ^{18}F fluorodeoxyglucose (FDG). Hibernating myocardium will be highlighted as areas still metabolizing but without any registerable flow. Cyclotron needed.

• Thallium-201 scanning with rest/redistribution study and late reinjection. This is an alternative to PET scanning and is much more widely available.

In one study, > 50% patients with coronary disease and poor LV function were found to have hibernating myocardium on PET scanning.

Myocardial stunning

This is prolonged but reversible LV dysfunction in the absence of ischaemia. Following total occlusion of a vessel with subsequent reopening, LV function gradually returns towards normal. This delayed recovery of regional wall motion occurs after prolonged inflations at PTCA, in unstable angina and possibly during non-transmural infarction.

5.2 Management of angina

This involves alteration of life style, exclusion or treatment of precipitating factors, drug treatment and possibly surgery or angioplasty if medical treatment fails.

Alteration of lifestyle

This involves a reduction of physical activity at work and in the home. It may require a change in job (heavy goods vehicle drivers, airline pilots, divers) or a change within employment (miners, furniture removers, etc.). Smoking must be stopped. Weight reduction may be needed. Many activities (e.g. gardening, sex) can be continued with medical treatment and nitrates taken prophylactically.

Driving may be continued provided that traffic does not induce angina, that angina is stable, and that it is a private car only. Vocational driving licence holders (formerly HGV and PSV licences) should not drive their vehicles and should inform the DVLC (pages 531–532).

Rarely, attention to climate or altitude may help. Patients may be helped by moving to warmer climates during winter months.

Flight as an airline passenger is not contraindicated provided that angina is stable. The airline medical personnel should be informed before the flight, the patient should not carry heavy luggage and should be well insured for hospital care abroad.

Vigorous competitive sports should be stopped (e.g. squash, rugby). Regular daily exercise within the anginal threshold is important. Swimming is allowed if angina is stable. Patients should not swim alone, should not dive into cold water and should get into the water within their depth. Heated pools are obviously preferable.

Skiing is not recommended (high altitude, physical effort, cold air and emotional factors).

Exclusion and treatment of precipitating factors

These include anaemia, high-output states, thyrotoxicosis, etc. diabetes mellitus, hypercholesterolaemia.

The most important cardiac precipitating factors are hypertension, obstruction to LV outflow, aortic valve stenosis, HCM, paroxysmal arrhythmias.

Angina in aortic valve stenosis may be cured by aortic valve replacement. Patients with angina and aortic regurgitation should have a VDRL/TPHA checked (ostial stenosis). Twenty-four hour ECG monitoring should be performed if the history suggests arrhythmias precipitating angina.

Investigation and medical treatment

Exercise testing is performed on patients with stable angina provided that there are no contraindications (see **12.2**). This helps confirm the diagnosis, assess the severity of symptoms and is a guide to the need for coronary angiography. Patients who cannot complete Stage 2 of the standard Bruce protocol because of symptoms or who develop positive ST changes, hypotension or arrhythmias need angiography.

Drug therapy involves three groups of drugs: nitrates, beta-blocking

agents and calcium antagonists. Additional diuretic or antihypertensive therapy may be needed. Stable angina is treated initially with a beta-blocking agent and glyceryl trinitrate. Calcium antagonists or long-acting nitrates are the drugs of first choice when beta-blockers are contraindicated, i.e.
- low-output state, borderline LVF
- Prinzmetal's variant angina
- high-degree AV block
- severe peripheral vascular disease, claudication, gangrene
- asthma, moderate or severe bronchospasm
- depressive psychosis in the history
- Raynaud's phenomenon.

Unstable angina is controlled initially medically and then investigated with a view to surgery. Nocturnal or decubitus angina may respond to a diuretic taken in the evening or a calcium antagonist taken at night.

5.3 Beta-blocking agents (Figure 5.3)

Choice of beta-blocker

The table (pages 152–153) shows the currently available agents in the UK. Personal preference and experience mainly dictate the choice. Most of the ancillary properties of beta-blockers e.g. membrane-stabilizing effect, intrinsic sympathomimetic activity (ISA) matter little clinically. Drugs with ISA prevent a resting bradycardia. The membrane-stabilizing effect (quinidine-like) may play a role in the anti-arrhythmic action, as may the reduction in platelet stickiness that occurs with beta-blockade. Additional non-cardiac conditions are considered in the choice.

- Patients with cool peripheries, peripheral vascular disease, diabetes mellitus or mild bronchospasm should start with a cardioselective drug such as bisoprolol or celiprolol (which contains in addition beta-2-agonist properties). In patients with airways obstruction, start on a small dose and monitor peak flows at least twice daily.
- Patients complaining of bad dreams (e.g. on propranolol) should receive a non-fat-soluble drug (atenolol, nadolol or sotalol).
- Hypertensive patients may be best managed with a single-dose schedule taken in the morning (atenolol, sustained-action metoprolol, propranolol). Alternatively they should start labetalol, a combined alpha- and beta-receptor antagonist. Many beta-blockers can be used as single-dose schedules for hypertension. More frequent dose schedules are usually required for angina.
- Renal failure. Choose a beta-blocker with hepatic excretion (e.g. propranolol, labetalol, carvedilol) but at a lower dose than in patients

Table of beta-blocking agents

Drug (trade name/s)	Fat-soluble	Cardio-selective	ISA	Plasma half-life (hours)	Plasma protein binding (%)	Elimination route	Starting oral dose for angina	? Single schedule for hypertension	Intravenous dose (slowly over 5 min)
Acebutolol (Sectral)	+	Yes	Yes	3	15	Hepatic 60% 1st pass renal	200 mg tds	200–400 mg od	10–50 mg
Atenolol (Tenormin)	–	Yes	No	6–9	10	Renal only	100 mg od	100 mg od	5–10 mg
Betaxolol (Kerlone)	–	Yes	No	15–22	50	Renal	10 mg od	Yes	—
Bisoprolol (Emcor, Monocor)	++	Yes	No	10–12	30	Renal 50% Hepatic 50%	10 mg od	Yes	—
Bucindolol*	++	No but alpha-1 blocker	No	3–4	90	Hepatic	50 mg od	100–200 mg od	—
Carteolol (Cartrol)	–	No	Yes	6–9	15	Mainly renal	10 mg od	Yes	—
Carvedilol (Eucardic)	++	No but alpha-1 blocker	No	6–7	95	Hepatic	12.5 mg bd	25–50 mg od	—

Drug (Trade name)									
Celiprolol (Celectolol)	+	Yes + beta-2	Yes	5–6	25	Hepatic and renal	200 mg od	Yes	—
Labetalol (Trandate)	++	No	No	3–4	85	Hepatic 90% metabolized	100 mg tds	No	50 mg, repeated if necessary
Metoprolol (Lopresor, Betaloc)	+	Yes	No	3	15	Hepatic and renal	50–100 mg tds	Durules 200 mg od	5–10 mg
Nacolol (Corgard)	–	No	No	16–24	20	Renal only	40 mg od	40–80 mg od	—
Oxprenolol (Trasicor)	+	No	Yes	2	75	Hepatic	40 mg tds	Slow oxprenolol 160 mg od	1–10 mg
Penbutolol (Lasipressin)	+++	No	Yes	4–5	80	Hepatic	20 mg od	Yes	—
Pindolol (Visken)	–	No	Yes	3–4	50	Hepatic and renal	5 mg tds	No	—
Propranolol (Inderal)	+++	No	No	3–6	90	Hepatic 95% 1st pass metabolism	40 mg tds	Propranolol LA 160 mg od	1–10 mg
Sotalol (Betacardone Sotacor)	–	No	No	12–15	5	Renal only	80 mg bd	No	10–20 mg
Timolol (Betim, Blockadren)	±	No	No	4–6	65	Hepatic and renal	10 mg bd	No	0.5–1 mg

*Bucindolol is not yet available in the UK.

with normal renal function. Reduction in cardiac output lowers renal plasma flow and may cause a deterioration in renal function.
- Elderly patients. Start with a very low dose (e.g. propranolol 10 mg bd, or metoprolol 25 mg bd).
- Liver disease. First pass metabolism occurs with fat-soluble drugs (e.g. propranolol, labetolol, acebutolol). Patients with liver disease should have the dose of fat-soluble drugs reduced or switched to a non-fat-soluble drug (e.g. pindolol, nadolol), which is excreted only by the kidneys.
- Heart failure (see page 242). Interest is growing in the use of beta-blockade in patients with mild-to-moderate heart failure. Carvedilol and bucindolol are non-selective beta-blockers with additional alpha-1 blocking activity. Introduced slowly at very low dose, improvement in LV function has been demonstrated in some patients, but some patients have deteriorated and have been withdrawn from the trials. Identifying which patients are suitable is a problem and beta-blockade cannot be recommended yet in heart failure.
- Diabetes mellitus is not a contraindication to beta-blockade, even if the patient is on insulin. Beta-blockade prevents the sympathetic reaction to hypoglycaemia. Muscle glycogenolysis is mediated via beta-2-receptors. Hence the cardioselective drugs are preferable in diabetic patients.
- Pregnancy. The evidence that beta-blockade during pregnancy results in small-for-dates babies is largely retrospective. Prospective trials have shown that beta-blockade as treatment for hypertension in pregnancy confers a benefit to the fetus compared with methyldopa or hydralazine.
- Overdose of beta-blocking agents is treated by intravenous beta-agonists in competitive doses, e.g. dobutamine (10–15 µg/kg/min or more as required) or atropine 1.2 mg i.v. (Complete AV block may occur and not be reversed by atropine.) Temporary pacing is often necessary.

5.4 Nitrates (Figure 5.4)

Sublingual preparations

Preparations	Effective time
Glyceryl trinitrate 0.5 mg	10 s–30 min
Isosorbide dinitrate 5 mg	10 s–1 h
Pentaerythritol tetranitrate 10 mg	10 s–45 min

Isosorbide dinitrate preparations dissolve particularly quickly in the mouth and are often preferred by patients to standard glyceryl trinitrate (GTN). Nitrates may relieve the pain of oesophageal spasm and renal or biliary colic.

They are contraindicated in angina due to HCM because they increase the outflow tract gradient.

Patients should be informed of the following.
- To renew the tablets every 6 months. Shelf life is limited.
- A GTN spray may be preferred.
- To take them prophylactically and concurrently.
- Tablets taken in hot atmospheres may induce postural hypotension or even syncope.
- To expect a headache and/or facial flushing. If these symptoms are intolerable, GTN may be swallowed and absorption is reduced. The tablet may of course be spat out. Isosorbide is absorbed from mouth and gut.
- The tablets are not addictive. Tolerance is not a problem. Patients should not limit their intake to a fixed number daily. (Methaemoglobinaemia is possible with very high tablet consumption but is rare in clinical practice.)
- Chewing the tablets will speed absorption in severe angina.

Patients on additional beta-blocking therapy will not develop a reflex tachycardia.

Care must be taken on prescribing nitrates to patients with cerebral arteriosclerosis. Hypotension may provoke cerebral ischaemia.

Amyl nitrite

Ampoules of amyl nitrite are used in echocardiography or in the catheter laboratory to provoke outflow tract gradients in patients with labile LVOTO. They cause headaches to both patients and operators and are only used diagnostically.

Transdermal nitrates

Nitropaste 2% (Percutol, Nitro Bid)

This ointment is absorbed through the skin and has a prolonged action (3–4 hours). Ointment is usually contained in 30 or 60 g tubes and 2.5 cm is squeezed on to the chest and covered by an occlusive plaster. Absorption occurs and if the patient becomes hypotensive or develops severe headache it can be wiped off. It is rather messy and dosage control is uncertain.

Oral nitrates (longer acting than GTN sublingually)

Drug	Preparation marketed	Tablet strengths	Dose used
Glyceryl trinitrate	Nitrocontin	2.6 mg, 6.4 mg	2.6–6.4 mg bd or tds with either
	Sustac	2.6 mg, 6.4 mg	
Isosorbide dinitrate	Cedocard	5 mg	5–20 mg bd to tds
	Cedocard Retard	20 mg	20 mg bd with either
	Isoket Retard	20 mg	
	Isordil	5 mg, 10 mg, 30 mg	5–30 mg tds to 4 hourly
	Isordil Tembids	40 mg	40 mg bd or tds
	Soni-Slo	20 mg	20 mg bd or tds
	Sorbid SA	40 mg	40–80 mg bd
	Sorbitrate	5 mg, 10 mg, 20 mg	5–20 mg bd to tds
	Vascardin	10 mg	10–20 mg bd to tds
Pentaerythritol tetranitrate	Cardiacap	30 mg	30 mg bd
	Mycardol	30 mg	30 mg bd
	Peritrate	10 mg	20–60 mg tds
	Peritrate SA	80 mg	80 mg bd
Isosorbide mononitrate	Elantan	10 mg, 20 mg, 40 mg	10 mg bd to 40 mg tds
	Elantan LA 25 or 50	25 mg 50 mg	25 mg or 50 mg od
	Isotrate 20	20 mg	20 mg bd or tds
	Ismo 10, 20 or 40	10 mg, 20 mg, 40 mg	10 mg bd to 40 mg tds
	Monit LS	10 mg	10 mg bd or tds
	Monit	20 mg	20–40 mg bd or tds
	Monit SR	40 mg	40 mg od
	Mono-Cedocard	20 mg, 40 mg	20–40 mg bd or tds
	Imdur	60 mg	60 mg od

Nitrate patches

These are preparations of GTN contained beneath a small plaster with a rate-limiting membrane that controls its release. Two sizes are available and two different brands.

1 Transiderm-Nitro 5 and 10: GTN content 25 and 50 mg, respectively.

2 Deponit 5 and 10: GTN content 16 and 32 mg, respectively.

In 24 hours 5 or 10 mg of GTN is absorbed for either brand, depending on patch size. Only one plaster is needed daily. The plaster is waterproof. It should be removed at night unless the patient suffers from nocturnal angina.

With both transdermal preparations it is important to make sure that the area of skin used each day is different. Inflamed, cracked or icthyotic skin should be avoided (too rapid absorption). Skin sensitivity is not common.

Steady-state plasma levels can be achieved with the once-daily preparation (0.1–0.2 ng/ml) which, although much lower than oral therapy, has been shown to reduce the number of anginal attacks per day.

Nitrate sprays

Many patients find these quicker and more convenient than GTN tablets. Coronitro and Nitrolingual Spray both dispense 0.4 mg of GTN with each squirt. Approximately 200 puffs are available per dispenser.

Oral nitrates

The drugs considered in this section are longer acting than sublingual nitroglycerine (see table on page 156. Isosorbide mononitrate preparations have the theoretical advantage over the dinitrate preparations in that the mononitrate does not require first-pass metabolism in the liver and bioavailability is thus greater. Both preparations are valuable and the few trials done suggest GTN requirements were less with the mononitrate.

Nitrate tolerance

In many patients, tolerance to nitrate therapy develops quite rapidly. Mechanisms that have been suggested to cause this are:

• activation of renin–angiotensin system. If this is the cause it should be blocked by captopril but there is evidence that captopril does not prevent nitrate tolerance in patients with congestive cardiac failure. Activation of the renin–angiotensin system has also been said to account for the rebound phenomenon (vasoconstriction occurring on nitrate withdrawal)

- plasma volume expansion. This may develop during nitrate therapy. It may also be partly responsible for nitrate tolerance.
- Depletion of sulphydryl (—SH) groups in vascular smooth muscle (see Figure 5.1). Administration of *N*-acetylcysteine has been shown to reduce nitrate tolerance and may well prove to be useful in the future if a palatable way of administering it orally is found.

Tolerance can be avoided by arranging therapy to provide a nitrate-free period during the 24-hour cycle. Oral nitrates should not be given after 6 p.m. in the evening and nitrate patches should be removed also. A nitrate-free period at night can be achieved in this way.

Intravenous nitrates

Both preparations below are very similar in action and are comparable in price:
- glyceryl trinitrate/nitroglycerine (Tridil); 0.5 mg/ml in 10 ml ampoules
- isosorbide dinitrate (Cedocard i.v. or Isoket); both are 1 mg/ml in 10 ml ampoules.

Indications

Intravenous nitrates are used in the following situations.
- Crescendo or unstable angina not responding to medical treatment orally.
- Left ventricular failure and pulmonary oedema. This may be secondary to acute mitral regurgitation, ruptured ventricular septum, etc.
- Accelerated hypertension (malignant hypertension), although nitroprusside is a better drug in this condition, having more arterial vasodilator properties.
- During and after coronary artery bypass surgery. Hypertensive episodes following cardiac surgery.
- During cardiac catheterization: intracoronary injection of nitroglycerine or isosorbide may be necessary if chest pain is associated with ST segment elevation (i.e. coronary spasm or impending myocardial infarction).
- As a prophylactic measure during PTCA (see **5.7** page 169).

Problems and difficulties with i.v. nitrates

Direct measurement of arterial pressure may be necessary. Pulmonary artery wedge (PAW) pressure or PA pressure can also be monitored by a Swan–Ganz catheter.

Hypotension may occur with excessive dosage. The infusion should be stopped, the legs elevated and if necessary plasma expansion/ volume replacement given.

Side-effects. Palpitations, giddiness, nausea, retching, sweating, headache, restlessness, muscle twitching have all been seen.

Drug incompatibility. Both nitroglycerine and isosorbide i.v. are incompatible with PVC infusion bags or giving sets. Up to 30% potency may be lost within 1 hour. Polyethylene or glass is not a problem, see table for examples.

Incompatible PVC	Compatible polyethylene
Viaflex (Travenol)	Polyfusor (Boots)
Steriflex (Boots)	Bottlepak/Flatpak (Dylade)

The drugs can be given either by drip infusion or by infusion pump using a glass syringe or rigid plastic syringe and polyethylene tubing.

Patient incompatibihty. Intravenous nitrates are best avoided in:
• pregnancy
• uncorrected hypovolaemia
• patients with closed-angle glaucoma
• anaemic or hypotensive patients
• patients with severe cerebrovascular disease.

Nitroglycerine dose calculation

Nitroglycerine (Tridil). 10 ml ampoules contain either 0.5 mg/ml (5 mg ampoule) or 5 mg/ml (50 mg ampoule).
Single-strength preparation: add 1 × 5 mg ampoule to 40 ml
   5% dextrose or 1 × 50 mg ampoule to 490 ml 5% dextrose
   (concentration = 100 µg/ml).
Double-strength preparation: add 2 × 5 mg ampoules to 30 ml
   5% dextrose or 2 × 50 mg ampoules to 480 ml 5% dextrose
   (concentration = 200 µg/ml).
Start at 10 µg/min. Increase every 20–30 min by 20 µg/min until effect
   is achieved. To maximum 400 µg/min. Usual range needed
   10–30 µg/min.

Isosorbide dinitrate (ISDN) dose calculation

Isosorbide dinitrate (Cedocard i.v. or Isoket). Both are 1 mg/ml in 10 ml ampoules. Isoket also as 50 mg in 50 ml ampoules for use in an infusion pump. Add 5 × 10 ml ampoules (50 mg) to 450 ml 5% dextrose. Mixture concentration = 1 mg in 10 ml. Start at 10 ml

Nitroglycerine

Dose (µg/min)	Paediatric microdrops/min	Dextrose (ml/24 hour)
Single-strength preparation: *(concentration 100 µg/ml)*		
10	6	144
20	12	288
30	18	432
40	24	576
50	30	720
60	36	864
70	42	1008
80	48	1152
90	54	1296
100	60	1440
Double-strength preparation *(concentration 200 µg/ml)*		
120	36	864
140	42	1008
160	48	1152
180	54	1296
200	60	1440

Isosorbide dinitrate

Dose ISDN (mg/hour)	(µg/min)	Paediatric microdrops/min	Dextrose (ml/24 hour)
Using above mixture (5 × 10 ml in 450 ml 5% dextrose)			
1	17	10	240
2	33	20	480
3	50	30	720
4	67	40	960
5	83	50	1200
6	100	60	1440
Using double-strength mixture (10 x 10 ml ampoules in 400 ml 5% dextrose)			
7	117	35	840
8	133	40	960
9	150	45	1080
10	167	50	1200

Note: Paediatric microdrops: 60 drops/ml. Standard drops: 15 drops/ml. Paediatric microdrops make calculations easier, e.g. 30 microdrops/min = 30 ml/hour.

(1 mg)/hour, i.e. 10 paediatric microdrops/min. Usual range needed is 1–7 mg/hour. In severe cases 10 mg/hour may be needed.

Nicorandil

This is a new drug consists of two components: a nitrate and a potassium-channel opener. It is of use in stable angina and side-effects and precautions are as for nitrates. Headache is the commonest side-effect. Dose is 10–20 mg bd. Half-life is 1 hour. It should be avoided in hypotensive patients, paediatrics, pregnancy and lactating patients. It is a relatively weak drug and unlikely to have much effect in patients who are already on a long-acting nitrate, but worth a try in refractory angina.

5.5 Calcium antagonists

A group of drugs which share the property of inhibition of calcium influx during phase 2 of the cardiac action potential (plateau phase). Calcium enters the cell via two types of voltage-dependent calcium channel (L and T) in myocardial and vascular smooth muscle. These channels are voltage dependent as calcium influx occurs only during depolarization. The inward movement of calcium ions triggers further calcium release from the sarcoplasmic reticulum which in turn triggers the contractile proteins (excitation–contraction coupling). Hence some calcium antagonists may have a negative inotropic effect. Inhibition of the calcium channel in vascular smooth muscle cells causes muscle cell relaxation and vessel dilatation. Conventional calcium antagonists block the L-type channel. The T-type channel blocked by Mibefradil (soon to be avaliable in the UK) is important in the sinus and AV node: Mibefradil should slow the heart rate without a negative inotropic effect and hopefully this will prove of value in both angina and cardiac failure. Beta-agonists increase calcium influx via a receptor-operated channel and this is not inhibited by calcium antagonists.

The increasing number of calcium antagonists have varying properties and some seem to have a predilection for certain vascular beds. The drugs have a wide variety of chemical structures and the nature of the voltage-dependent channel and how the drugs block it, are imperfectly understood. There is an overlap in drug effects but the table overleaf outlines the more specific uses of the drugs.

Although the degree of negative inotropism varies, all calcium antagonists should be used with great care in patients with a history of left ventricular failure or large hearts on the CXR and verapamil definitely avoided.

Effect	Drug	Condition
Negative inotropic effect	Verapamil	HCM Hypertension
Effect on AV node conduction	Verapamil	SVT. Fast AF or flutter Fascicular tachycardia
Systemic vasodilatation	Dihydropyridines	Hypertension Raynaud's phenomenon Aortic regurgitation
Pulmonary vasodilatation	High-dose nifedipine or diltiazem	Primary pulmonary hypertension
Coronary vasodilatation	All	Stable angina Microvascular angina Coronary spasm ? Diastolic dysfunction
Cerebral vasodilatation	Nimodipine	Subarachnoid haemorrhage

There is considerable interest in the fact that calcium antagonists can help suppress the development of atheroma in cholesterol-fed rabbits. Preliminary work in humans suggests that calcium antagonists may help delay the development of coronary disease (nifedipine 20 mg qds in the INTACT study over a 3-year period and diltiazem 30–90 mg tds in heart-transplant recipients). The three most commonly used calcium antagonists in the UK are verapamil, nifedipine and diltiazem.

Nifedipine (dihydropyridine group)
Useful in all types of angina, especially when beta-blockade is contraindicated. It can be used synergistically with beta-blockade. It dilates both coronary and systemic vessels and is useful in systemic hypertension. It is of great value in Raynaud's phenomenon but of very limited value in intermittent claudication. Not to be used in pregnancy and should be avoided in women who may wish to become pregnant. Its vasodilating properties result in a warm generalized flush from 30 min to 1 hour after taking the drug, and a reflex tachycardia. It is of no value in supraventricular or junctional tachycardia.

Side-effects: Flushing and tachycardia, ankle and leg oedema gradually developing during the day. This does not respond well to diuretics and is better managed with advice about posture and support stockings, if necessary. Pruritus. (Avoid in inflammatory skin disease.) Gum hyperplasia. Some patients notice a diuretic effect.

Dose: Use slow-release preparation only for maintenance. Start with 10–20 mg bd after meals up to a maximum of 40 mg daily. The short-acting capsules (5 mg or 10 mg) may be chewed in acute angina and the drug is absorbed through the buccal mucosa. The capsule contents can be squeezed into the mouth of a patient with acute hypertension or coronary spasm during or after cardiac catheterization. An intracoronary preparation is available: 0.2 mg given i.c. will help prevent coronary spasm during PTCA.

Contraindications to dihydropyridine drugs (nifedipine group)
- Severe aortic stenosis.
- HCM.
- Pregnancy.
- Women of childbearing age unless using reliable contraception.
- Poor LV function.
- Unstable angina as a sole agent: must be used with beta-blocker.

Diltiazem (benzothiazepine group)
This drug is a potent coronary vasodilator but has less effect on dilating peripheral vascular beds. It causes less flushing and reflex tachycardia than nifedipine. Like nifedipine it can be used synergistically with beta-blockade. It increases AV nodal refractoriness and can be used for supraventricular tachycardia. It also appears to have an antiplatelet effect, which may be shared by other calcium antagonists. It is useful in the first-line treatment of angina where beta-blockade is unsuitable. The three commonest calcium antagonists (diltiazem, nifedipine and verapamil) all increase coronary blood flow.

Side-effects: These are few and the drug is well tolerated. A small number of patients develop an irritating skin rash, which resolves when the drug is stopped. Rarely, a more serious exfoliative dermatitis and epidermal necrolysis have been reported.

Dose: Orally 60–120 mg tds. An i.v. preparation is not generally available yet. Slow-release preparations, 90 mg bd or 120–240 mg od.

Verapamil (phenylalkylamine group)
Although introduced initially as a drug for angina, it has become very valuable in the treatment of supraventricular and junctional tachycardia

because of its effect on AV nodal conduction. It can be used as an alternative to beta-blockade but should be avoided in patients on beta-blockers unless they are under close supervision, have good LV function and no conduction defect. It is useful in decubitus angina. It has a negative inotropic effect and should be used with great care in patients with a history of LVF in the past, or a large heart on the CXR. Reduce the dose in liver disease.

It is of value in the acute management of supraventricular (narrow complex) tachycardia but has been superseded by adenosine, which is safer and better. (See **7.12**, page 322). It will increase the degree of AV block in atrial fibrillation and atrial flutter with fast ventricular rates, and can be used with digoxin in the chronic management of these arrhythmias. Given i.v. in atrial flutter with a fast ventricular rate, it will slow the ventricular rate allowing the flutter waves to appear more clearly. Carotid sinus massage may abort an attack of supraventricular tachycardia after or during verapamil administration even if it did not do so before it.

Side-effects: Constipation is the main drawback with verapamil. Haemorrhoids may be the result.

Dose: Orally. Initially 80 mg tds increasing to 120 mg tds. A slow-release preparation is available (e.g. for hypertensive patients) 240 mg od as a single dose. Intravenously 5–10 mg. Repeat in 30 min if necessary. ECG monitoring is essential during verapamil administration i.v.

Verapamil should be avoided in:
- Patients on beta-blocking agents unless under close supervision and LV function is good.
- Sino-atrial disease.
- Patients with AV block.
- Possible digoxin toxicity.
- Hypotensive patients.
- AF and WPW syndrome (see pages 339–345).
- Wide complex tachycardias. These may be VT rather than SVT with aberrant conduction. Verapamil given to patients with VT may produce hypotension and asystole.

Other calcium antagonists
There are a large number of second-generation calcium antagonists of the dihydropyridine group (nifedipine analogues) on the market, with

an increasing emphasis on long-acting drugs such as amlodipine or nisoldipine or slow-release preparations of nifedipine, verapamil or diltiazem, which need to be taken once or at most twice daily. There is very little to choose between the increasing number of calcium antagonists whose properties differ only slightly.

Nimodipine
More selective for cerebral vessels and of value following sub-arachnoid haemorrhage increasing flow to poorly perfused areas. Dose is 1 mg/hour for 2 hours i.v. then 2 mg/hour (or 60 mg 4-hourly for 21 days). Infusion must be protected from light.

Amlodipine
Longest-acting calcium antagonist with half-life 35–50 hours. Once-a-day preparation starting with 5 mg od for angina or hypertension. Maximum dose 10 mg od. Slow absorption and 90% metabolized. No need to reduce dose in renal disease but care in liver disease. The PRAISE study showed that it was safe in patients with severe heart failure, and was useful in treating coexisting angina or hypertension in this group. It appeared to be of particular benefit in improving the prognosis in patients with dilated cardiomyopathy.

Nicardipine
Short-acting water-soluble drug, which is highly protein bound and has weaker negative inotropic action than nifedipine. It is not light sensitive. Dose: 20 mg tds up to 40 mg tds. Approximately 30% first-pass metabolism. Dose reduced in both liver and renal disease. Increases digoxin levels.

Felodipine
High vascular selectivity. Half-life 8 hours. Very similar to nifedipine. Dose: start 5 mg bd, up to 10 mg tds. For hypertension and/or angina. In the VHeFT III trial it was shown to be no better than enalapril and did not improve survival in patients with heart failure although it was shown to produce a fall in BP and a rise in LV ejection fraction.

Isradipine
Another dihydropyridine more specific for vascular smooth muscle than the myocardium. Extensive first pass metabolism with approx. 20% bioavailability. 95% protein bound. Pronounced diuretic effect. Dose: 2.5 mg bd up to 10 mg bd. Half-life 8 hours.

Nisoldipine

A drug with high vascular selectivity available as a slow-release coat-core preparation. It has been shown to be safe in patients with moderate left ventricular dysfunction with no negative inotropic effect. Dose is 10–30 mg od on an empty stomach. Its predilection for the coronary vascular bed results in few peripheral side-effects compared with nifedipine.

Long-term safety of calcium antagonists

Since 1995 there has been a great deal of unrest in both the medical and popular press regarding the long-term safety of calcium antagonists based on meta-analysis of 16 pooled trials by Furberg and Psaty. This suggested that high-dose short-acting nifedipine (80 mg daily) carried a threefold long-term mortality risk compared with placebo. It was suggested that this might have been due to arrhythmias induced by activation of the sympathetic nervous system secondary to acute vasodilatation. Other concerns have been expressed relating to gastrointestinal bleeding and malignancy. What came out of all the furore was:
• there were considerable dispute about the analysis methods
• the 80 mg dose of nifedipine exceeded the manufacturer's recommendations.
• there were virtually no long-term prospective data.
And in practical terms:
• nifedipine is not a recommended drug for acute myocardial infarction
• short-acting calcium antagonists of any type should be avoided, particularly short-acting dihydropyridines except in the management of acute hypertension or coronary spasm
• the third generation of calcium antagonists now have long half-lives or are slow-release preparations. Nifedipine is also available in slow release format and considered perfectly safe as shown in the prospective STONE study of treating long-term elderly hypertensives.

5.6 Management of unstable angina

It is now well established that patients with unstable angina should be managed medically until the symptoms have settled. They are then investigated by coronary angiography with a view to possible angioplasty or surgery. Patients who do not settle on medical treatment require urgent investigation.

Unstable angina:
- angina occurring with increasing frequency or severity
- angina occurring at rest, or more frequently at night
- angina not relieved quickly with nitroglycerine
- associated with ST depression on the ECG.

Investigation, angioplasty or surgery in the unstable phase carries only a very slightly higher risk than when undertaken in stable angina.

Stage 1

Complete bed rest. Light sedation. Restricted visitors. Analgesia as required (diamorphine 2.5–5.0 mg i.v./i.m. prn 4 hourly. Drug therapy is started immediately.

- *Beta-blockade*, e.g. Propranolol 40 mg tds. Beta-blockade is avoided if there is any evidence of coronary spasm (labile ST segments during pain with some ST elevation) as this avoids unopposed alpha effects on coronary arteries in patients with spasm.
- *Diltiazem slow release*, 90–180 mg bd. One trial suggested that nifedipine should not be used without a beta-blocker in unstable angina. Calcium antagonists have not been shown to reduce mortality in unstable angina when used alone but are considered safe and useful as synergistic agents with a beta-blocker.
- *Nitrates*. Start with oral isosorbide mononitrate slow-release 60 mg od. Additional GTN spray or tablets available as required. If the angina does not settle rapidly switch to i.v. nitrates: e.g. isosorbide dinitrate starting at 2 mg/h up to 10 mg/h if necessary.
- *Soluble aspirin*, 75–150 mg daily. Aspirin has been shown to reduce the incidence of myocardial infarction and death in unstable angina. It inhibits platelet cyclooxygenase, reducing synthesis of thromboxane A_2 and platelet adhesiveness. This may help to reduce microthrombi formation on an atherosclerotic plaque, which are known from angioscopy studies to be part of the syndrome of unstable angina.
- *Heparin*. Low-molecular-weight heparins, e.g. dalteparin (Fragmin) and enoxaparin (Clexane) have a longer half-life than unfractionated heparin and are given subcutaneously twice daily. Dalteparin has been shown in the FRISC study to reduce the incidence of new myocardial infarction and death in patients already taking aspirin in unstable angina. Dose is 120 IU/kg body weight twice daily subcutaneously for 1 week followed by once daily. Enoxaparin has been shown to be superior to unfractionated heparin when given with aspirin in unstable angina (the ESSENCE trial). There are several advantages of low-molecular-weight heparins to i.v. standard unfractionated heparin. No

monitoring of coagulation is required as standard clotting tests are unaffected (e.g. activated partial thromboplastin time, APTT), antifactor Xa activity is higher, administration is easier and can be continued at home for patients waiting for revascularization, and the incidence of thrombocytopenia and osteoporosis seems to be less than with i.v. heparin.

Thrombolysis is not on this list and has not yet been shown to carry any benefit in patients with unstable angina or non-Q wave infarction.

Stage 2
Coronary arteriography. This is usually performed when symptoms have settled, but may be required urgently if pain continues. Patients should be referred to a centre able to do this, preferably sedated and with i.v. isosorbide dinitrate running. Approximately 7–10% of patients will have left main stem stenosis, about 70% will have left anterior descending stenosis, < 3% will have coronary spasm and a few will have normal coronary arteries (< 10%).

Stage 3
This depends on the coronary arteriographic findings, the facilities available and the expertise of the investigator. The options are:
• percutaneous transluminal coronary angioplasty (PTCA)
• coronary artery bypass surgery (CABG)
• continue medical treatment
• intra-aortic balloon pumping (IABP).

PTCA is proving very valuable in unstable angina. The history is often short and the lesion if a single one is often soft: ideal for angioplasty. In unstable angina stand-by facilities for coronary artery bypass surgery are necessary.

IABP is rarely used in unstable angina except as a holding mechanism prior to surgery or to move the patient to a surgical centre. The balloon can be inserted percutaneously without the need for X-ray screening. IABP is very useful in the short term for controlling pain. Difficult or high-risk angioplasty can be performed with the balloon pump working. (See **6.4**, page 255.)

Medical treatment is reserved for patients with normal coronary arteries, or those with dominantly coronary spasm. A very few patients with unstable angina will have severe diffuse coronary disease that is considered inoperable. These patients must also be managed medically.

Patients with normal coronaries or spasm will continue calcium antagonists and nitrates with soluble aspirin, but their beta-blocking agent is stopped.

In spite of the enormous contribution of PTCA, it is still in the patient's best interest, initially, to manage unstable angina medically if possible. The infarction rate for medically treated patients (without PTCA) is about 14–18%. It is expected that the addition of PTCA will lower this figure.

Future trends

Risk markers

There is increasing evidence that inflammatory markers are raised in unstable angina and have prognostic value. C-reactive protein (CRP), serum amyloid A protein (both acute phase proteins) and interleukin 6 levels from macrophages and T cells are raised in unstable angina and the higher the level the worse the prognosis. These raised markers must reflect inflammatory cell infiltrate into the atheromatous plaque. Aspirins greatest effect is in patients with higher CRP levels. Cardiac troponin T is also a risk marker in unstable angina.

Platelet IIb/IIIa antagonists

The value of aspirin and the finding of microthrombi on culprit lesions in unstable angina have led to studies using more specific platelet anatagonists. Antibodies to the platelet glycoprotein IIb/IIIa receptor help prevent platelet adhesion and subsequent degranulation. c7E3 is a monoclonal antibody to this receptor studied in the EPIC trial in patients with unstable angina undergoing PTCA. There was a reduced acute complication rate and a reduced need for revascularization at 6 months in patients receiving c7E3, but at the expense of more bleeding complications.

A newer IIb/IIIa receptor antagonist, tirofiban, a non-immunogenic peptide, has been studied in the PRISM trial in patients with unstable angina. Given i.v. it proved better than i.v. heparin in reducing the incidence of new myocardial infarction or death, with minimal increase in bleeding complications.

There appears to be considerable potential in this group of drugs but an orally active form is badly needed.

5.7 Percutaneous transluminal coronary angioplasty (PTCA)

First peformed in humans in 1977, this has now become a standard technique in cardiology offering some patients a real alternative to conventional coronary artery bypass surgery.

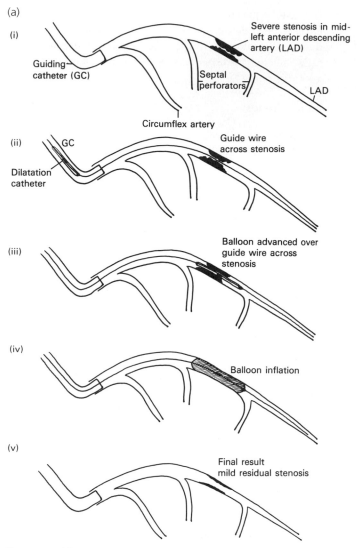

Figure 5.5 (a) Stages in coronary angioplasty: (i) the guiding catheter (GC) is positioned in the ostium of the left coronary artery (LCA). Angiography shows a severe stenosis in the mid-anterior descending artery. (ii) A guide wire (0.014–0.018 inch) is positioned across the stenosis. The balloon catheter (dilatation catheter) remains in the shaft of the guiding catheter. (iii) The dilatation catheter is advanced across the stenosis. (iv) The balloon is inflated. (v) The balloon and guide wire are withdrawn for the final angiogram. In the LAD, a coronary stent is then deployed (Figure 5.5b), or in any other vessel with a suboptimal result.

PTCA is performed in the catheter laboratory under local anaesthetic and sedation only. The technique is illustrated in Figure 5.5 and can be performed via the femoral, brachial or radial artery route. Rapid advances in equipment design have enabled cardiologists to attack more difficult and more numerous lesions. Initially the technique was applied to single-vessel disease but multivessel dilatation is now common.

In the UK in 1995, the PTCA rate was 304 per million population as against a minimum recommended target of 400 per million. These figures are still much lower than many European countries due probably to a lack of staff and facilities as well as perhaps to the conservative views of some community physicians. Stent implantation rates are rising fast. In 1995, 27% PTCA procedures involved stenting. Many centres are now implanting stents in > 70% cases.

Many trials have now compared PTCA with CABG, all showing similar results. PTCA is as effective as surgery initially in relieving angina with a similar mortality. Morbidity is lower with PTCA than with CABG

(b)

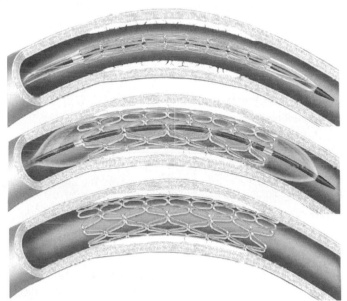

Figure 5.5 (b) Coronary stent deployment. In the top panel the balloon is advanced across a predilated stenosis (as in Figure 5.5a) with the stent premounted on the balloon. In the middle panel, the balloon is inflated expanding the stent, and compressing it into the arterial wall. In the bottom panel, the balloon and wire are withdrawn leaving the stent fully expanded.

and the patient returns to work quicker. Overall costs are still cheaper with PTCA. However the need for re-investigation or re-intervention is much higher with PTCA (38% in the UK RITA trial) due to restenosis. All these comparative trials were in the present era.

Indications
- Anyone being considered for CABG. Are their lesions suitable for PTCA?
- Patients with refractory angina who are not fit for CABG on account of other medical reasons (e.g. renal failure, severe lung disease).
- The elderly.
- Patients who have already had CABG. Stenosis in a native vessel, internal mammary artery or vein graft.
- Severe varicose veins.
- Major clotting disorders.
- Very poor LV function.
- Intolerance to medical therapy.
- Post-thrombolysis: in patients with severe stenoses, symptoms or positive stress tests.
- Acute myocardial infarction if catheter laboratory immediately available (see page 188).

Relative contraindications
- Left main stem disease.
- Very tortuous coronary vessels.
- Multiple restenoses.
- Diffuse proximal coronary disease with bypassable vessels.
- Total occlusion of an important vessel for > 6 months.
- Three previous PTCAs.
- Diabetic patients with multivessel disease. The BARI trial showed these patients were best managed surgically.

None of these are absolute and depend on the skill and experience of the operator.

Suitable lesions
Some lesions are definitely easier than others and the table on page 173 outlines characteristics which make lesions easy or difficult, low risk or higher risk.

Risks and complications
In experienced hands the risks of PTCA parallel those of coronary artery bypass surgery. The risks are slightly higher for multivessel disease

Easier lesions: lower risk	More difficult lesions: higher risk
Single-vessel disease	Multivessel disease
Good LV function	Poor LV function
Young patient	Old patient
Short history of angina	Long history of angina
Discrete } Softer	Longer stenosis } Rough
Smooth concentric } lesions	Rough ulcerated } harder
stenosis	eccentric stenosis } lesions
Non-calcified	Calcified
Proximal part of vessel	Distal part of vessel
No side branch involved	Side branches involved or
Left anterior descending artery	bifurcation stenosis
	Right or circumflex vessels

(MVD) than single-vessel disease (SVD) and slightly greater still in patients with unstable angina. The table shows the present percentage risks (figures are percentages; from 1991 British Cardiovascular Intervention Society).

- *Mortality*. This is thus approximately 1 in 200 or 0.5%.
- *Acute coronary occlusion*. In 2.5%, due to acute dissection or thrombus or both. About half the cases can be dealt with in the laboratory by redilatation using a perfusion balloon (which allows distal blood flow while the balloon is inflated). Alternatively most centres prefer the deployment of a coronary stent, which compresses the dissection flap back against the arterial wall. Use of these techniques has lowered the acute referral rate for coronary bypass surgery.

	SVD	MVD	Unstable angina	Overall
Death	0.43	0.5	0.7	0.48
Emergency CABG	2.6	2.2	3.3	2.57
Myocardial infarction	1.4	1.6	2.5	1.59

- *Damage to coronary artery at site other than dilatation site*. For example, ostial dissection with guiding catheter; perforation of the coronary artery is very rare.
- *Guide-wire fracture*. Distal fragment has to be removed surgically.
- *Side-branch occlusion*. This may reverse spontaneously. Risks of this can be reduced using a 'two-wire' technique, or more rarely a pair of balloons: the kissing balloon technique.
- *Distal vessel emboli*. This is probably much more common than is generally realized, involving micro-emboli into tiny distal vessels. More

serious occlusion of the larger vessels can occur due to distal movement of thrombus or atheromatous material. Vigorous heparinization during the procedure is mandatory. PTCA of acutely embolized vessels may be necessary.

• *Complications of arterial catheterization.* The guiding catheter is slightly larger than a conventional coronary catheter. Haematoma and false aneurysm formation at the femoral puncture site may occur. More serious is the possibility of systemic emboli from within the guiding catheter itself if heparinization is inadequate.

Successful PTCA

This is judged primarily angiographically. A reduction in the stenosis by > 20% was judged by Gruntzig as a primary success. Most PTCA procedures reduce the stenosis by considerably more. The vessel may look rather shaggy following PTCA, but it quickly remodels itself, and provided there is a good lumen, with a good perfusion pressure, there is usually no problem. Remodelling occurs in the subsequent 3 months. The advent of coronary stents has largely solved the problems of dissection flaps seen in the prestent era.

Preparation of the patient

The operator must explain the entire procedure to the patient. Most patients will already be familiar with the catheter laboratory, having had previous coronary angiography. Diagrams (e.g. Figure 5.5) help in the explanation. Important points that should be included are listed.

• The procedure takes a little longer than coronary angiography, but in many respects is very similar. There will be no hot flush (no need for repeat LV angiography). There is no need for a general anaesthetic A sheath will be left in the patient's groin for a few hours after PTCA.

• The patient should expect angina during balloon inflation and should tell the operator if he or she gets it.

• The possible need for emergency coronary bypass surgery (< 2%).

• The very small mortality risk (< 0.5%).

• The possible need for one or more intracoronary stents (50–70% cases). Particularly likely for PTCAs of the LAD and by-pass grafts. One per cent risk of subacute stent thrombosis.

• The possible need to repeat the procedure in the next 6 months (approximately 15–20% clinical restenosis requiring re-intervention without stenting). If the vessel is stented reintervention is probably needed in < 10% now.

• The patient will spend the night after the procedure in the CCU.

- The operator should obtain the patient's consent on a special consent form.

The house physician must help organize the drug regime, group and save serum, etc. He or she should have observed coronary angioplasty to answer patient's questions. A standard regime is:

- stop beta-blocking agents 48 hours prior to PTCA if angina is stable. This is done to try and reduce any tendency to coronary spasm during PTCA
- soluble aspirin 75–150 mg daily
- oral nitrates and a calcium antagonist in standard doses.

On the morning of the procedure:

- starve the patient for 4 hours prior to PTCA
- group and save serum
- premedication as for conventional cardiac catheter. Additional sedation may be given in the catheter laboratory if necessary.

Management of the patient following PTCA

The patient is monitored overnight in the coronary care unit and can usually go home the following day.

- Careful monitoring of blood pressure is necessary. It is important to avoid hypotension with excess sedation, analgesia and nitrates all causing a fall in systemic pressure and hence a drop in coronary perfusion pressure. This could potentiate the development of acute coronary occlusion. A fall in systemic pressure below 90 mmHg should be corrected by i.v. dextran 40 (which may help prevent red cell sludging), or i.v. Haemaccel or Gelofusine. In addition atropine 0.6–1.2 mg i.v. may be needed if the patient is bradycardic.
- No further heparin is given once the patient leaves the catheter laboratory except in unusual circumstances where the procedure was complicated by thrombus or unresolved dissection in which case it may be continued overnight.
- Stent cases. No extra heparin is needed, and the regime is as for ordinary balloon PTCA.

Many centres use additional ticlopidine 250 mg bd for 4 weeks as well as soluble aspirin 150 mg daily in stent cases. Ticlopidine inhibits ADP-induced platelet aggregation and platelet serotonin release but is not available in the UK on prescription (named-patient basis only in hospitals). It takes about 72 hours to reach its maximum effect. Patients are given a 4-week supply and told to have a full blood count at 2 weeks as the drug causes leukopenia in about 0.7% cases. There is no advantage or need for warfarin over this simple aspirin and ticlopidine regime. Some units are using aspirin alone. The use of clopidogrel, a similar drug to ticlopidine but faster acting, is under study.

- Sheaths are removed after 4–6 hours with straightforward cases. If the patient is on heparin this is stopped 2 hours previously. The ACT (activated clotting time) should be checked prior to sheath removal with a Haemochron and should be < 150 s (normal 100 s). Alternatively the sheaths are removed the following morning. Sheath removal is painful, as the local anaesthetic has worn off. Patients may develop an acute vagal episode and it is sensible to premedicate them: i.v. atropine 0.6 mg + i.v. Diazemuls 10–20 mg. Some patients develop oozing around the sheath, and this may necessitate its removal earlier than planned.
- A post-PTCA ECG is taken as soon as practical.
- Acute occlusion of the dilated vessel is suggested by the development of chest pain and rapidly rising ST segments over the relevant leads. This is a medical emergency and is usually managed by transferring the patient back to the catheter laboratory for a repeat PTCA procedure as soon as possible. If the first PTCA was particularly complex or difficult, the operator may opt for emergency coronary by-pass surgery. Intravenous thrombolysis is a third possibility, but there may be bleeding problems with the large arterial sheath *in situ*.
- Discharge home. The patient should take soluble aspirin 75–150 mg daily indefinitely. If stented then ticlopidine 250 mg bd is often also prescribed for 4 weeks only (see above). Beta-blocking agents and calcium antagonists can usually be stopped unless the patient is hypertensive. Follow up is at 1 month and 6 months. Exercise testing and thallium-201 scanning may be needed for patients who redevelop symptoms and coronary angiography where indicated. Patients must not drive for 72 hours post-PTCA.

Restenosis

Denuded endothelium stimulates platelet accretion, release of platelet-derived growth factor (PDGF) and many others. These reach the media within 24 hours and stimulate smooth muscle cell proliferation. These cells then migrate through into the intima and rapidly cause restenosis. The restenotic lesion is thus due to fibrocellular proliferation and not lipid deposition.

It is recognised that this occurs in 20–30% of all cases undergoing PTCA, usually within the first 6 months. Only about 15% of patients actually require redilatation. Few centres perform routine repeat coronary angiography and restenosis is suggested by the development of angina again or the recurrence of a positive treadmill test.

The only drug regime found to reduce restenosis as assessed by the need for re-intervention (CABG or PTCA) or myocardial infarction or death has been the use of monoclonal antibody to the platelet glycoprotein IIb/IIIa receptor (c7E3) in the EPIC trial. This was only tested in patients with unstable angina or impending infarction and did cause an increased haemorrhagic risk at the time of the PTCA. Restenosis has not been prevented by any other antiplatelet regime (including aspirin), calcium antagonists, ACE inhibitors, self-administered subcutaneous heparin, oral anticoagulation or omega-3 fatty acid supplements.

Two stent trials (BENESTENT and STRESS) have both shown a reduction in restenosis in stented patients compared with ordinary balloon angioplasty (angiographic restenosis reduced from 32% to 20% at 7 months in the BENESTENT trial).

Factors reported to be associated with restenosis are:
- inadequate initial dilatation, e.g. balloon undersizing
- high inflation pressures at initial PTCA (> 7 atm)
- male sex
- PTCA of vein bypass graft
- smoking
- variant angina
- multivessel disease
- long stenoses
- diabetes
- complex dissection and vessel trauma at first dilatation
- ostial lesions
- proximal LAD lesions.

Restenosis is dealt with by repeat PTCA. The lesion may be smoother and not ulcerated compared with the initial dilatation, and the procedure often easier with a lower complication rate. Restenosis within a stent can also be dealt with by balloon dilatation or by rotablation (see below).

Two other avenues of animal research in restenosis prevention are particularly exciting. The first is in the use of radioactive stents (Brachytherapy). These emit beta or gamma irradiation and completely prevent smooth muscle cell hyperplasia. Transluminal irradiation is already being tried in man following stent deployment. The second is using a variety of gene-transfection techniques, e.g. coating the outside of a traumatized rat carotid artery with a gel containing antisense oligonucleotide to c-*myb*, a proto-oncogene also completely prevents restenosis. Delivering a gene locally inside a coronary artery using a non-replicating adenoviral vector is now a possibility. Keeping it at the site of angioplasty is a problem.

Newer technology
There is a variety of new technology to help the interventionist with difficult stenoses or occlusions.
• *Coronary angioscopy*. This has been used intra-operatively to examine the vessel in unstable angina and the effects of PTCA. Angioscopy is now starting in the catheter laboratory and will greatly improve our understanding of the effects of PTCA on the vessel wall.
• *Intravascular ultrasound*. (IVUS). Special monorail solid-state intracoronary catheters are available using 20 or 40 MHz transducers mounted cylindrically in a phased array pattern. They are expensive as they are used for one patient only. Imaging before and after the PTCA gives extra information regarding tissue characterization and dissection not avaliable at angiography, e.g. IVUS often shows more calcification in a lesion than had been suspected at angiography.

IVUS has proved very useful in coronary stenting as it is important to ensure that the stent struts are fully deployed against the arterial wall. This can only be detected with IVUS.

Finally ultrasound ablation of coronary lesions is starting experimentally and has been used in humans successfully.
• *Directional coronary atherectomy (DCA)*. This device is placed across the stenosis via a conventional guide wire and punches out slivers of atheroma, which can be examined histologically and from which smooth muscle cells, etc. can be grown. Atherectomy is used for bulky and eccentric lesions in large vessels (> 3.0 mm). It is not suitable for tortuous arteries and the circumflex vessel can be difficult. The design of the 'atherocath' is improving fast. Unfortunately two trials (CAVEAT and CCAT) have shown that elective atherectomy is inferior to conventional balloon angioplasty, with a higher cost, a greater myocardial infarction rate and acute closure rate. DCA remains useful for bulky eccentric lesions particularly in the main LAD, but restenosis rates are similar to balloon angioplasty.
• *Laser technology*. The expense and problems with control of the laser beam have reduced the popularity of this technique. Excimer laser angioplasty can tackle difficult long stenoses, ostial lesions and total occlusions not possible with conventional balloon dilatation.
• *Rotablation*. This is a diamond studded burr rotating at 150 000–

200 000 r.p.m. over a special guide wire. It is valuable for long lesions and diffuse disease, as well as tough or calcified lesions. It can be used in smaller vessels where stenting is less successful and to deal with in-stent restenosis. Pulverized microscopic debris migrates distally and can cause coronary spasm. Patients receive an infusion of nitrates and verapamil to prevent this and temporary pacing is often necessary.

• *Coronary stents.* These are fast revolutionizing coronary angioplasty being used in 27% of all UK angioplasty procedures in 1995. In many centres the figure is > 70%. They are expensive (approximately £800 each) but have been shown to reduce restenosis (see above). The stent is delivered to the lesion over a conventional balloon. More than one can be put into the same vessel – in series – and side branches remain patent. High pressure inflation (16–20 atm) is employed after stent deployment to ensure good stent strut apposition against the arterial wall. A wide variety of designs (coil or mesh stents) and lengths (6–49 mm) are available. They are stainless steel, tantalum, nitinol or platinum and only just visible on X-ray screening.

Stents are particularly indicated for dilatation of the LAD, vein graft lesions and ostial lesions (where the restenosis rate is so high). They should be used for bulky and ulcerated lesions as an elective procedure. They are best reserved for vessels > 3.0 mm diameter if possible. As well as compressing plaque, they prevent elastic recoil at the site of dilatation.

One of their great benefits is in the bail-out situation of acute occlusion occurring during conventional balloon PTCA. They hold back a dissection flap and usually the need for emergency CABG is avoided.

Post-stent management is now much simplified. Anticoagulation with heparin or warfarin is unnecessary once the patient has left the catheter laboratory. Patients just receive aspirin and ticlopidine (see Management, page 175). Aspirin for life and ticlopidine for 4 weeks.

Choice of PTCA or surgery (CABG) for stable angina

The RITA trial has shown that both forms of treatment are very successful in relieving angina with very low rates of mortality or myocardial infarction. However, patients treated with PTCA are more likely to get angina again, need anti-anginal medication and require further hospital admission for repeat coronary angiography and/or repeat PTCA. Assuming some form of intervention is needed, generally patients with single-vessel disease are managed with PTCA if possible. Patients with two-vessel disease can be managed with either technique, depending on the nature of the lesions, and patients with three-vessel disease or long-standing occlusions are managed with coronary by-pass surgery. Diabetic patients should be considered for surgery rather than PTCA (high restenosis rate with PTCA).

5.8 Myocardial infarction

Mortality untreated is approximately 40% in the first 4 weeks and 50% of these patients die within the first 2 hours of symptoms. The great delay in getting patients to hospital is generally due to the delay in the patient recognizing the importance of his or her symptoms.

Mobile coronary care units developed in Brighton and Belfast in the UK have shown how successful they can be, possibly by:
• reduction of transport deaths
• resuscitation of on site VF
• possible reduction of infarct size by early treatment of arrhythmias, although this will be impossible to prove
• reduction of the time taken to reach a coronary care unit
• early administration of thrombolysis (see page 194).

Education of lay people in cardiac resuscitation has proved very valuable (e.g. in Seattle) and static coronary care units (e.g. in sports stadia) are being developed.

Hospital mortality has dramatically halved in the last few years with the advent of thrombolysis, aspirin, etc. and now runs at about 10%.

Pathology
Approximately 90% of patients with a transmural infarct have total occlusion of the relevant coronary artery (as visualized by angiography) within 4 hours of pain onset. Incidence decreases with time (possibly due to relaxation of additional spasm or recanalization). The majority of occlusive thrombi are associated with intimal plaque rupture and haemorrhage into the plaque.

A small proportion of patients will have normal coronary arteries. Emboli or spasm must be the prime mechanisms in these cases.

Home or hospital care?
Since the original work of Mather and his colleagues in 1971, numerous publications have appeared extolling the virtues of both home and hospital care for myocardial infarction.

Since 50% of patients who are going to die do so within 2 hours of their symptoms, home care may be considered where:

- time from onset of symptoms is > 6 hours
- the patient is warm, well perfused, out of pain and normotensive
- there are no signs of LVF
- there is no history of diabetes
- the cardiac rhythm is stable.

The wishes of the patient and his or her relatives are considered, the social circumstances, the availability and proximity of a coronary care unit, and the available transport facilities.

Immediate treatment in the home

Analgesia: diamorphine is the drug of choice. It should be given i.v. (2.5–5.0 mg) in case subsequent thrombolysis is given.
Metoclopramide 10 mg i.v. or i.m. or cyclizine 50 mg i.m. or orally should be administered as an anti-emetic. Both opiates and myocardial infarction cause vomiting. Cyclizine is more sedative than metoclopramide. Numerous other anti-emetics are available. Metoclopramide has the additional advantage of speeding gastric emptying and increasing the tone of the cardia (oesophagogastric junction).

Oxygen at 5 l/min.

Bradycardia (sinus or junctional) is treated with atropine 0.6 mg i.v. repeated to a maximum of 3.0 mg.

Lignocaine at 300 mg i.m. in the absence of bradycardia, hypotension or shock may be given for frequent multifocal ventricular extrasystoles, salvos of ventricular tachycardia, etc. or prior to transfer to hospital.

Intravenous frusemide is given to the patient in acute pulmonary oedema (also has a venodilator effect). Dose 40–80 mg initially i.v. It should not be given for a raised JVP in the presence of an inferior infarct unless the patient is also in pulmonary oedema.

Diagnosis

This may pose a great problem, and there are no absolutely accepted criteria. Diagnosis is based on the following:

- typical history
- ECG changes
- cardiac enzyme elevation
- postmortem evidence.

Other criteria which may help but are less reliable include the following:

- physical signs, e.g. new high dyskinetic apex, pericardial rub

- fever developing 48 hours after the pain
- elevated WBC and ESR
- myocardial scintigraphy. Not positive until 48 hours postinfarction, e.g. hot-spot scanning using isotopes taken up into dead/dying cells (e.g. imidodiphosphate) or cold-spot scanning using potassium analogues taken up by living cardiac cells (e.g. thallium).

The table on page 183 shows the criteria modified from WHO analysis.

Summary of changes (for examples see **12.1**)

1 *Pathological Q waves.* New Q waves are the hallmark of so-called transmural infarction. In standard leads pathological Q wave should be not less than 25% of the R wave and 0.04 s in duration with negative T waves. In precordial leads pathological Q waves should be associated with ORS duration < 0.1 s (i.e. not LBBB), and with negative or biphasic T waves. Q waves in V_4 or V_5 should be > 0.4 mV and in V_6 > 0.2 mV.

Large Q waves occur also with hypertrophy and fibrosis (e.g. HCM), and infiltration (e.g. amyloidosis). It is most valuable to be able to establish that the Q waves are new. Q waves also occur in the chest leads in corrected transposition.

2 *Injury current/ST segment elevation.* ST-segment elevation should persist preferably for 24 hours. (Transient ST-segment elevation occurs with Prinzmetal's angina.) It usually appears within 24 hours of a transmural infarct, and returns to isoelectric baseline in < 2 weeks. Persisting ST segment elevation at > 1 month suggests LV aneurysm.

3 *Reciprocal ST-segment depression.* This is thought to reflect a 'mirror image' of electrical activity on the opposite non-infarcted wall. It is not thought that reciprocal ST-segment depression indicates additional ischaemia and coronary disease in the relevant territory.

4 *T-wave inversion.* By itself it is not diagnostic of infarction. (Occurs in the normal heart in some patients with catecholamine stimulation, reversed by beta-blockade.)

Steep symmetrical T-wave inversion may occur without new Q-wave development either in ventricular hypertrophy or in 'subendocardial' infarction. Enzyme elevation is necessary to confirm infarction in the absence of new Q waves.

Localization of infarcts from ECG

- Anterolateral: Q waves in I, aVL, and V3–6. ST elevation with T inversion in I and aVL.
- Anteroseptal: Q waves in V2 and V3 (but often none in lateral precordial or standard leads) with ST elevation and T inversion.

Criteria for diagnosis of myocardial infarction

	Definite	Probable	Possible
History	Severe, typically cardiac pain lasting ≥ 20 min and unrelieved by nitrates	As in definite category	Atypical chest pain A sense of suffocation or indigestion. General malaise History of syncope History of acute dyspnoea or CCF
ECG	New Q waves in at least two ECGs ST-segment elevation persisting for 24 hours, > 2 mm in precordial lead, > 1 mm in standard leads	Either definite ECG changes or →	Transient ST-segment elevation T-wave inversion only No new Q waves
Cardiac enzymes	Rise to more than twice normal	Definite enzyme changes	Rise to less than twice normal

....

- Antero-apical: Q wave in I with ST elevation. Apparent right-axis deviation. May be Qs in V3–4.
- Inferior (diaphragmatic): 0 waves in II, III aVF with ST elevation and T inversion. Additional ST elevation in V4R suggests RV infarction.
- True posterior: tall R waves in V1 and V2 (exclude RV hypertrophy, Type A WPW syndrome and RBBB) with negative ST depression in V1–3. This can be confirmed by the oesophageal lead.

Changes on ECG not diagnostic of infarction, but which may be ischaemic:

- ST-segment depression
- transient ST-segment elevation (e.g. spasm)
- axis shift – left or right
- transient T-wave inversion (Figures 5.6 and 12.10)
- increase in R wave voltage (e.g. on exercise testing; Figure 12.17)
- LBBB or RBBB
- 1°, 2° or 3° AV block
- tachyarrhythmias
- transient tall peaked T waves

Cardiac enzymes

CPK (creatine phosphokinase). MB isoenzyme. The most specific cardiac enzyme. Rises and falls within the first 72 hours. Cumulative CPK

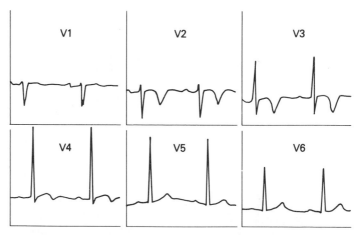

Figure 5.6 ECG chest leads in a man with a tight LAD stenosis and history of severe chest pain lasting 30 min. No pathological Q waves. Enzyme elevation needed to confirm infarction. This ECG returned completely to normal following angioplasty.

concentrations have been used to estimate infarct size. Peak concentration 24 hours postinfarction. Other isoenzymes of CPK are CPK–MM (skeletal muscle) and CPK-BB (brain and kidney). Very small amounts of CPK–MB also occur in small intestine, tongue and diaphragm.

Recent analysis of CPK–MB isoforms has helped discriminate true myocardial infarction at the very early stage of 4–6 hours when thrombolysis may be needed. CPK–MB has two isoforms: MB_1 from serum and MB_2 from myocardial tissue. The normal ratio is 1.0. A ratio of $MB_2/MB_1 > 1.5$ is diagnostic of myocardial damage. This raised ratio occurs before total CPK–MB is elevated by conventional testing.

SGOT (serum glutamic–oxaloacetic transaminase, also known as aspartate aminotransferase). Less specific than CPK–MB. Rises and falls within 4–6 days. Peak concentration at 24 hours. SGOT is also elevated in liver disease hepatic congestion), pulmonary embolism, skeletal muscle injury, shock or i.m. injections.

LDH (lactic dehydrogenase). Again not cardio-specific. Peaks about 4–5 days postinfarction, and may take 2 weeks to return to baseline. LDH also elevated in: haemolysis, leukaemia, megaloblastic anaemia, renal disease, plus all the false-positive causes of elevated SGOT.

The LDH false-positives can be separated by isoenzyme electrophoretic studies. LDH_1, cardiac, red cells; LDH_4 and LDH_5, liver and skeletal muscle.

HBD (hydroxybutyrate dehydrogenase). This is really measuring the activity of LDH_1 isoenzyme and is often used instead of LDH analysis and isoenzyme differentiation.

Myoglobin. Although not strictly an enzyme, peak levels of serum myoglobin occur before peak CPK–MB activity. It is also excreted in the urine. It is not clinically useful (due to its skeletal muscle origin).

Troponin T. A new immunodiagnostic test is now available to detect this myofibrillar protein which appears to be a specific marker for myocardial infarction. Levels of troponin T remain raised for up to 2 weeks following infarction, much longer than CPK (2–3 days). It appears to have prognostic value in patients admitted with unstable angina, raised levels indicating a high likelihood of subsequent infarction.

Non-Q-wave (subendocardial) infarction

A total coronary occlusion usually produces a transmural Q-wave infarct. Incomplete thrombosis or early lysis in a coronary artery produces a non-Q-wave infarct. The diagnosis of a subendocardial infarct is based on a typical history of chest pain, ECG changes (ST-segment elevation, ST depression or T-wave inversion) plus enzyme elevation which is often mild compared with transmural Q-wave infarction. See Figures 5.6 and 12.10.

Generally it is an incomplete and small infarct. It may be due to diffuse three-vessel disease or a single severe stenosis in a large artery. In either case it may occur early in the course of a Q-wave infarct, before the vessel is totally occluded. Frequently it progresses to a Q-wave infarct within a year. Subendocardial infarcts account for about 20–30% of all infarcts.

Relevance of diagnosis to subsequent course and prognosis

It is very important to follow up and investigate patients with a non-Q-wave infarct. The subsequent course and prognosis differ sharply from Q-wave infarction.
• Low hospital mortality: approximately 2% (12–18% in Q-wave infarcts).
• High late (1 year) mortality, particularly with evidence of early extension: (approximately 65% versus 34% in Q-wave infarcts).
• ST-segment depression at diagnosis more dangerous than ST elevation.
• High incidence of arrhythmias, 24-hour ECG monitoring needed.
• More incidence of post-infarct angina than following Q-wave infarction.
• LV function may improve transiently following a non-Q-wave infarct. If segmental wall motion can be shown to improve, then that area is at high risk for a full thickness infarct subsequently.

Immediate treatment in the hospital

It is important that patients with suspected myocardial infarction receive immediate treatment in accident and emergency departments with a fast-track system to get them quickly to the coronary care unit (CCU) where thrombolysis can be started if appropriate. Immediate measures in casualty should include:
• rapid assessment of the patient, e.g. ?shock, hypotension, signs of LVF or RVF, heart murmurs
• establish i.v. access

....

- 12-lead ECG
- give:
  oral aspirin 150 mg and daily thereafter if no contraindications. O_2
  40% if no history of chronic obstructive airways disease diamorphine
  2.5–5.0 mg i.v. and repeat as necessary to control pain
  metoclopramide 10 mg i.v.
  GTN spray × 2 if not hypotensive
- portable CXR (or in CCU)
- arrange for transfer to CCU
- take blood for urgent U and E, glucose, CPK, HBD and FBC.
Repeat bloods at 24 and 48 hours
- if delayed in getting patient to CCU start thrombolysis in casualty
- thrombolytic therapy. This is considered in detail in **5.9**.

It is important that thrombolysis is not delayed due to logistic
problems of getting the patient transferred from casualty to CCU.
Many casualty departments start thrombolysis after the ECG and CXR
are done and before transfer.

In CCU consider additional therapy.

- *Beta-blockade.* Beta-blocking agents without intrinsic
sympathomimetic activity have been shown to reduce mortality and
subsequent cardiac events. Probably reduces early mortality by
preventing cardiac rupture. (Analysis of ISIS 1 data.) Use atenolol 5 mg
i.v., metoprolol or propranolol 5 mg i.v. Then continue orally
thereafter. Contraindicated in patients with pulmonary oedema, third
sound gallop, peripheral ischaemia and asthma.
- *Heparin.* This is still controversial. Low subcutaneous dose (5000
units bd) helps prevent deep-vein thrombosis. High subcutaneous dose
(12 500 units bd) helps prevent mural thrombus, but does slightly
increase risk of cerebral haemorrhage. Many units use i.v. heparin after
tissue plasminogen activator (tPA) for 24 hours in an attempt to
improve coronary patency. Generally i.v. heparin should be given to
patients with large infarcts, those who are slow to mobilize, with heart
failure, etc.

  Dose: 5000 units as an initial bolus then 1000 units/hour. Check
APTT at 2–4 × control (see also page 167 for alternative use of low
molecular weight heparin).
- *Intravenous nitrates.* These are used for selected patients only: those
with left ventricular failure or continuing pain, e.g. isosorbide dinitrate
starting at 2.0 mg i.v./hour. See nitrates, **5.4**.
- *ACE inhibitors.* The SAVE trial has shown that captopril started 3–16
days after a myocardial infarction in patients with abnormal left

ventricular function helps reduce long-term mortality (17%), recurrent heart failure and re-infarction (24%). This is independent of other agents above and thrombolysis. Captopril appears to reduce left ventricular dilatation with beneficial effects on left ventricular remodelling. The CONSENSUS II trial was unable to show similar beneficial effects with enalapril, possibly because the drug was started too early and was not confined to patients with poor LV function. Therefore on present evidence use captopril starting at 6.25 mg tds on the fourth post-infarct day aiming to reach 25 mg tds by hospital discharge. Select patients particularly with:

large infarcts

heart failure

large heart on CXR

anterior Q waves on ECG

LVEF < 40% on echocardiography or MUGA scanning.

• *Magnesium.* Evidence from the LIMIT 2 study from Leicester suggested that i.v. magnesium given within 24 hours after acute infarction reduced mortality by 24%. Data from the much larger ISIS 4 trial completely refutes this and there is no indication for routine use of magnesium now. It should be considered in cases of resistant or recurrent VT.

Dose: 8 mmol in 20 ml 5% dextrose over 20 min, followed by 65 mmol in 100 ml 5% dextrose over 24 hours.

Contraindications to magnesium: AV block, renal failure (creatinine > 300 mmol/l), severe bradycardia.

• Calcium antagonists. The evidence that these are beneficial early after infarction is skimpy and they are best avoided particularly if LV function is impaired. One trial suggested a benefit with diltiazem if LV function was normal, and the Danish verapamil trial (DAVITT II) with verapamil started 4–5 days postinfarct suggested a benefit if LV function was normal.

Role of immediate angioplasty without thrombolysis

Until 1993 it was accepted that PTCA in acute infarction could be delayed until 2–3 weeks after thrombolysis and performed only in those with evidence of continuing ischaemia or a positive stress test (page 169).

The PRAMI trial has suggested that immediate PTCA without thrombolysis can successfully reduce re-infarction, death and intracranial bleeding compared with conventional thrombolysis. Myocardial salvage appears similar with either technique.

The logistical difficulties in providing an immediate PTCA service for acute myocardial infarction are considerable, and in spite of the results of the PRAMI study, almost all hospitals will continue to use conventional thrombolysis in acute infarction.

Postinfarct management

Early investigation is necessary, with exercise testing and coronary angiography. PTCA is useful for suitable lesions, or coronary surgery for patients with diffuse three-vessel disease.

Medical management alone is unsatisfactory, but if no other facilities are available, treatment with soluble aspirin and beta-blockade is recommended for patients with good LV function, and aspirin and captopril for poor LV function.

Early hospital discharge

Selection of a low-risk group of patients has allowed early discharge from hospital at about 1 week following infarction. If there have been no complications at the end of the fourth day, then there are unlikely to be any. Using an early discharge policy will very rarely result in the release of a patient who later develops problems. Early follow up is necessary.

Patients who should not be discharged early are those with:
- pulmonary oedema or evidence of LVF
- further chest pain after admission
- diabetes
- arrhythmias
- conduction defects: 2° or 3° AV block, bifascicular block
- persistent fever.

Common sense and the patient's social circumstances are all important.

Early investigation

Treadmill exercise testing has been performed as little as 1 week after uncomplicated infarcts and is useful in assessing the severity of coronary artery disease, and the 1-year prognosis.

Most centres now exercise patients before returning them to work and perform coronary angiography on young patients or those with strongly positive tests and poor exercise tolerance. There is no need to discontinue beta-blockage prior to the tests.

Advice to the coronary patient prior to hospital discharge

This should be also re-inforced at the first outpatient visit 4 weeks later.

Work. The patient should consider returning to work if possible 2 months after a myocardial infarct. In a few cases this time may be shortened. A return to full-time work is the single most important item in a patient's recovery. A few occupations, however, cannot be restarted following infarction: public service vehicle drivers, heavy goods vehicle drivers, airline pilots or air traffic control personnel, divers.

Several occupations should be considered hazardous for the postinfarct patient, e.g. furniture removers, scaffolders, bricklayers, dockers, miners, steelworkers, and if possible the patient should be advised to seek a lighter job.

Exercise. Regular daily exercise is encouraged. The patient should be recommended to take initially two short walks (15–20 min) daily, with prophylactic GTN if necessary. This distance should be increased weekly. Instructions for swimming, etc. are as with angina (page 150).

Weight. Weight control is important and is often difficult when giving up smoking.

Smoking. Should be stopped.

Diet. A diet that does not produce weight gain is the most important factor. A high-fibre diet with vegetables and cereals should be encouraged. Vitamins C and E are anti-oxidants and help prevent oxidation of LDL cholesterol in the blood vessel wall. The CHAOS trial from Cambridge used 400–800 mg vitamin E/day and reduced cardiac events by 77% but surprisingly had no effect on cardiac mortality. Vitamin E supplementation can be recommended, but there is no evidence yet that it lowers mortality.

Reduction in saturated fats is important in secondary prevention. Three studies (4S, CARE and WOSCOPS) have provided strong evidence for both primary and secondary prevention in coronary disease and emphasized the importance of lowering even only slightly elevated serum cholesterol. See section on hyperlipidaemias (page 209).

Sex. This should be discussed. Intercourse is probably best avoided for 1 month only after myocardial infarction. GTN prophylaxis and beta-blockade will help patients who suffer with angina on intercourse, but beta-blockade may cause impotence. A relatively passive role in intercourse should be encouraged initially.

Contraception. The Pill should be discouraged and alternative methods suggested for the female patient.

Alcohol. Regular evening alcohol intake in moderation is perfectly satisfactory (e.g. two glasses of wine or a double whisky). Several pints of beer, however, should be discouraged because of its water-load effect.

Travel. Travel abroad should be discouraged for the first 2 months, but may be unavoidable (see angina).

Secondary prevention

There is enough evidence now to recommend soluble aspirin 150 mg daily and a routine beta-blocker, both of which have been independently shown to reduce subsequent cardiac events. Meta-analysis of seven randomized prospective trials has shown an overall reduction in mortality of 21% and a reduction in re-infarction of 31% in patients taking aspirin. The aspirin and beta-blocker are continued indefinitely as late withdrawal of the beta-blocker has been shown to cause a late rise in mortality in both metoprolol and timolol trials. Beta blockage reduces re-infarction by about 25%. Beta-1 receptor blockade is important, and a cardioselective drug can be used. Avoid beta-blockers with intrinsic sympathomimetic activity (e.g. oxprenolol). There have been positive trials with timolol, propranolol, atenolol and metoprolol.

There is concern that aspirin intake in the over 75-year-old age group may increase the risk of cerebral haemorrhage and prophylactic aspirin is best avoided in the long term in this group.

Long-term calcium antagonists are of doubtful value. There has been a positive trial for both diltiazem and verapamil, but only if LV function was normal. Generally they should only be used if the patient has angina.

ACE inhibitors such as captopril should be used in the long term in patients with large hearts or poor LV function (reduction in both future heart failure and further myocardial infarction). The largest tolerable dose is recommended: 25–50 mg tds.

Long-term oral magnesium is of no benefit.

Warfarin should only be used for patients in AF, those with left ventricular thrombus visualized on echocardiography, or those with an LV aneurysm or grossly dilated hypokinetic ventricles. Warfarin is less effective than aspirin at preventing recurrent ischaemic events following successful thrombolysis.

Outpatient follow up after myocardial infarction

The first outpatient visit 4 weeks following an infarct is very important. Symptoms must be assessed. Risk stratification, secondary prevention and the possible need for rehabilitation must be considered with a view to getting the patient back to work and to a normal life.

Symptoms

Angina is treated medically initially (page 149) and the patient is put on the waiting list for coronary arteriography. Priority is given for those at greater risk. See risk stratification, below.

Dyspnoea is most commonly due to poor LV function which is assessed clinically and on echocardiography. Mitral regurgitation, a possible VSD or developing LV aneurysm must be picked up, as must possible additional anaemia, airways obstruction, etc. Occasionally patient's symptoms are misinterpreted by the physician as dyspnoea when they are in fact complaining of angina. Dyspnoea due to poor LV function is treated with ACE inhibitors and diuretics (page 230).

Palpitation. See **7.10** page 314. 24-hour monitoring is necessary. Isolated ventricular ectopics and non-sustained VT do not necessarily need treatment unless associated with poor LV function. Avoid Class 1 anti-arrhythmic agents (higher mortality than placebo in the CAST study). Ensure the serum potassium is > 4.0 mmol/l.

Occasional ventricular ectopics should be ignored and the patient reassured. Frequent ectopics (> 10/hour) with good LV function are managed with β-blockade if the patient is symptomatic. If LV function is poor start with an ACE inhibitor which also helps keep the potassium up.

Non-sustained VT (bursts of < 30 s). Refer for coronary angiography and treat those with poor LV function with an ACE inhibitor and amiodarone. Sustained VT merits urgent admission and coronary arteriography. Patients are revascularized where possible (either PTCA or CABG) and subsequently restudied with Holter monitoring and treadmill testing. Patients who are not suitable for revascularization are considered for an implantable cardioverter defibrillator (ICD) or amiodarone (see page 291).

Risk stratification

It is important to determine which patients are at high risk of sudden death or re-infarction as they need coronary angiography during the first admission or as soon after as is practical.

Those particularly at risk are:
- history of previous myocardial infarction
- age > 75 years
- diabetic patients
- resting tachycardia > 100/min
- poor LV function as evidenced by:
  clinical signs; systolic blood pressure < 100 mmHg
  echocardiography LVEF < 40%
  MUGA scanning
  large heart on CXR (CTR > 50%)
- unstable angina; rest or nocturnal angina unrelieved by GTN
- documented VT (sustained > 30 s)
- positive treadmill testing, unable to complete Stage 2 of the Bruce protocol, 7 METS (add 6 min for the modified Bruce protocol, a gentler test for the post-infarct patient)
- frequent episodes of silent ischaemia on 24-hour monitoring
- depression of heart rate variability.

Unfortunately studies of afterpotentials (which are theoretically linked with ventricular arrhythmias) on the signal-averaged ECG following infarction have not yielded as valuable prognostic information as was initially hoped.

Of all of these the single most useful variable is the left ventricular function.

Myocardial infarction with normal coronary arteries

Definite Q-wave infarcts occasionally occur in patients who have normal coronary angiograms at subsequent investigation. It is not always possible to provide an explanation but probable considerations are:
- coronary spasm
- coronary emboli
- recanalization following coronary thrombosis
- thyrotoxicosis
- coronary arteritis
- prothrombotic state.

Spontaneous thrombus developing in a normal artery is rare but may indicate a hypercoagulable or prothrombotic state. It may occur in heavy smokers, women on the Pill and polycythaemic patients. Haematological help is needed but investigations which should be considered include:

- full blood count
- platelet count
- prothrombin time, partial thromboplastin time and thrombin time
- platelet aggregation to ADP ?Spontaneous aggregation of platelets in platelet-rich plasma
- lupus anticoagulant, check dilute Russell viper time
- anticardiolipin antibody
- antithrombin III deficiency
- protein C deficiency
- protein S deficiency
- activated protein C resistance (factor V Leiden)
- homocystinuria/hyperhomocystinaemia.

The haematologist will want the patient off asprin for at least 2 weeks before all these tests can be done, and they are best organized in outpatients about a month after the infarct.

 ## 5.9 Coronary thrombolysis

It is now well established that thrombolysis has an important part to play in acute myocardial infarction. Several studies have shown a significant reduction in early (1 month) and late (1 year) mortality in those patients receiving thrombolytic agents even up to 12 hours of onset of pain.

The pre-existing high-grade stenosis in the coronary artery suddenly becomes occluded by thrombus, usually secondary to plaque rupture. The cause of plaque rupture remains unknown. Acute occlusion of the coronary artery results in myocardial infarction in the dependent territory. Coronary angiography at the time of acute infarction shows total occlusion of the relevant vessel in 90–100% of cases. Progressive myocardial damage develops and becomes irreversible at 6 hours. The aim of thrombolysis is to produce reperfusion of the distal artery. The high-grade stenosis may have to be dealt with by coronary angioplasty on a subsequent occasion.

Thrombolytic agents
Non-specific thrombolytic agent: streptokinase (Kabikinase).
Fibrin-specific agents:
- rt-PA: recombinant tissue plasminogen activator. Alteplase (Actilyse). single-chain (double-chain duteplase no longer marketed), half-life 4–7 min

- APSAC (anisoylated plasminogen streptokinase activator complex) i.v. half-life 90 min. Anistreplase (Eminase)
- prourokinase: inactive precursor of urokinase
- urokinase (Ukidan)
- Streptokinase is the agent routinely used at present in the UK. Cost of treatment is approximately £83 per patient. It can be given either i.v. or via the coronary artery catheter. Disadvantages are that it causes a systemic lytic state and depletes fibrinogen and alpha-2 antiplasmin levels.

It is antigenic and often causes a fever and allergic reaction (see Complications). APSAC, tPA and urokinase are likely to cost more than £470 per patient. They have the advantage of working only at the site of the thrombus, and deplete fibrinogen and alpha-2 antiplasmin levels less. Approximately 25% of patients will receive tPA (see page 199). See Figure 5.7

Indications for thrombolysis

- Patients with a typical history of cardiac pain within the previous 24 hours and ST segment elevation on the ECG. There should be 1 mm ST elevation in standard leads or at least ≥ 2 mm ST elevation in adjacent chest leads.
- Chest pain plus LBBB on ECG.

If the ECG is doubtful on arrival, thrombolysis should be withheld and the ECG repeated at 15 and 30 min. Thrombolysis should not be given if the ECG remains normal. There is as yet no evidence that

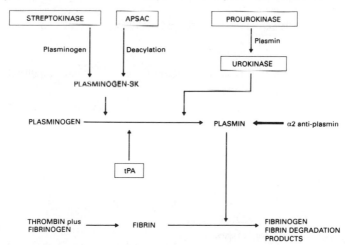

Figure 5.7 Thrombolytic agents: site of action.

patients with isolated ST depression benefit from thrombolysis even though they may represent true posterior infarction.

Patients whose pain started 12–24 hours previously should receive thrombolysis only if they are in continuing pain or if their general condition is deteriorating.

Patients with unstable angina should not receive thrombolysis unless thrombus is seen in a coronary artery at angiography.

Special benefit
Trials have so far shown that the following groups particularly benefit from thrombolysis:
- anterior infarction
- pronounced ST elevation
- the elderly > 75 years
- poor LV function or LBBB, systolic pressure < 100 mmHg
- very early administration (within the first hour of symptoms): 'the golden hour'.

Contraindications to thrombolysis
- Recent CVA (in last 6 months).
- Recent gastrointestinal bleed.
- Haemorrhagic diathesis or warfarin therapy.
- Recent abdominal surgery, neurosurgery, eye surgery, liver biopsy, dental extraction, lumbar puncture within 1 month.
- Pregnancy or postpartum.
- Trauma.
- Aortic dissection, beware wide mediastinum on CXR, or the absent pulse.
- Aortic aneurysm.
- LV aneurysm containing thrombus (Figure 5.8) (see complications).
- Prolonged cardiopulmonary resuscitation.

Although not absolute contraindications care should be taken in patients with:
- liver or renal disease
- menstrual bleeding
- i.m. injections in casualty
- ulcerative colitis
- severe hypertension, blood pressure > 200/100
- heart block requiring pacing
- diabetic retinopathy.

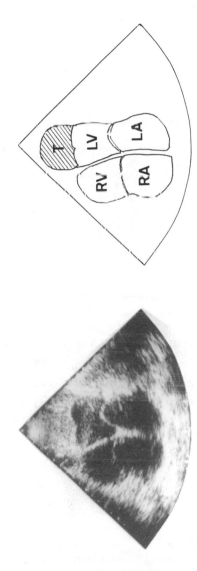

Figure 5.8 Transthoracic echocardiogram in a man with an anterior infarct, showing, in the apical four chamber view, extensive apical thrombus (T). This patient should not receive thrombolysis.

It is important to note that cardiogenic shock and advanced age are not contraindications to thrombolysis.

Administration

Prior to streptokinase administration, the patient should receive hydrocortisone 100 mg i.v. and chlorpheniramine 10 mg i.v. The need for this prophylactic anti-allergic regime is debated. It is sensible to consider it in any patient with a history of a recent sore throat. Streptokinase is given i.v. 1.5 million units in 100–200 ml N saline over 60 min.

Summary of commonly used thrombolytic agents (see page 199 for choice)

	tPA	Streptokinase	APSAC
Intravenous dose	80-100 mg	1.5 million units	30 mg
Infusion time	90 min or 3 hours	1 hour	5 min
Half-life	4 min	30 min	90 min
Storage	Room temperature	Room temperature	Refrigerator
Source	Recombinant human protein	Bacterial	Bacterial + human plasma
Anaphylaxis	Nil	0.1%	0.1%
Allergic reaction	Nil	2–3%	2–3%

Intracoronary streptokinase is rarely given now as the advantages over the intravenous route are minimal and the logistics much more difficult. The intracoronary dose is 10 000 units stat followed by an infusion of 4000 units/min for 60 to 120 min. APSAC is given as 30 units i.v. over 5 min.

Accelerated ('front loaded') tPA

This regime was used in one arm of the GUSTO trial. The full dose of tPA is given over 90 min with two-thirds of the dose given in the first 30min. Dose regime: 15 mg bolus. Then 0.75 mg/kg over 30 min (not to exceed 50 mg). Then 0.5 mg/kg over 60 min (not to exceed 35 mg). Heparin dose: 5000 unit bolus followed by 1000 U/hour. Most benefit: anterior infarcts within 4 hours. Use this regime within six hours of symptoms; beyond this time dose is 40 mg i.v. over the first hour and 40 mg over the next 2 hours.

Role of heparin

The ISIS 3 trial showed no advantage in mortality reduction in using heparin with any of the three agents in addition to aspirin. Heparin has not been shown to reduce mortality nor fortunately to increase strokes. The GUSTO trial showed a benefit of heparin only with the accelerated tPA regime and this is the only indication for additional heparin in thrombolysis. Heparin is not used routinely after streptokinase.

Choice of thrombolytic agent

Although results from the GUSTO trial show a slight benefit in mortality reduction in patients receiving accelerated tPA, streptokinase is the thrombolytic agent of choice. The ISIS 3 trial showed no clear benefit for tPA (3 hour infusion regime not accelerated) over streptokinase. tPA and anistreplase are more expensive and any additional benefit in mortality reduction is small (1%). The short administration time for anistreplase means that it will probably become the agent of choice for prehospital thrombolysis.

Accelerated tPA should be considered the agent of choice if:
- previous streptokinase or anistreplase therapy, as neutralizing antibodies are still present in about 30% of patients even after 1 year and persist for at least 4 years. Neither drug should be repeated beyond the fourth day of first administration
- recent streptococcal infection
- large anterior infarcts if presenting within 4 hours.
- hypotension. Systolic pressures < 100 mmHg
- likely need for temporary pacing (tPA has shortest half-life).

Reperfusion

This occurs in untreated control patients spontaneously in about 20%. Reperfusion occurs in approximately 50–70% of patients who receive thrombolysis within 4 hours of pain onset. The greatest improvement occurs in patients treated within 2 hours. It has also been shown that fibrin-specific thrombolytic agents (e.g. rt-PA) are superior to streptokinase in producing reperfusion but only marginally superior in reducing overall mortality. Early reperfusion reduces infarct size and helps preserve LV function. In the large majority of patients who receive intravenous therapy, successful reperfusion is marked by a rapid improvement in chest pain and a fall in ST segment (Figure 5.9). Occasionally reperfusion arrhythmias occur due to washout of toxic metabolites. They are not an indication to stop the thrombolytic agent. The commonest is a short run of accelerated idioventricular rhythm but VT or VF may occur (as they may after successful PTCA). Washout also results in a brisker rise in CPK levels. Peak CPK levels may be higher than in non-thrombolysed patients but the total area under the CPK/time curve (a measurement of total myocardial damage) will be less.

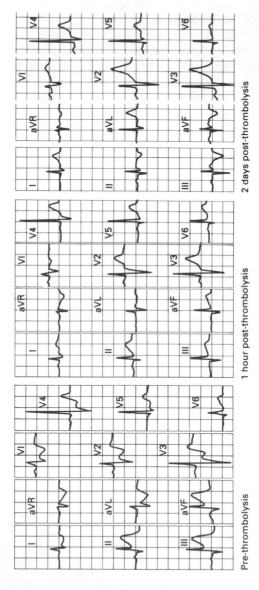

Pre-thrombolysis

1 hour post-thrombolysis

2 days post-thrombolysis

Figure 5.9 Rapid evolution of ST segment changes with thrombolysis. Acute inferior infarction in a 47-year-old man receiving 1.5 million units streptokinase within 2.5 hours of onset of chest pain. Left panel: marked inferior ST segment elevation with reciprocal ST depression in anteroseptal leads. Middle panel: there is rapid improvement in the ST segments within 1 hour of completing streptokinase. Right panel: by 2 days the ST segments are isoelectric.

Myocardial stunning occurs after reperfusion. It is delayed functional recovery. Poor LV function post-thrombolysis may not be permanent.

Re-occlusion
Exact rates of re-occlusion are unknown, as coronary angiographic data are not available in large numbers. It is probable that 25% of patients re-occlude within 3 months of thrombolysis unless the residual stenosis is dealt with by angioplasty.

Complications
• *Haemorrhage.* This is by far the biggest problem. It affects 7–10% of patients receiving streptokinase. Bleeding from drip sites and i.m. injection sites is common and a large i.m. haematoma can develop from simple i.m. analgesic injections. Transfusion is occasionally required. General practitioners and accident and emergency physicians should be encouraged to give analgesic injections i.v. to patients who are likely to be candidates for thrombolysis. More serious bleeding complications include haematemesis and melaena from occult peptic ulcers and cerebral haemorrhage.
  Bleeding from a drip site is treated with local pressure. More severe bleeding complications require transfusion, and possible fresh frozen plasma or cryoprecipitate. Very rarely the streptokinase can be reversed by slow i.v. infusion of tranexamic acid 10 mg/kg body weight.
• *Allergic reactions.* These are common with streptokinase. A low-grade fever and rash are common. Nausea, vomiting, headaches and flushing are also reported. A few patients who receive APSAC develop a vasculitis resembling Henoch–Schönlein purpura. This is usually self-limiting after a few days. Bronchospasm has also been reported with APSAC. One of the advantages of rt-PA is that it does not cause allergic reactions and is the agent of choice in patients who have already had a course of streptokinase in the past.
• *Systemic emboli.* Lysis of preformed thrombus within the left atrium, left ventricle or great vessels may result in systemic embolism. Aortic aneurysm and left ventricular aneurysm containing thrombus, however old, are contraindications to thrombolysis (see Figure 5.8).
• *Cerebrovascular bleeds.* Thrombolysis results in a slight increase in the incidence of intracerebral bleeds. The risk is 0.3% for streptokinase, 0.6% for tPA and 0.7% for anistreplase. The risk is small and should not influence the use of thrombolytics even in the elderly.
• *Early hazard.* This is the definite but slight increase in mortality in the first day in patients receiving thrombolysis. It is probably due to cardiac

rupture causing electromechanical dissociation. It is more common in the elderly, those receiving thrombolysis late and in patients who have had previous infarctions. Beta-blockade possibly reduces cardiac rupture, but a trial of thrombolysis with and without beta-blockade has not been performed.

Subsequent management

Following successful thrombolysis, patients who need PTCA must be identified. This requires exercise testing in those patients who are pain-free. Patients who continue to get angina following thrombolysis, or who have positive exercise tests at low work load, need coronary angiography. The proportion of patients who are likely to need PTCA following thrombolysis is probably > 30%. The exact timing of PTCA after successful thrombolysis remains controversial. The increase in thrombolysis will put a greater burden on cardiac catheter laboratories, and facilities for performing PTCA may not be available close to the district hospital.

Future trends

Unfortunately research has been directed at finding newer and better thrombolytic agents with only marginal benefit over agents already available rather than directing attention at the real problem of getting patients treated < 90 min of symptom onset. This could be achieved by:

• more out-of-hospital thrombolysis will reduce time to administration. This involves education of the general public to recognize their symptoms plus the establishment of a rapid response and highly trained ambulance team. Thrombolytic therapy could also become much more the province of the general practitioner on the spot. This is particularly likely to be of value in rural communities. Drugs which can be given as a bolus (e.g. anistreplase or the newer reteplase) might be the agents of choice in this situation

• a shorter door to needle time for those patients brought into casualty who have not received thrombolysis in the community. This should be < 15 min in the Accident & Emergency department with a fast-track system for definite infarcts. The thrombolytic should be administered in casualty rather than waiting for the patient to be transferred to the CCU.

On the pharmacological side, some newer agents are listed below.

• *Lanoteplase*. nPA or novel plasminogen activator. Two domains deleted from wild-type rt-PA. This has a longer half life than rt-PA.

There is little comparative data yet.

• *Reteplase*. Three domains deleted from wild-type rt-PA. This can be given as two boluses 30 min apart. One trial has suggested better 90 min patency compared with rt-PA but 30-day mortality and complication rates were virtually identical. The two drugs are clearly very similar.

• *Recombinant staphylokinase*. This is more fibrin-specific than streptokinase and causes less fibrinogen depletion.

• *Platelet IIb/IIIa receptor antagonists*. Tirofiban, a non-immunogenic peptide, has been shown to be superior to heparin at prevention of infarction or death in patients with unstable angina or non-Q-wave infarcts (the PRISM trial). It remains to be seen whether the drug has advantages in Q-wave infarcts.

• The search continues for a better antithrombotic agent than heparin. Hirudin has been shown to be of no benefit over heparin. The addition of argatroban (a direct thrombin inhibitor) to streptokinase as adjunctive therapy has not been shown to carry any benefit at 30 days postinfarct. Attempts to increase the heparin dose in several trials has resulted in increased bleeding.

5.10 Complications of myocardial infarction

See separate sections for:

• Recurrent unstable angina (**5.6**, page 166).
• Bradycardias or heart block requiring pacing (**7.1**, page 271).
• Tachyarrhythmias; atrial or ventricular (**7.12–7.14**, page 315–339).
• Cardiac arrests (**6.6**, page 263).
• Left ventricular failure (**6.1**, page 221).

Sudden death

This can occur at any time following an infarct and is usually due to:

• acute cardiac rupture
• VF or fast prolonged VT degenerating to VF
• massive pulmonary embolism
• left main stem embolism from mural thrombus (rare).

Acute cardiac rupture occurs usually from about the fourth day to the tenth day postinfarction. Electromechanical dissociation is typical. (Good ECG with no output at all.) Very occasionally it is contained by the pericardium (see Tamponade, page 363). Analysis of the causes of death in beta-blocking trials and myocardial infarcts suggests beta-blockers reduce mortality in infarction by reducing the incidence of cardiac rupture, but the drug has to be given early – within the first 2 days.

Massive pulmonary embolism may also show electromechanical dissociation on the ECG.

Right ventricular failure (RVF)

This is less common than LVF but very important as it usually is either missed or wrongly treated.

It occurs primarily following inferior infarction and is usually transient. RV infarction is probable if V4R lead on ECG shows ST segment elevation.

Persistent RVF presents with high neck veins and hepatic congestion. In the acute stage in severe cases Swan–Ganz monitoring is required and may show low left-sided filling pressures with high right-sided pressures. Cardiac output may be improved by plasma expansion in careful regulated amounts, rather than diuretic therapy, which may make the situation worse.

The differential diagnosis is pulmonary embolism (page 396).

Pericarditis

This is often acute (within the first few days) and transient. It may occur with anterior or inferior infarcts. Pain is typically cardiac in distribution and relieved by sitting up or leaning forward. It is worse when lying flat. Inferior/diaphragmatic involvement may cause shoulder-tip pain. A pericardial or pleuropericardial rub may be heard, but the pain is so typical in character it should be suspected with the history alone. The ECG shows transient T-wave changes or 'saddle-shaped' ST-segment elevation (Figure 12.9).

Treatment is with non-steroidal anti-inflammatory agents (e.g. soluble aspirin, indomethacin, ibuprofen, etc.). Echocardiography should be performed frequently to check for an enlarging effusion. The ECG with an enlarging effusion shows progressive voltage reduction and sometimes electrical alternans (Figure 8.2).

Systemic embolism

From mural thrombus is more frequent following large infarctions and generally occurs 1–3 weeks postinfarct. Patients with large infarctions should be heparinized until fully mobile (e.g. for first week), but the evidence that anticoagulants improve mortality figures from acute infarcts is small and only possible with pooled trials.

Peripheral limb emboli may be removed surgically (e.g. Fogarty technique). Large mesenteric emboli are generally fatal. Coronary emboli may account for a small number of re-infarctions.

Pulmonary embolism (10.2, page 396)

This occurs due to a combination of:

- low cardiac output, poor peripheral flow and venous stasis if venous pressure is high
- prolonged bed rest
- haemoconcentration with diuretic therapy
- increased platelet stickiness.

Patients are thus mobilized early – within 48 hours of uncomplicated infarction to avoid pulmonary emboli – and discharged early. Patients who are likely to require several days bed rest should be heparinized until they are fully mobile.

Tamponade (8.2, page 363)

This occurs following sub-acute cardiac rupture in which the pericardium acts as a barrier. A false aneurysm may follow if the patient survives (Figure 5.10).

Examination may reveal raised neck veins filling on inspiration, with systolic 'x' descent. Small-volume pulse possibly with pulsus paradoxus (see Figure 8.1). Soft muffled heart sounds.

Cardiac rhythm quickly becomes slow, idionodal or ventricular bradycardia with no output (electromechanical dissociation).

Diagnosis can be confirmed by echocardiography. Needle aspiration may be of temporary benefit, but in the acute stage the condition is

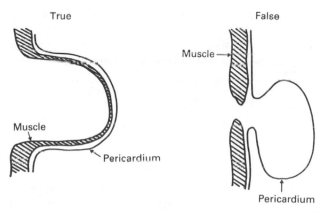

Figure 5.10 Ventricular aneurysm. Shows the difference between a true and a false ventricular aneurysm. The true aneurysm is lined by a thin layer of a muscle/scar tissue as well as pericardium. The false aneurysm is subacute cardiac rupture with only pericardium lining the aneurysm. It tends to have a narrower neck than a true aneurysm.

usually fatal unless urgent surgical repair is possible. (The false aneurysm has a narrow neck and can be repaired occasionally in the acute stage.)

Acute cardiac rupture is a common cause of sudden death following myocardial infarction.

Mitral regurgitation (see **3.3**, page 78)

Mild subvalvar mitral regurgitation is common following inferior or posterior infarction, due to papillary muscle dysfunction. It is often transient. The murmur is ejection in quality, often mid- or late systolic and heard at both apex and left sternal edge.

Severe mitral regurgitation is due to chordal rupture or papillary muscle infarction and rupture. Pulmonary oedema occurs rapidly, often with a small left atrium.

Physical signs: a loud pansystolic murmur at apex or left sternal edge with possible thrill. Systolic expansion of the left atrium may be confused with an RV heave.

Echocardiography may show chaotic movement of the posterior leaflet with anterior movement during diastole and fluttering.

Treatment depends on the patient's condition (see LVF, page 226). Diuretics and vasodilator therapy (nitroprusside) may hold the situation prior to mitral valve replacement, which may be life saving in the acute stage.

Acquired ventricular septal defect

Physical signs may be very similar to acute mitral regurgitation, however, acute pulmonary oedema is less prominent, and right-sided signs predominate in the early stages, with very high venous pressures. A VSD may occur with an anterior or inferior infarct.

	Mitral regurgitation	VSD
Infarct site	Inferior/posterior	Anterior
CXR	Acute pulmonary oedema	Pulmonary plethora
Dyspnoea	Severe orthopnoea and PND	Less dyspnoeic
JVP	May be normal	Raised
But:	Both may have pansystolic murmur and thrill at left sternal edge, parasternal heave (RV or LA +). Both may be in cardiogenic shock	

Without Echocardiography it may be impossible to differentiate acute VSD from mitral regurgitation. The table is a general guide only.

Swan–Ganz catheterization will confirm the diagnosis with a step-up in saturation in the right ventricle.

Echocardiography. This is proving very valuable in diagnosis. Pulsed or continuous wave Doppler ultrasound is necessary. The sample volume is scanned up the RV border of the septum in the four-chamber view and the Doppler signal is picked up at the site of the VSD. This technique may avoid the need for Swan–Ganz catheterization.

Treatment. Earlier attempts to control the situation with medical treatment for as long as possible are now considered inappropriate. Surgery is recommended early now. A double-patch technique either side of the septum may be needed to close the typical 'Swiss-cheese'-type defect. Recurrence of a small VSD post-operatively is not uncommon. Postero-inferior VSDs carry a higher mortality than antero-apical VSDs. RV function is an important predictor of survival.

This is a high-risk condition: 50% mortality within the first week.

LV aneurysm

Anterior
Is suspected clinically if the high paradoxical apex of an anterior infarct persists. The ECG shows persistent elevation of ST segments after 4–6 weeks.

The patient may have no symptoms. The diagnosis can be confirmed by:
- two-dimensional echocardiography
- multiple-gated acquisition (MUGA) scanning
- LV angiography.

Symptoms are commonly left ventricular failure or angina refractory to medical treatment. Occasionally patients develop recurrent ventricular tachycardia or systemic emboli.

Symptomatic patients are investigated with a view to left ventricular aneurysmectomy if the residual contractile segment function is adequate, and if medical treatment fails to control symptoms.

Inferior/posterior
This is less common than anterolateral aneurysm. It may be associated with considerable mitral regurgitation. False aneurysm may also occur inferoposteriorly.

Physical signs are less obvious, as there is no paradoxical apex.

Persistent ST elevation occurs on inferior leads. Investigation and indications for surgery are as with anterior aneurysms, but additional mitral valve replacement may be necessary.

Late malignant ventricular arrhythmias

Occurring 1–3 weeks after myocardial infarction, often at about 10 days, these are the cardiologist's nightmare: the patient having made an uneventful recovery, about to return home, suddenly collapses with VF.

Fortunately the problem is uncommon, even so patients with large infarcts should have 24-hour monitoring prior to discharge. Early exercise testing may point to patients at risk. Recently signal averaging of the standard 12-lead ECG has shown that patients at risk of late ventricular arrhythmias may show late or after-potentials. Signal averaging of ECGs is expensive and not generally available yet. See Risk Stratification, page 192.

The most easily avoidable cause is hypokalaemia from excessive diuretic therapy. Digoxin should be avoided in infarcts unless the patient is in AF.

Dressler's syndrome

Described in 1956, this is a syndrome of recurrent pericarditis, pleural effusions, fever, anaemia and high ESR. It occurs in about 1–5% of infarcts, usually 1–4 weeks following myocardial infarction. It is thought to be due to an auto-immune reaction to exposed myocardial antigens following infarction (and a similar illness may occur following cardiac surgery – also called the postcardiotomy syndrome). Anti-heart antibodies have been demonstrated, but are not useful clinically.

It is a chronic condition. Treatment in the first instance is with non-steroidal anti-inflammatory agents, or steroids in more severe or refractory cases. Steroids are said to increase the likelihood of LV aneurysm development, but the evidence for this is anecdotal.

Treatment may have to be continued for several months and patients observed when treatment is stopped or weaned off, as the syndrome may recur. Tamponade is rare.

Shoulder–hand syndrome

This is now rare following myocardial infarction, probably due to early mobilization. It develops from 2 weeks to 2 months postinfarct. It develops as stiffness and pain in the shoulder (usually left). Pain and swelling of the hand (becoming puffy and mottled).

A few late cases develop wasting of small muscles of the hand with irreversible contractures forming (like Dupuytren's).

Treatment is with mobilization, physiotherapy of hand and shoulder with analgesia. Hydrocortisone injections into the subacromial bursa may help. Systemic steroids are not used.

Depression
Occurs in up to one-third of postinfarct patients. It can be largely prevented by:
- a sensible encouraging approach from the doctor: worried doctors produce worried patients
- early mobilization
- predischarge advice about work, driving, sex, travel, etc.
- exercise programme and follow up to check that the patient is considering returning to work
- avoidance of antidepressant drugs if possible. If absolutely necessary mianserin, doxepin or lofepramine are said to have less cardiac effects than earlier tricyclics (amitriptyline or imipramine)
- cardiac rehabilitation course. There is renewed interest in this aspect of cardiac care. Unfortunately there is little evidence yet that it has long-term physical benefits, but there is no doubt that cardiac rehabilitation provides motivation, company, reassurance and carefully graded and medically supervised exercise.

Depression following infarction may result in denial of symptoms, with the patient too frightened to admit to any problems.

5.11 Management of hyperlipidaemias

Several large trials have confirmed that active reduction of serum cholesterol reduces the risk of death, myocardial infarction, the need for coronary intervention and stroke in patients with hypercholesterolaemia (see table, page 210).The risk of fatal or non-fatal myocardial infarction in the primary prevention (WOSCOPS) trial was reduced by about 30%. The reduction in the secondary prevention trials (4S and CARE studies) is similar. There was no increased risk of cancer or suicide in the treated groups. Meta-analysis of these trials has suggested that a 10% reduction in serum cholesterol results in a 20% reduction in mortality from cardiac disease and a 17% reduction in incidence of myocardial infarction. Aggressive lowering of cholesterol has also been shown to reduce the progression of disease in coronary vein grafts.

Results of three large cholesterol lowering trials. For references see page 525.

Trial	Drug	n	Time (years)	Reduction in total serum cholesterol (%)	Reduction in fatal or non-fatal myocardial infarctions (%)	Reduction in CVAs (%)	Reduction in need for CABG/PTCA (%)
4S	Simvastatin 20–40 mg od	4444	5.4	28	37	35	34
CARE	Pravastatin 40 mg od	4159	5	20	24	31	27
WOSCOPS Men only	Pravastatin 40 mg od	6595	4.9	20	31	11	37

Reduction of triglycerides is important in reducing episodes of pancreatitis and peripheral neuropathy in relevant cases, but has not yet been shown to reduce coronary risk in large trials.

Motivation of patients is important. The diet is unpleasant and rigid. Some drugs may have unpleasant side-effects and patients rarely feel better on medication. In addition the doctor rarely sees any immediate benefit and therapy is expensive. Patient compliance will be a problem.

Screening

Fasting blood is only needed for estimation of triglycerides. Patients should also avoid alcohol for 24 hours prior to the test. A random test is sufficient for cholesterol alone. The following groups of patients should be screened:

- family history of coronary disease, especially if < 50 years
- family history of hyperlipidaemia
- xanthomas
- xanthelasma or corneal arcus < 40 years (as these signs are less specific than xanthomas except in younger age groups)
- obesity
- hypertension
- history of myocardial infarct, CVA or intermittent claudication < 60 years.

Finger-prick testing kits are now available. They can be used in outpatients with the results available immediately. Care is required in sampling in order to get accurate results, and the reagent strips are not cheap.

If a random test is performed and a total cholesterol level of > 6.5 mmol/l is found, the test is repeated fasting with estimation of both low-density lipoprotein (LDL) and high-density lipoprotein (HDL) cholesterol and triglycerides. The ratio of HDL to LDL cholesterol is often calculated. A ratio of < 0.2 is considered a risk factor for coronary disease.

Secondary hyperlipidaemia

Dietary
- Excess dietary fat or calories.
- Excess alcohol.
- Anorexia nervosa.

Renal
- Nephrotic syndrome.

- Chronic renal failure.
- Long-term dialysis.

Endocrine
- Hypothyroidism.
- Poorly controlled diabetes.

Intestinal
- Biliary obstruction.
- Acute pancreatitis.

Drugs
- Steroids.
- Oral contraceptives.
- Thiazides.
- Non-selective beta-blockers.
- Isotretinoin (acne).

The drugs listed cause a rise in plasma triglycerides. HDL cholesterol rises with thiazides and the contraceptive pill, but falls with isotretinoin and non-selective beta-blockers. Women with a history of hyperlipidaemia, coronary or cerebrovascular disease should not take the oestrogen-containing Pill. Otherwise drug effects on lipids are not important.

Types of lipid measured (in decreasing order of size)

Chylomicrons. The largest lipid particle. Size > 800 Å. Formed in the small bowel mucosal cells and carried in the lymphatics and plasma. Consist mainly of triglyceride. This is removed in the peripheral tissue by the action of lipoprotein lipase. The remnant particles are reabsorbed by the liver.

VLDL. Very low-density lipoproteins. Size 300–800 Å. Synthesized in the liver. Endogenously synthesized triglyceride. Broken down by lipoprotein lipase to smaller LDL particles.

LDL. Low-density lipoproteins. Size 200 Å. Major carrier of cholesterol in the plasma. Derived from intravascular breakdown of VLDL particles. LDL is primarily removed by the liver from the circulation. Its removal depends on the available number of LDL receptors on the liver and peripheral cells. The receptors available partly depend on the need for intracellular cholesterol and on a genetic factor. Thus a reduction in the intrahepatic cholesterol pool (e.g. by bile acid depletion with cholestyramine) increases the number of LDL receptors on the hepatocyte membrane, resulting in an increased uptake of LDL by liver and peripheral cells and a fall in plasma LDL cholesterol. High levels of LDL cholesterol are associated with coronary disease (e.g. LDL > 5 mmol/l).

HDL. High-density lipoproteins. Size 100 Å. The smallest lipoprotein rich in phospholipid and carries about one-quarter total cholesterol. Secreted by the liver and also produced from chylomicron metabolism. Low levels of HDL are associated with coronary disease (e.g. < 1 mmol/l). Regular exercise increases HDL levels.

Apoproteins. There are at least ten different apoproteins that form an essential part of the lipoprotein particle. Each is specific for a type of lipoprotein or involved in lipid transport, enzyme activation or cellular uptake and receptor recognition.

Raised levels of some apoproteins have been shown to be better discriminators for the presence of coronary disease than their respective lipoproteins: e.g. raised levels of apoprotein A1 and apoB. Patients with levels of apoB > 125 mg% are at risk from coronary disease. Lipoprotein(a) known as Lp(a) is an LDL-like particle containing apoB100 and apo(a). Levels are raised in patients with coronary disease.

Normal lipid levels
Plasma lipid levels rise with age. These figures are a guide to patients under the age of 70 years:
* total cholesterol: 4.0–6.5 mmol/l (150–250 mg/100 ml)
* HDL cholesterol: 0.8–2.0 mmol/l
* LDL cholesterol: < 4.9 mmol/l
* triglycerides: 0.8–2.0 mmol/l (70–170 mg/100 ml).

The aim of treatment is to reduce the cholesterol to < 5.2 mmol/l and the LDL to < 2.5 mmol/l. Maximum reduction in saturated fat intake will only reduce the plasma cholesterol by a maximum of 15%. Patients with cholesterol levels > 6.5 mmol/l who are already on a low-cholesterol diet and who are under the age of 70 years should be considered for additional drug therapy. In particular, with statins so expensive it is important to concentrate on secondary prevention (e.g. patients with previous myocardial infarction or CABG). Top dose of statin therapy should lower total serum cholesterol by > 30%.

Treatment

Diet

Weight reduction, cutting back on alcohol intake and low-fat diet are the first stage in treatment. This means avoiding: egg yolks, butter, cream, lard and fatty meats. Reduce cheese intake, but cottage cheese allowed.

Substitute margarine for butter, vegetable oils for lard, chicken and turkey for red meat.

Encourage fish intake (avoid fish roe), vegetables and fibre.

Reduce red meat intake to 3 oz per day.

This diet will reduce both cholesterol and triglycerides. If still high on diet, then drug treatment is needed.

Drug therapy for hypercholesterolaemia (e.g. Type IIa)

Several drugs below may be needed in combination and only after dietary measures have been tried.

First choice: HMG Co-A reductase inhibitors, the statins. Five statins are available in the UK.

Drug	Daily dose range
Cerivastatin (Lipobay)	100–300 µg
Fluvastatin (Lescol)	20–80 mg
Simvastatin (Zocor)	10–40 mg
Pravastatin (Lipostat)	10–40 mg
Atorvastatin (Lipitor)	10–80 mg

In addition lovastatin (Mevacor) in the USA (dose 10–40 mg bd). They directly inhibit hepatic cholesterol synthesis. Hepatic LDL receptors are increased, HDL cholesterol is increased and triglycerides reduced slightly. Safe in renal disease (biliary excretion only). They are well-tolerated drugs and by far the most palatable in hypercholesterolaemia. The drugs vary in potency and cost and there are no back to back trials. Fluvastatin is probably the weakest but also is cheap compared with atorvastatin which is probably the most potent but also the most expensive at top dose.

Side-effects: These are both idiosyncratic and dose-related. Minor elevation in liver transaminases. Rarely a problem. Stop the statin if liver enzymes exceed three times normal or if the patient develops muscle pain. Rhabdomyolysis with greatly raised CPK levels is fortunately rare, but the risk increased slightly if the statin is combined with a fibrate or nicotinic acid. If the drugs are combined start with low doses of both and follow up closely.

Avoid statins in: liver disease, alcoholism, pregnancy, lactation, immunosuppression with cyclosporin (rhabdomyolysis risk). Increased, HDL cholesterol is increased and triglyceride levels reduced slightly. Dose 10 mg nocte. Maximum effect in 4–6 weeks. Dose can be increased to ≤ 40 mg nocte. Safe in renal disease (biliary excretion only). It is a well-tolerated drug and by far the most palatable in hypercholesterolaemia.

Second choice: anion exchange resins. Cholestyramine 4–8 g tds. Colestipol 5-10 g tds. These bind the bile acids in the small bowel preventing their reabsorption in distal 200 cm of the terminal ileum. The intra-hepatic bile salt pool is reduced, there is an increase in LDL receptors on the hepatocyte and more cholesterol is absorbed from the plasma to synthesize more bile salts

Side-effects are:
- constipation, bloating, flatulence, haemorrhoids, even intestinal obstruction
- fat-soluble vitamin supplementation may be needed (i.e. A, D, E, K)
- drug absorption reduced; e.g. digoxin, thyroxine, warfarin, dose may need increasing.

Third choice: nicotinic acid. Dose 100 mg tds. Gradually increasing to 1 g tds. Reduces hepatic VLDL synthesis. Inhibits release of FFA from fat cells. Reduces LDL synthesis by reducing synthesis of apoprotein B in the liver.

Side-effects may limit its use. These are:
- flushing soon after taking the drug (reduced by adding small dose of aspirin)
- nausea, abdominal discomfort, diarrhoea
- rarely, itching, hyperpigmentation, acanthosis nigricans, macular oedema
- rise in serum alkaline phosphatase, liver enzymes, uric acid and glucose.

Avoid nicotinic acid in: liver disease, gout, history of recent peptic ulcer.

Fourth choice: fibrates. Primarily drugs for hypertriglyceridaemia. They activate lipoprotein lipase and increase the number of hepatic LDL receptors. They partly inhibit HMG Co-A reductase also. HDL levels are increased slightly.

- Bezafibrate (Bezalip): 200 mg tds after meals, or mono-preparation (Bezalip mono) 400 mg od.
- Gemfibrozil (Lopid): 600 mg bd.
- Clofibrate (Atromid-S): 500 mg tds after meals. Hardly used now except for hypertriglyceridaemia with pancreatitis risk.

Problems with fibrates are:
- nausea, abdominal discomfort occasionally
- risk of gallstones due to increased excretion of cholesterol in bile
- potentiates warfarin: reduction in warfarin dose necessary
- avoid in liver or renal disease
- risk of rhabdomyolysis if combined with statins.

Fifth choice. Drugs rarely used now: D-thyroxine, probucol, neomycin.

Drug therapy for hypertriglyceridaemia (e.g. Types I, III, IV and V)

First choice: fibrates. See above. The best single drug type for high triglycerides.

Second choice: nicotinic acid. See above.

Third choice: marine oil supplementation. Inhibit hepatic VLDL synthesis. Fish oils providing 5–20 g omega-3 fatty acids daily lower triglycerides. They are expensive (approximately £40.00 per month on low dosage).

Fourth choice. Consider low-fat diet with MCT (medium chain triglyceride) supplementation.

Other forms of treatment for hypercholesterolaemia
In patients with homozygous hypercholesterolaemia high levels of cholesterol (15–30 mmol/l) may not be reduced satisfactorily on diet and combination drug therapy. These patients are usually children and further options to be considered are:
- plasma exchanges every 2–3 weeks
- plasma exchange using an LDL immunoabsorber column
- surgery:
Resection of distal 200 cm of ileum or bypassing this segment: preventing reabsorbtion of bile acids.
Portacaval shunt.

Frederickson classification of primary hyperlipidaemia types

Type	Frequency	Lipoprotein abnormality	Triglyceride and cholesterol	Clinical features
I	Rare	Chylomicrons+++ Plasma lipaemic LDL↓ VLDL →	Triglyceride+++ Cholesterol+	Abdominal pain Hepatosplenomegaly Pancreatitis Eruptive xanthomata
IIa	Common	LDL+++ VLDL →	Cholesterol+++	Premature atheroma Tendon xanthomata
IIb	Common	LDL++ VLDL+	Cholesterol++ Triglyceride+	As in Type IIa
III	Uncommon	VLDL+ Remnants+ Abnormal apolipoprotein E	Cholesterol++ Triglyceride++	Diabetes, gout Premature atheroma Orange palmar crease Eruptive xanthomata
IV	Common	VLDL+ LDL →	Triglyceride++	May have diabetes, gout, obesity, premature vascular disease
V	Uncommon	VLDL++ Chylomicrons++ Plasma lipaemic LDL↓	Triglyceride++ Cholesterol +	Pancreatitis Hepatosplenomegaly Diabetes, gout Eruptive xanthomata

Other terms commonly used to describe subtypes:

Type I: Familial hypertriglyceridaemia or chylomicronaemia. Lipoprotein lipase deficiency.

Type IIa: Familial or primary hypercholesterolaemia. This may be homozygous presenting in childhood with angina, myocardial infarction or aortic stenosis. More commonly it is heterozygous (1 in 500 of the population) presenting in early adult life.

Type IIb or IV: Familial combined hyperlipidaemia.

Type III: Broad B hyperlipoproteinaemia.

Type IV: Endogenous hypertriglyceridaemia.

Liver and heart transplantation. The liver transplant provides new LDL receptors and the heart transplant is necessary, as severe premature coronary disease develops in the first few years of life. These are highly specialized procedures requiring referral to a specialist centre.
• gene therapy. Recently three patients have been treated with a gene for the LDL receptor transfected into cultured hepatocytes (the hepatocytes cultured from the patient's own left hepatic lobe). This in time may prove the most effective form of treatment.

Regression of coronary lesions on treatment

Theoretically, getting lipid out of coronary plaques should make them more solid – reducing their growth and making them more stable. There is growing clinical evidence that this is the case.

Vigorous therapy to lower serum LDL cholesterol either with drugs (e.g. with lovastatin and colestipol, or niacin and colestipol – the FATS study) or with partial ileal bypass (the POSCH study) in six separate trials has been shown to delay progression of coronary lesions on angiography, or reduce clinical events. In some cases regression of coronary lesions was seen. In the ileal bypass trial (POSCH) there was a highly significant reduction in non-fatal coronary events, and the need for PTCA or CABG in the ileal bypass group compared with controls.

Although combination therapy trials have shown a fall in LDL they have produced a mean stenosis regression of only 1–2%. In contrast, there has been a striking reduction in cardiovascular events such as myocardial infarction, death, or the need for revascularization by $\geq 50\%$. As well as changing the plaque composition, reducing the number of foam cells, thickening the fibrous cap, etc. cholesterol lowering can improve endothelial function and EDRF release. Studies of coronary flow in patients who have had successful lowering of their cholesterol have shown a reduction or loss of a vasoconstrictor response in the epicardial coronaries to acetylcholine. Lipid lowering improves endothelial vasomotor function.

6 Cardiac Failure

Cardiac failure occurs when cardiac output and blood pressure are inadequate for the body's requirements. The incidence increases with age and carries a poor prognosis. In the Framingham study the 5-year mortality was 62% for men and 42% for women. In the USA it probably affects 3 million patients with 200 000 deaths annually. Only three patients in the CONSENSUS 1 trial published 10 years ago are still alive. In the UK cardiac failure accounts for 5% of all hospital admissions with an estimated cost to the NHS of £360 million annually.

Left and right ventricular failure may occur independently or together as congestive cardiac failure (CCF). The terms 'forward' and 'backward' failure refer to symptoms and signs relating to a poor cardiac output (forward failure) or venous congestion (backward failure). The normal cardiac index is 2.5–4.0 l/min/m². In CCF this may fail to ≤ 1.0 l/min/m².

High-output failure is an uncommon condition in which a high cardiac output (often > 10 l/min) is associated with failure symptoms and signs such as pulmonary oedema. It may occur in sepsis, thyrotoxicosis, large AV fistula, chronic anaemia, beri-beri and in severe Paget's disease of bone.

6.1 Concepts of treatment

Aetiology

- Coronary artery disease.
- Hypertension.
- Valve disease.
- Cardiomyopathy. dilated ➔ hypertrophic.
- Infiltrative: e.g. amyloid, sarcoid, iron, rarely malignant.
- Infective: e.g. viral myocarditis rheumatic myocarditis, sepsis, infective endocarditis with myocarditis.
- Collagen vascular disease.
- Drug induced e.g. Adriamycin, Daunorubicin, 5-fluorouracil.
- Metabolic and endocrine: e.g. myxoedema thyrotoxicosis, acromegaly, phaeochromocytoma.
- Toxins: e.g. alcohol.
- Radiation: e.g. myocardial fibrosis following radiotherapy for breast carcinoma.
- Nutritional: e.g. beri-beri, kwashiorkor, pellagra.
- Inherited: e.g. Fabry's disease, muscular dystrophies, Friedreich's ataxia, glycogen storage diseases.
- Hypersensitivity, anaphylactic shock.

....

- Cardiac transplant rejection.
- Incessant tachycardia.
- Miscellaneous: trauma, etc.
  By far the commonest causes in the western world are coronary disease and hypertension. Several of the insults listed above also affect the pericardium at the same time: e.g. radiation, viral, bacterial and rheumatic carditis. Ventricular dilatation will lead to functional mitral and/or tricuspid regurgitation.

Symptoms
Depend on which ventricle is primarily affected, the severity of the damage and the aetiology.

Left ventricular failure
Fatigue and increasingly limited exercise tolerance, exhaustion after even minor tasks, dyspnoea in all its stages (see page 4), orthopnoea and paroxysmal nocturnal dyspnoea. Dry nocturnal cough, cold peripheries, palpitation, angina, giddiness or syncope on effort. Leaden sensation in legs on walking. Systemic embolism. Nocturia and reversed diurnal rhythms. Weight loss, muscle wasting and eventual cachexia.

Right ventricular failure
Peripheral oedema increasing to thigh and sacral oedema, ascites and anasarca. Abdominal distension with ascites. Hepatic pain, especially on effort. Nausea and anorexia. Facial engorgement. Pulsation in face and neck (tricuspid regurgitation). Distended and even pulsatile varicose veins. Epistaxes.

NB To all these should be added the common side-effects of treatment: e.g. nausea and anorexia (digoxin), gout, impotence, diabetes mellitus, hypokalaemic weakness (thiazide diuretics), postural hypotension (diuretics and all afterload-reducing agents), dry nocturnal cough and abnormal taste (ACE inhibitors), headache and migraine (nitrates).

Psychological
Depression is very common. Many patients have to give up work, and may get into financial difficulty at a time when they feel too ill to cope with their problems. All sports, hobbies such as gardening, and often sex have to be abandoned. Impotence is common even in the absence of thiazides. Foreign travel becomes difficult and can be hazardous. It is hardly surprising patients get depressed.

....

Signs to look for

• An exhausted ill-looking patient. Dyspnoeic at rest or after minor effort.
• Cool hands and feet with peripheral cyanosis. Muscle wasting.
• Blood pressure: low systolic pressure with low pulse pressure. Check no paradox.
• Raised JVP. Prominent systolic wave of TR. Kussmaul's sign should be negative. Prominent 'x' and 'y' descents in restrictive cardiomyopathy. Prominent veins over shoulders, chest, abdomen and legs.
• Low volume pulse. Resting tachycardia. Possible pulsus alternans (see Figure 6.1). May be in fast AF. Check for possible anacrotic pulse in occult aortic stenosis.
• Displaced apex with LV dilatation. Thrusting apex of hypertensive heart failure. May have high diffuse paradoxical apex of LV aneurysm. Systolic apical thrill in ruptured mitral chordae. Double apex of LV hypertrophy in sinus rhythm.
• RV heave in pulmonary hypertension or with TR. Severe MR may produce a sensation similar to an RV heave due to systolic expansion of the LA.
• Auscultation. S_3 gallop is the most important sign of all. Signs of organic aortic or mitral valve disease. May just have functional mitral and/or tricuspid pansystolic murmurs. In low-output states, murmur of severe aortic stenosis may not be heard. Loud honking systolic murmur of torn mitral xenograft or diastolic murmur of torn aortic xenograft. More continuous murmur of ruptured sinus of Valsalva.
• Smooth hepatomegaly. Pulsatile liver with TR.
• Ascites with TR and RVF.
• Leg oedema. Check sacral pad. Oedema is more easily seen round the lower back than on anterior abdominal wall.
• Ventilation pattern: hyperventilation if in acute pulmonary oedema. Cheyne–Stokes ventilation in a sedated patient with a very low output state.
• Chest: bilateral basal effusions. Expiratory wheeze. Bubbly cough. Fine basal crepitations are an unreliable sign of pulmonary oedema.
In addition check for signs of possible infective endocarditis (see Chapter 9).

Differential diagnosis

Pulmonary oedema
Mitral stenosis, cor triatriatum and atrial myxoma may all present in

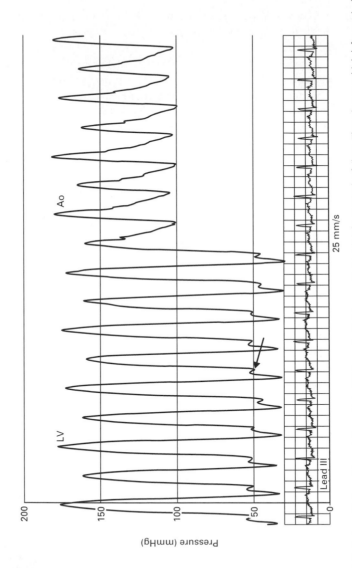

Figure 6.1 Catheter withdrawal from left ventricle (LV) to aorta (Ao) in a patient with left ventricular failure. There is a very high left ventricular end-diastolic pressure (LVEDP) arrowed of 50 mmHg. There is also pulsus alternans in the peak LV pressure and the aortic pressure trace.

pulmonary oedema with perfectly normal ventricular function. The murmurs may be very difficult to hear in an acutely breathless patient. Echocardiography is diagnostic.

Pulmonary oedema may occur with low LA pressures with sepsis, noxious gas inhalation, severe myxoedema, hypoalbuminaemia, head injury, subarachnoid haemorrhage or adult respiratory distress syndrome.

RV failure

The most important differential is from pericardial constriction. This is covered in **8.3**. Also consider SVC obstruction (non-pulsatile neck veins), malignant ascites with liver secondaries and pelvic nodes causing lymphatic obstruction, and leg oedema.

Treatment

The concept of treating both acute left ventricular failure and chronic congestive cardiac failure with afterload reduction is now firmly established. In heart failure there is an inappropriately raised systemic vascular resistance due to a combination of sympathetic overdrive and activation of the renin–angiotensin system. Neuroendocrine activation results in raised levels of angiotensin II, noradrenaline and arginine vasopressin (antidiuretic hormone, ADH). Endothelin levels (released from vascular endothelium) are also raised in heart failure contributing to the vasoconstriction. The use of inotropes on top of this vasoconstriction may increase afterload and cardiac work still further.

Raised levels of atrial natriuretic peptide (ANP) also occur in heart failure. ANP promotes a natriuresis, arterial and venous dilatation and inhibits ADH and aldosterone release. However, its effects are overwhelmed by the other neuroendocrine activation mechanisms described above.

The use of inotropes to flog a failing heart raises problems other than increasing cardiac work:
- no oral agent other than digoxin has been shown to be safe and effective in long-term trials
- increased myocardial oxygen consumption
- possible increase in infarct size
- arrhythmias with increased myocardial excitability (beta-1 effect)
- increased heart rate with shorter diastolic coronary flow
- possible vasoconstrictor effect on coronary arterioles (alpha effect)
- central-line administration needed with most drugs.

In view of these, heart failure is managed with bed rest, diuretics and vasodilating agents. Vasodilators are divided into three groups.

1 *Venodilators.* Reduce preload by dating venous capacitance vessels, e.g. nitrates, some diuretics. They lower filling pressures without initially much improvement in stroke volume. At higher doses they also become arterial dilators.

2 *Arterial dilators.* Reduce afterload. Dilate arterial resistance vessels, e.g. hydralazine. They improve stroke volume without much reduction in filling pressure or pulmonary venous pressure.

3 *Combined arterial and venous dilators.* Drugs such as nitroprusside and alpha-blocking agents. These improve stroke volume and reduce filling pressure. They are very useful in LVF.

A wide variety of vasodilating drugs is now available (see table, page 228).

Choice of vasodilators

Left ventricular failure (acute) with pulmonary oedema with normotension

For example, acute mitral regurgitation, septal infarction with VSD. Acute infarction in normotensive patient:
- nitroprusside: if full haemodynamic monitoring available, with
- frusemide i.v.

If no monitoring facilities available other than ECG:
- frusemide i.v. + isosorbide dinitrate i.v., then
- oral isosorbide dinitrate plus ACE inhibitor + oral diuretic as the patient improves.

The great majority of patients with LVF can be managed with this regime without the need for arterial pressure monitoring.

Low-output states

Hypotensive, cool, oligaemic patients (so-called 'forward failure').
- Dopamine (see inotropes section), monitoring haemodynamics. Once normotension is restored addition of nitroprusside may be beneficial. Alternatively dobutamine if urine output satisfactory.

Chronic congestive cardiac failure (oral therapy only) in combination

- Frusemide (+ amiloride) if hypokalaemic.
- ACE inhibitor, especially if hypertensive.
- Long-acting nitrate once or twice daily.
- Digoxin if in AF, large heart on CXR or audible S_3.

- Warfarin if large heart or in AF.
- No added salt to food (allow a little for cooking in most cases).

The systolic arterial pressure and renal function will dictate the dose of ACE inhibitor possible and whether the patient will tolerate other vasodilators such as nitrates. The aim should always be to maximize the vasodilator therapy and to use the minimal amount of diuretics possible. However, some patients will need quite vigorous diuretic therapy to cope with systemic oedema.

For refractory oedema not responding to increasing doses of i.v. frusemide, consider:

- two-dimensional echo to exclude pericardial collection or constriction
- fluid restriction to 1500 ml daily
- a frusemide drip at 2 mg/min for 2 hours
- oral metolazone 2.5 mg up to 10 mg daily
- low-dose dopamine through a central line: 5–10 µg/kg/min
- haemofiltration.

Prazosin has not been included because of its tachyphylactic problem and hypotensive first-dose effect. Hydralazine is less used now, as tachyphylaxis is also a problem, the lupus syndrome may occur in doses > 150 mg/day (see page 234). and ACE inhibitors have been shown to be superior in the VHeFT II study. Calcium antagonists should be avoided. The ACE inhibitors have revolutionized the treatment of chronic congestive cardiac failure following the demonstration of reduced mortality in the CONSENSUS trial in patients taking enalapril.

Drugs in acute LVF

Intravenous nitrates
See **5.4**.

Intravenous sodium nitroprusside (SNP)
Controlled infusion of nitroprusside is of great value in the treatment of acute LVF (e.g. ruptured chordae), the management of hypertensive crises and the postcardiac surgical control of hypertension. It can be used to lower blood pressure in aortic dissection prior to surgery.

Its great advantage is its rapid onset and equally rapid cessation of action on switching the infusion off. A computerized feedback technique is available in which automatic control of the SNP infusion rate is governed by the arterial pressure.

It is a potent dilator of arteries and veins by acting locally on vascular smooth muscle.

Vasodilating drugs in heart failure

Drug	Arterial dilator	Venous dilator	Oral dose	i.v. dose (adult)	Side-effects other than hypotension
Captopril	++	+	6.25–50 mg tds	–	Dry cough. Loss of taste. Abdominal pain. Stomatitis. Leukopenia. Proteinuria. Hyperkalaemia. Rashes
Diazoxide	++	+	100 mg tds	150 mg at 5–10 min intervals	Diabetes mellitus. Action i.v. not sustained. Fluid retention
Hydralazine	+++	–	25 mg tds to 150 mg qds	20 mg over 5 min (0.3 mg/kg)	Lupoid reaction (> 200 mg/day). Fluid retention. Tachyphylaxis
Isosorbide dinitrate	(+)	+++	10 mg 6 hourly to 30 mg 4 hourly	1–7 mg/hour	Headaches. Nausea
Minoxidil	++	+	2.5 mg bd to 10 mg tds	–	Hirsutism. Gut disturbances. Fluid retention. Breast tenderness
Nitroprusside	+++	+++	–	1–6 µg/kg/min	Cyanide toxicity. Metabolic acidosis. Hypothyroidism
Phentolamine	+++	+	50 mg qds	5–10 mg i.v. stat 10–20 µg/kg/min	Diarrhoea. Flushing. Tachycardia
Phenoxybenzamine	+++	+	10 mg nocte to 30 mg bd	10–40 mg slowly i.v.	Paralytic ileus – dry mouth. Impotence
Prazosin	++	++	0.5 mg test dose 1–10 mg tds	–	First-dose syncope. Drowsiness. Impotence. Tachyphylaxis
Salbutamol	+	(+)	4–8 mg tds	10–40 µg/min	Tremor. Hyperglycaemia. Apparent hypokalaemia
Trimetaphan	++	+	–	3 mg/min	Tachycardia

Infusion preparation:

1 *Weak solution.* Dissolve 50 mg sodium nitroprusside (SNP) (Nipride) in 2 ml 5% dextrose; add this to 500 ml 5% dextrose. Infusion strength 100 mg/l (100 µg/ml). Start at 1 µg/kg/min (40–70 µg/min usually). Maximum infusion rate 400 µg/min.

Wrap infusion bottle/paediatric giving set/infusion line in aluminium foil to protect from light.

Renew infusion every 4 hours. Must be in a separate line from bicarbonate.

2 *Strong solution.* This is often easier to manage clinically and involves smaller volume load. Add 50 mg SNP to 100 ml 5% dextrose solution (in paediatric giving set) = 500 µg/ml. Then 6 dpm (paediatric microdrops) = 50 µg/min; 12 dpm = 100 µg/min; 30 dpm = 250 µg/min, etc.

Cyanide toxicity

Over 90% cyanide released from nitroprusside is bound by erythrocytes. Cyanide free in plasma is freely diffusible and causes a cytotoxic hypoxia by inhibition of cytochromic oxidase. Cyanide is slowly metabolized to thiocyanate.

• Toxicity is related more to the rate of infusion than to total dose, but care must be taken once a total dose of 50 mg is exceeded.

• Plasma cyanide or thiocyanate levels are not necessarily a reliable guide to toxicity.

• A metabolic acidosis (arterial lactate from anaerobic metabolism) occurs with cyanide toxicity, but may not necessarily be due to it. However, it is the easiest guide to nitroprusside dose and usually reverses quickly when the infusion is stopped.

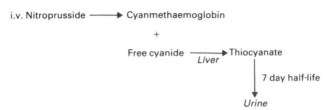

Summmary of nitroprusside infusion

• Monitor arterial and preferably PAW pressure.
• Frequent measurement of acid–base balance.
• Keep levels as below (if assays available):
  plasma cyanide < 3 µmol/l

plasma thiocyanate < 100 µg/ml
red cell cyanide < 75 µg/100 ml.
• Max. infusion rate < 400 µg/min (approximately 5-6 µg/kg/min in adults)
   Toxic levels of thiocyanate may, cause hypothyroidism. If possible, nitroprusside infusion should not be used for > 48 hours. Hydroxycobalamin infusion given at the same time as SNP infusion reduces plasma cyanide levels (forming cyanocobalamin). This infusion also has to be protected from light. Dose of B_{12} = 25 mg/hour (mixture of 100 mg B_{12} in 100 ml 5% dextrose).

Emergency treatment of cyanide toxicity
• Amyl nitrite inhalation or isosorbide dinitrate i.v. (increase methaemoglobin).
• Sodium thiosulphate injections.
• Bicarbonate for lactic acidosis.
• Hydroxycobalamin infusion.

Drugs in chronic congestive cardiac failure

Angiotensin-converting enzyme inhibitors (ACE inhibitors)
A group of drugs that inhibit the conversion of inactive angiotensin I to the powerful vasoconstrictor angiotensin II. At present there are ten ACE inhibitors available in the UK, but there will be many more in the next few years. The profound vasoconstrictor effect of angiotensin II is reduced. They work in congestive cardiac failure where other drugs have failed and have a sustained action. They may be useful even when plasma renin activity is low. This may be mediated by reduction of bradykinin degradation and activation of prostaglandin production.

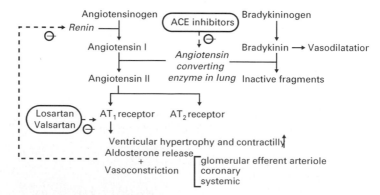

Figure 6.2 Angiotensin actions and sites of drug inhibition.

Some are pro-drugs converted in the liver to the active metabolite (e.g. enalapril, cilazapril) and this may delay onset of action following an oral dose. At present there seems little to choose between all these long-acting drugs.

Starting therapy with ACE inhibitors

Hypertensive patients can be safely started on ACE inhibitors as outpatients with the first dose taken on going to bed at night. They should be warned of possible initial postural hypotension. A small dose of a long-acting ACE inhibitor (e.g. enalapril 2.5 mg or lisinopril 2.5 mg) can be used safely.

Patients with congestive cardiac failure are best started on ACE inhibitors under close supervision in hospital. Again the first dose is given at night and captopril, the only short-acting drug, should be used. It is important that the patient is not hypovolaemic, and if on diuretics with invisible neck veins then the diuretic should be stopped for 48 hours prior to starting the captopril. Once the patient is comfortably established on captopril the drug can be switched to a longer-acting agent.

Problems and side-effects with ACE inhibitors

• *Hypotension.* This is the commonest problem, especially with the first dose. Severe hypotension can result in a neurological deficit or renal failure. It is important to make sure patients are not hypovolaemic or severely hyponatraemic (excess diuretics) before starting treatment. May need i.v. N saline.

• *Chronic cough.* This is the commonest and most irritating side-effect of ACE inhibitors and possessed by all the drugs. It is one of the chief reasons for dose limitation. It is probably due to bradykinin levels increased by ACE inhibition. It responds to a reduction in dose, but not often to cough suppressants.

• *Loss of taste.* This or abnormal taste (dysgeusia) may be due to the —SH (sulphydryl) group in some drugs. Apthous ulcers may develop.

• *Hyperkalaemia.* Due to a reduction in aldosterone. Care needed with potassium-retaining diuretics.

• *Deteriorating renal function.* This may be due to hypotension and 'prerenal failure'. In hypertensive patients with pretreatment normal renal function, who suddenly deteriorate on ACE inhibitors, consider renal artery stenosis. Deteriorating renal function is the commonest long-term reason for restricting or reducing the dose. Careful monitoring of blood urea and creatinine needed.

ACE inhibitors

Drug (proprietary name/s)	Starting dose	Maximum dose	Doses daily	Pro-drug	Half-life (hours)	Metabolism and excretion
Captopril (Capoten, Acepril)	6.25 mg tds	50 mg tds	3	No	3	Has —SH group. Liver and kidney. Rapid onset action
Enalapril (Innovace)	2.5 mg od	40 mg od	1	Yes	6	No —SH group. Liver to active enalaprilat
Lisinopril (Carace, Zestril)	2.5 mg od	40 mg od	1	No	12	No —SH group. Renal excretion only, unchanged
Cilazapril (Vascace)	0.5 mg od	5 mg od	1	Yes	9	Liver to active cilazaprilat. Renal excretion only unchanged
Fosinopril (Staril)	10 mg od	40 mg od	1	Yes	11	Liver to active fosinoprilat. Liver and kidney excretion
Moexipril (Perdix)	7.5 mg od	30 mg od	1	Yes	14	Liver to active moexiprilat. Renal and faecal excretion
Perindopril (Coversyl)	2 mg od	8 mg od	1	Yes	25	Liver to active perindoprilat. Renal excretion
Trandalopril (Gopten Odrik)	0.5 mg od	4 mg od	1	Yes	16–24	Liver to trandaloprilat Renal and faecal excretion
Quinapril (Accupro)	2.5 mg od	40 mg od	1	Yes	4	Liver to active quinalprilat
Ramipril (Tritace)	1.25 mg od	10 mg od	1	Yes	15	Binding to tissue ACE ++. Renal and hepatic excretion

- *Urticaria and angioneurotic oedema.*
- *Rarely: proteinuria, leukopenia, fatigue, exhaustion.*
- *False positive urine test for ketones (captopril).*

There is little evidence to suggest that ACE inhibitors without the —SH group (e.g. enalapril and lisinopril) may have less side-effects, e.g. with taste problems, than captopril. There is no rebound hypertension on stopping ACE inhibitors.

Contraindications to ACE-inhibitor treatment

- Severe renal failure, serum creatinine > 300 μmol/l.
- Hyperkalaemia.
- Hypovolaemia.
- Hyponatraemia.
- Pregnancy or lactating mothers.
- LV outflow obstruction.
- Hypotension, peak systolic pressures < 90 mmHg.
- Cor pulmonale.
- Renal artery stenosis.

Use with other drugs

ACE inhibitors can be safely used with digoxin and diuretics (care with volume and sodium depletion). Potassium-retaining diuretics are reduced or stopped. The drugs may be used with other hypotensive agents if necessary, e.g. nitrates and beta-blockers. The effect is synergistic.

Management of hyperkalaemia

- Discontinue potassium-sparing diuretics, potassium supplements, ACE inhibitors, angiotensin II receptor antagonists, non-steroidal anti-inflammatory agents and salt substitutes.
- Restrict intake of fresh fruit, fruit juice and vegetables (rich in potassium).
- Add 12 units soluble insulin (Actrapid) to 50 ml of 50% glucose and infuse over 15 min. This temporarily should lower the serum K^+ by 1 mmol/l for about 2 h. If K^+ is still > 6.5 mmol/l repeat the regime and contact the renal team.
- Check arterial blood gases for a metabolic acidosis. If base excess > −5 give 50 ml sodium bicarbonate 8.4% slowly i.v. and repeat blood gases. Dose may need repeating.
- If ECG changes of hyperkalaemia present (page 450) give calcium chloride 10 ml of 10% slowly i.v. but not in the same line or vein as sodium bicarbonate.

• Consider calcium resonium 15 g tds orally or 30 g enema (8% w/w calcium). This causes constipation and a laxative, e.g. co-danthramer must be given also.

Drugs in asymptomatic LV dysfunction

ACE inhibitors started in asymptomatic patients with mediocre left ventricular function (LVEF < 35%) help prevent the development of clinical heart failure and reduce long-term mortality slightly (8% in the SOLVD trial using enalapril). Patients with large hearts on the CXR or poor ejection fractions should be started on ACE inhibitors whether or not they have symptoms.

Angiotensin-receptor antagonists (AT$_1$-receptor antagonists)

Figure 6.2 shows the difference in site of action of these drugs compared with ACE inhibitors. Bradykinin is a vasodilator and thought to be responsible for the ACE inhibitor cough. Its degradation is not inhibited by AT$_1$-receptor antagonists. Hence theoretically these drugs might not be quite as effective as ACE inhibitors in heart failure. Losartan has been shown to improve haemodynamics in CCF and one trial in elderly patients with cardiac failure suggested that losartan was superior to captopril. More trials are needed and at the moment losartan or valsartan should be used in CCF when patients are unable to tolerate the ACE inhibitors' cough.

Drugs of second choice in heart failure

Hydralazine

This drug causes arteriolar vasodilatation and a rise in stroke volume. Its inotropic effect may be primary or secondary to vasodilatation. It does not reduce pulmonary capillary wedge pressure or systemic venous pressure to any great extent. In heart failure a compensatory reflex tachycardia does not necessarily occur.

Starting oral dose is 25 mg tds (half-life 2–8 hours). It is acetylated in the liver, and excreted in the urine.

The lupus syndrome. Is more likely to develop in patients who:
• receive > 200 mg daily (check ANF and LE cells)
• are slow acetylators
• have histocompatibility locus DR4.

However, the lupus syndrome may occur on doses < 200 mg daily. Positive ANF is not an indication to stop the drug, as it occurs in

30–60% patients receiving hydralazine for ≥ 3 years, but lupus occurs in only 1–3%. The lupus syndrome is less common in black patients. It is fully but slowly reversible on stopping the drug.

Tachyphylaxis. Unfortunately, recent reports suggest that long-term tolerance to the drug occurs, possibly due to reduction in the number of receptor sites in the arterial wall, or to a change in receptor itself.

Benefit from acute administration may not persist and a change of drug may be necessary. The drug may cause fluid retention and should be used with a diuretic.

Parenteral administration. Is possible in emergency situations (e.g. severe hypertension, pre-eclampsia). The drug can be given i.m. (20 mg) or slowly i.v. (20 mg slowly over 5 min).

Prazosin

Acts on alpha-1 receptors in the vessel wall and causes arterial and venous dilatation. Unfortunately tachyphylaxis is a problem.

Initial dose is 0.5 mg taken on going to bed. In spite of this a few patients develop first-dose syncope which limits its use. If the test dose is taken satisfactorily then the patient is started on 1 mg tds.

The drug is well absorbed following oral administration (half-life 3–4 hours). It is probably more useful in hypertension than chronic heart failure.

Care should be taken in using nitrites with prazosin, as both are powerful venodilators and may cause syncope when taken together. Although prazosin reduces systemic vascular resistance, renal plasma flow is reduced and fluid retention may result.

Salbutamol

This beta-2-agonist causes arterial dilatation, an increase in stroke index, but also an increase in heart rate. It does not restore normotension in the hypotensive patient with LVF. It is not suitable for the patient in acute pulmonary oedema.

It causes tremor. It shifts potassium into the cells and causes an apparent hypokalaemia. It causes restlessness and insomnia.

Alpha-blocking agents

Phenoxybenzamine, phentolamine. These drugs can be used in the management of acute LVF, but nitroprusside is better owing to its more pronounced venodilating properties.

They are more useful in hypertensive crises or management of phaeochromocytoma. Phenoxybenzamine may be of some use in coping with severe Raynaud's phenomenon.

Of these two drugs, phentolamine may be the more useful in heart failure by having a weak inotropic effect (noradrenaline release) as well as alpha-blocking properties.

Diazoxide. Is rarely used now in hypertension or LVF. Acute intravenous administration (150–300 mg) causes a sudden fall in blood pressure, but the fall is not sustained and the dose needs to be repeated in 10–15 min. Chronic use causes diabetes mellitus. It also causes fluid retention. Infusion of diazoxide is not as hypotensive as bolus administration.

Minoxidil. This drug causes salt and water retention and is not suitable for chronic heart failure. It is more useful in hypertension and must be given with a diuretic. Hirsutism limits its use to men. Reflex tachycardia requires additional beta-blockade. The drug has a long half-life (1–4 days) and can be given as a single oral dose daily (starting 5 mg od) initially.

6.2 Digoxin

Controversy regarding the value of digoxin in patients with cardiac failure continues even 210 years after its discovery by Withering. The large DIG mortality trial showed digoxin reduced deaths or hospital admissions due to heart failure but did not reduce overall mortality in a randomized trial against placebo of 7700 patients in whom digoxin levels were measured. This disparity may have possibly been due to an increase in arrhythmic deaths in the digoxin group. The benefit of digoxin appears to be on symptomatic improvement rather than mortality reduction.

Action
Digoxin is thought to inhibit the action of sarcolemmal membrane Na^+/K^+-ATPase, inhibiting the sodium pump. This allows greater influx of sodium and displacement of bound intracellular calcium. The increase in calcium availability exerts the inotropic effect. Other effects of digoxin are:
- AV node refractory period prolonged
- AV node conduction slowed

- mild peripheral vasoconstriction (arteries and veins)
- vagotonic effect
- automaticity increased (myocardial excitability)
- possible acceleration of bypass conduction in WPW syndrome.
  Its inotropic effect is much weaker than sympathomimetic inotropes.

Indications

Congestive cardiac failure with atrial fibrillation
This is the classic situation for digoxin. Its effect on the AV node slows ventricular response to fast AF, and its positive inotropic effect helps the dilated failing left ventricle increase its stroke volume.

Control of chronic atrial fibrillation (e.g. mitral valve disease)
The drug is used for its effect on the AV node, however, in some cases additional therapy with a beta-blocker or verapamil may be needed

Management of paroxysmal atrial fibrillation
Digoxin is of no value in the mangement of paroxysmal AF unless the episodes are frequent and prolonged when it may help control ventricular rate when it occurs. The most effective drug is amiodarone, but side-effects limit its use. Flecainide or propafenone should be considered as alternatives and are effective at reducing frequency and length of episodes. Quinidine is rarely used now (see page 352).

Heart failure in children
Digoxin is still the mainstay of therapy.

Congestive cardiac failure and sinus rhythm
Several studies have claimed that digoxin is of benefit in this situation and that the effect is sustained. The presence of a third sound is a strong correlate of a good response to digoxin. However, not all patients benefit from digoxin and in a group of patients already on the drug, about one-third deteriorate when it is withdrawn.

Thus digoxin is not the drug of first choice in CCF with sinus rhythm. If bed rest, diuretics and vasodilators do not achieve or maintain an improvement, digoxin should be tried. It is likely to help in patients who:

- have a third sound with a large heart
- do not have valvar obstruction.

Once heart failure has been controlled and the heart is smaller, digoxin may be withdrawn under supervision.

Conditions for which digoxin is no longer the drug choice

- supraventricular tachycardia. This is better managed with i.v. verapamil or adenosine.
- Sino-atrial disease. This is probably better managed with beta-blockade, amiodarone and/or pacing.
- Cor pulmonale. There are no studies to show it helps. The side-effects of digoxin could be dangerous. It can be used only if the patient is in AF.
- Myocardial infarction, unless the patient is in AF.
- Valvar or subvalvar aortic stenosis, unless the patient is in uncontrolled AF. Digoxin will increase the gradient in muscular subaortic obstruction (HCM).
- Hypertensive heart failure. This is better managed with after-load reduction.

Contraindications

- WPW syndrome.
- Hypertrophic cardiomyopathy, unless in AF with end-stage LV dilatation.
- Second- or third-degree AV block. Chronic first-degree AV block is not a contraindication to digoxin, although acute prolongation of the PR interval (e.g. myocardial infarction, infective endocarditis) is more dangerous and patients should be monitored carefully.
- Severe renal failure (creatinine clearance < 10 ml/min).
- Patients with recurrent ventricular arrhythmias.
- Prior to DC cardioversion.
- Cardiac amyloidosis.

Digitalization

Acute intravenous

This is not often necessary and the patient should be normokalaemic. Use digoxin 0.25 mg i.v. 2 hourly until effect is achieved, usually 0.75–1 mg is required. Using intermittent doses of 0.25 mg i.v. is safer than a bolus dose of 0.75–1 mg over 30 min. Following control of the fast AF, the patient is maintained on 0.125 mg i.v. as required 4 hourly.

Oral

The loading dose depends on lean body mass, as skeletal muscle binds digoxin. It is only necessary if a rapid result is required. Often patients can be started on the maintenance dose. Loading dose is 1.0–1.5 mg orally for a 70-kg adult; maintenance dose depends on renal function and is 0.25 mg. Larger doses ($\leq$ 0.5 mg daily) may be required, but care must be taken and, with larger doses, plasma levels are helpful.

A useful compromise in the absence of an emergency is to use: digoxin 0.25 mg bd for 2 days then 0.25 mg od. Digoxin can be given i.m. if necessary, but not s.c. (very irritant).

Plasma levels

Normal level for satisfactory therapeutic effect is 0.8–2 ng/ml (1–2.5 nmol/l). Blood is taken 6–8 hours after an oral dose. Serum half-life is 30 hours. However, the level should never be used as more than a guide and the clinical effect must be taken into consideration, i.e. levels > 2 ng/ml do not necessarily mean digoxin toxicity unless the patient's condition or ECG is consistent with this.

Very high plasma levels are associated with acute i.v. administration (e.g. $\leq$ 100 ng/ml), but these levels are transient and not toxic.

If the required effect is not achieved with plasma levels of 3–4 ng/ml then additional therapy with beta-blockade or verapamil should be used.

Approximately 20–40% of digoxin is bound to plasma proteins. Most digoxin is excreted unchanged by the kidney both by filtration and active tubular secretion. About 10% is excreted in the stools, and a smaller percentage metabolized in the liver

Reduction in digoxin dose

This is required in the following situations:
• Symptoms of digoxin toxicity: anorexia, nausea, vomiting, xanthopsia (very rare), neurological symptoms (paraesthesiae, fits, mental confusion), gynaecomastia, etc.
• ECG changes: junctional bradycardia, ventricular bigeminy, salvos of ventricular ectopics or paroxysmal VT. 2° or 3° AV block. Paroxysmal atrial tachycardia with varying block (PATB) may be a sign of digoxin toxicity in patients who are fully digitalized. The digoxin effect on the ECG is not an indication to reduce the dose.
• Other drug therapy. Several drugs increase plasma digoxin levels, possibly by protein displacement, reduced renal clearance or diminished distribution to the tissues. In several cases the cause is unknown.

Drugs increasing plasma digoxin are:

quinidine } reduced renal clearance
captopril }

amiodarone ⎫
propafenone ⎪
verapamil ⎬ displacement from protein binding
nifedipine ⎪
nitrendipine ⎭

erythromycin ⎫ reduction in gastrointestinal bacteria which
tetracycline ⎭ convert digoxin to inactive dihydrodigoxin.

Patients on any of these drugs should be on half the expected digoxin dose.

• Development of renal failure. Plasma digoxin levels may help. Digitoxin does not need dose reduction in renal failure. If the creatinine clearance is < 10 ml/min it is probably better to avoid digoxin altogether. Dose 10–25 ml/min, 0.0625–0.125 mg daily; 25–50 ml/min, 0.125 mg/0.25 mg alternate days; 50 ml/min, 0.25 mg daily. Cardiac glycosides are not removed by dialysis.

• The elderly require a smaller dose of digoxin. The paediatric 0.0625 mg tablets are small and blue and easily recognizable. If digoxin is necessary they can usually be managed on 0.0625–0.125 mg/day.

• Increased sensitivity to digoxin occurs in the following conditions and dose reduction may be necessary: hypokalaemia; hypercalcaemia; hypoxia; chronic pulmonary disease; hypomagnesaemia (e.g. chronic diarrhoea or prolonged diuresis); hypothyroidism.

Increase in digoxin dose

This may be needed in patients taking:

• cholestyramine: binds digoxin to the resin

• phenytoin ⎫ increased hepatic metabolism
• rifampicin ⎭

• sulphasalazine ⎫
• neomycin ⎬ delayed absorption
• malabsorption syndromes ⎭

• cancer chemotherapy: damage to gut mucosa may delay absorption.

Children

Paediatric digoxin elixir (lime flavour) contains 0.05 mg/ml. Children tend to need more digoxin than their small weight would suggest. Digitalizing dose is 0.01 mg/kg 6 hourly until therapeutic effect is obtained; maintenance dose is 0.01 mg/kg/day. Toxicity in children: sinus bradycardia, vomiting, drowsiness. AV block is not as common as in adults.

Digoxin overdose

The development of digoxin antibodies has made a great difference to the therapy of digoxin overdose. Infusion of the antibody fragment Fab (raised in sheep) rapidly reverses the toxic effects of digoxin. The dose is calculated from the plasma digoxin concentration assuming an interval of > 6 hours from ingestion.

Digoxin load (mg) = plasma concentration (ng/ml) x body weight (kg) x 0.0056. Antibody load needed (mg) = 60 x digoxin body load. If digitoxin has been ingested the factor 0.00056 is used not 0.0056.

The Fab fragments are excreted in the urine (half-life 16 hours). With reduction in serum digoxin, hypokalaemia may result as potassium goes back into the cells. Hypersensitivity and anaphylactic reaction are a theoretical possibility as this is a sheep protein.

Drug trade name: Digibind; 40 mg of Fab fragments/vial.

6.3 Inotropic sympathomimetic drugs

Most inotropic drugs work by increasing the level of intracellular cyclic AMP, which with intracellular calcium promotes contractility. The increase in cyclic AMP may be achieved by:
- stimulation of beta-receptors, i.e.

beta-1: isoprenaline, dobutamine, dopamine, ibopamine, xamoterol
beta-2: salbutamol, terbutaline, pirbuterol, prenalterol, dopexamine
- stimulation of glucagon receptor: glucagon
- stimulation of H_2-receptor; histamine
- inhibition of phosphodiesterase, the enzyme which converts cyclic AMP to inactive 5'-AMP. There are many drugs in this group, e.g.

bipyridines: amrinone, milrinone
imidazoles: enoximone, piroximone, imidazopyridine, sulmazole
xanthine derivatives: caffeine, aminophylline.

Other inotropes that do not work by increasing cyclic AMP
- Digoxin (see **6.2**).
- Alpha-agonists: stimulate postsynaptic alpha-receptors in the myocardium without increasing cyclic AMP: noradrenaline, adrenaline, high-dose dopamine (via noradrenaline).
- Calcium sensitizers: increasing the sensitivity of troponin to calcium: pimobendan.
- Enhancing sodium influx resulting in increased delivery of calcium to the myofilaments: vesnarinone.

....

Many of these drugs are under development. A few have been tried as oral agents in some countries in the long-term management of cardiac failure: e.g. xamoterol, ibopamine, enoximone, milrinone.

Downregulation of beta-receptors and beta-blockade in heart failure

The normal myocardium contains both beta-1- and beta-2-receptors in a ratio of about 4 : 1. In heart failure this ratio is reduced or reversed as the number of beta-1-receptors falls. This may be due to chronic high levels of circulating noradrenaline. Beta-1-agonists will therefore have less effect, and treatment with beta-2-agonists should assume more importance. Unfortunately beta-2-agonists have not proved of much help either in heart failure.

Attempts with low-dose beta-blocking agents that partially block the beta-1-receptor have been tried in patients with heart failure to try and overcome this downregulation. Xamoterol, a drug with intrinsic sympathomimetic activity, caused a deterioration in moderate or severe heart failure. Recent trials of carvedilol and bucindolol, drugs with vasodilating properties due to alpha-1 blocking activity, have shown an improvement in LV function (bucindolol) and a reduction in mortality in heart failure (carvedilol). However, several patients deteriorated on starting beta-blockade, and the case for beta-blockers in heart failure is not yet proved.

Beta-blockade should only be attempted in hospital in patients with mild or moderate heart failure starting with very small doses of beta-blocker. The dose should only be increased once a week.

Dopamine

The precursor of noradrenaline, dopamine has become a standard drug in the management of cardiogenic shock and low-output left ventricular failure secondary to myocardial infarction. It is also used in septic shock and postcardiac surgery.

It acts on several different receptors with activity changing with increasing dose.

Dose 1.0–5.0 µg/kg/min. Dopaminergic (DA_1) receptors activated resulting in dilatation of coronary, renal, cerebral and splanchnic beds. This is called the 'renal' dose of dopamine. Other sympathomimetics only increase renal blood flow by increasing cardiac output. Dopamine has this unique action on the renal vascular bed. Dopaminergic (DA_2) receptors activated in the periphery which inhibit presynaptic release of noradrenaline: causing vasodilatation.

Dose 5.0–10.0 µg/kg/min. Beta-receptors activated. The inotropic dose. Beta-1 activation increases contractility. Heart rate is increased probably more than by dobutamine. Beta-2 activation helps vasodilatation. Doses > 10 µg/kg/min are likely to cause arrhythmias. Dose > 15.0 µg/kg/min. Alpha-receptors activated. The drug also releases noradrenaline from myocardial adrenergic nerve terminals. Vasoconstrictive doses of dopamine are not beneficial. Renal blood flow falls.

Addition of nitroprusside or an alpha-blocking agent helps prevent this.

Precautions
As with all sympathomimetic agents except dobutamine, the drug must be given by a central line. Peripheral administration causes vasoconstriction and skin necrosis. This can be reversed by injections of subcutaneous phentolamine (5–10 mg phentolamine in 10–15 ml saline).
- The drug is inactivated by bicarbonate or other alkaline solutions.
- Dopamine is metabolized by β-hydroxylase and monoamine oxidase. It is contraindicated in patients on MAOIs.
- It is contraindicated in phaeochromocytoma, ventricular arrhythmias.

Dopamine infusion preparation
Four ampoules of dopamine (Intropin) each of 200 mg are added to 500 ml 5% dextrose. Using paediatric giving set (60 microdrops = 1 ml) infusion strength: 1 microdrop = 26.7 µg dopamine.

Infusion rate chart (microdrops/min)

Weight of patient (kg)	Dopamine dose (µg/kg/min)					
	2	5	10	15	20	25
30	2	6	12	18	23	29
40	3	8	16	23	31	39
50	4	10	20	29	39	49
60	5	12	23	35	47	58
70	5	14	27	41	55	68
80	6	16	31	47	62	78
90	7	18	35	53	70	88
100	8	20	39	58	78	97

Dobutamine
This synthetic inotrope is structurally similar to dopamine, but differs from it in several respects (see table of inotropes, page 246). It does

not activate dopaminergic receptors, and does not cause local release of noradrenaline from myocardial stores. Its advantage over dopamine is its lack of chronotropic effect at low doses, where it seems to be an exclusive inotrope. Also dobutamine can be given via a peripheral line if there is no central line available. Dopamine must never be given via a peripheral line.

Dobutamine is a racemic mixture of L- and D-dobutamine. D-Dobutamine is a potent beta-1 agonist, and L-dobutamine a potent alpha-agonist with weak beta-1 and beta-2 action. As with all beta-1 agonists, dobutamine may be liable to downregulation.

Both dopamine and dobutamine have their advocates. Crossover studies have suggested:
• heart rate lower with dobutamine for same increase in cardiac output
• pulmonary wedge pressure lower with dobutamine
• fewer ventricular ectopics
• more sustained action over 24 hours.

Its alpha-effects are less than noradrenaline and its beta-2 effects less than isoprenaline.

Precautions are the same as for dopamine. Both drugs have very short half-lives (e.g. dobutamine approximately 2.5 min). Of the two drugs dobutamine and dopamine, the former is probably the superior inotrope.

Second-line sympathomimetic drugs

Isoprenaline

Is rarely used as an inotrope now unless an increase in heart rate is required. Junctional bradycardia, transient second-degree AV block or sinus bradycardia unresponsive to atropine following myocardial infarction or cardiac surgery will be helped by isoprenaline, and may obviate the need for temporary pacing. However, the risk of increased myocardial excitability must be considered. It reduces systemic vascular resistance and dilates skeletal and splanchnic vessels (beta-2 effect), which is not where the flow is needed.

Dose and infusion preparation. (Various strengths available, e.g. 0.1 mg/ml, 1 mg/ml.) Add 2 mg isoprenaline to 500 ml 5% dextrose: mixture strength = 4 µg/ml. Start infusion at 1 µg/min = 15 microdrops/min. Increase dose as required, generally up to 10 µg/min.

Adrenaline

There is still a place for adrenaline infusion when other inotropes have failed. It has a mixed beta- and alpha-receptor activity.

Infusion preparation: 5 ml of 1 : 1000 adrenaline (= 5 mg) in 500 ml 5% dextrose; mixture = 10 µg/ml. Start at 1–2 µg/min (6–12 paediatric microdrops/min).

Glucagon

This activates adenyl-cyclase by a mechanism separate from the beta-1 myocardial receptor. It can be used in beta-blocked patients. It is not a powerful inotrope, does not have a sustained effect and causes hyperglycaemia, hypokalaemia and nausea. It is expensive and of little value in left ventricular failure or cardiogenic shock. It is of more use in treating hypoglycaemia.

Dose 1–5 mg slowly i.v. repeated after 30 min. Infusion rate is 1–7.5 mg/hour.

Choice of parenteral inotrope

In low-output states with oliguria (< 30 ml/hour) low-dose dopamine is the drug of choice. If urine output is > 30 ml/hour then dobutamine is preferable. In hypotensive states with pulmonary oedema, a combination of dopamine or dobutamine with nitroprusside should be tried. Dopamine and dobutamine may be employed together using the 'renal' dose of dopamine and dobutamine as the inotrope.

Other inotropes

1 *Dopexamine.* An alternative to dopamine but also only available as an i.v. preparation. Stimulates DA_1 dopamine receptors (renal vessels dilate). And strong beta-2 agonist. Weak beta-1 agonist. Also inhibits noradrenaline release (DA_2 receptor). It is thus a potent vasodilator plus the effects of dopamine. Dose: start at 0.5 µg/kg/min. Try to avoid doses > 4 µg/kg/min, as tachycardia and hypotension occur at high doses.

2 *Ibopamine.* The only oral inotrope available related to dopamine. Hydrolysed in plasma to epinine (methyldopamine). Little increase in heart rate at standard doses. Diuretic effect with DA_1- and DA_2- receptor activation, i.e. the drug is a renal and peripheral vasodilator. Dose 50–100 mg tds (becoming inotropic at > 800 mg daily). The

Inotropic sympathomimetic drugs

Drug and receptor affected	Increase heart rate β_1-effect	Myocardial release of noradrenaline	Peripheral vasoconstriction α-effect	Peripheral vasodilatation β_2-effect	Renal blood flow Dopaminergic	Dose i.v.
Dopamine Dopaminergic, β_1 α at high dose	++	++	– to ++	++ Low doses	++	Renal dose: 1–5.0 µg/kg/min; Inotropic dose: 5.0–10 µg/kg/min; Constricting dose > 15 µg/kg/min
Dopexamine DA_1 and β_1 (β_2 small)	++	+	–	++	++	0.5–6.0 µg/kg/min
Dobutamine β_1 (β_2 small)	+	–	– to +	++	–	2.5–15.0 µg/kg/min; Low dose – inotropic; High dose – inotropic + chronotropic
Salbutamol β_1 (β_2 small)	++	–	–	++	–	10–40 µg/min (≤ 0.5 µg/kg/min)
Isoprenaline β_1 and β_2	+++	–	–	+++	–	1–10 µg/min
Adrenaline $\beta_1 > \beta_2$ (α small)	+++	+	+	–	–	1–12 µg/min
Noradrenaline α (β small)	– or +	++	+++	–	–	1–12 µg/min

multicentre European trial (PRIME II) of ibopamine 100 mg tds versus placebo in heart failure was terminated early due to more deaths in the ibopamine group. The adverse effect was particularly noted in severe heart failure or in those patients on amiodarone therapy. There seems to be nothing to recommend this drug in heart failure.

3 *Xamoterol.* A partial beta-1 agonist increasing contractility. At the same time it blocks the effects of high endogenous catecholamines on the beta-1 receptor. It is said to lower LV diastolic pressure by improving relaxation. In a single controlled trial it has been shown to be superior to digoxin in patients with mild-to-moderate heart failure.

Xamoterol should be avoided in severe acute LVF or moderate or severe chronic CCF as there is a risk that the beta-blocking activity may cause a deterioration. It should also be avoided in patients with airways obstruction. It is compatible with other drugs in heart failure.

Hopes that the drug might prove useful in sino-atrial disease have unfortunately not been realized.

It can thus only be used in mild heart failure – a condition for which we already have better agents.

Dose: 200 mg bd. Reduce in renal failure.

4 *Enoximone.* Phosphodiesterase (PDE) inhibitor, once available as an oral preparation in some countries. Preliminary trials showed a sustained benefit in LV ejection fraction, exercise tolerance and symptoms. However, one small trial showed a high withdrawal rate and only a transient improvement. The concern of a pro-arrhythmic effect as with other PDE inhibitors remains (see milrinone below). Can be used as an i.v. preparation with dobutamine. The oral preparation has been withdrawn. Parenteral dose: 90 μg/kg/min over 30 min, then 5–20 μg/kg/min. Dose not to exceed 24 mg/kg over 24 hours.

5 *Milrinone.* Phosphodiesterase inhibitor, much more potent than amrinone and available orally. In one trial it was found to be inferior to digoxin, and in the PROMISE trial, treating patients with severe heart failure, the mortality rate with milrinone was 28% higher than with placebo and the trial was stopped early.

6 *Pimobendan.* This inotrope works by sensitizing the myofibril to cytosolic calcium and is also a modest phosphodiesterase inhibitor. In a multicentre European trial exercise duration was increased slightly after 24 weeks therapy but functional status, quality of life or VO_{2max} were not improved. There was a trend to an increased mortality in the pimobendan group.

On present evidence phosphodiesterase inhibitors cannot be recommended for the long-term management of cardiac failure with a possible pro-arrhythmic effect, while their use in the short-term management of acute left ventricular failure remains valuable. The long-term results of other oral inotropes are awaited, but for the moment we continue with digoxin, vasodilators and ACE inhibitors.

Possible future directions

Endothelin-receptor antagonists
Endothelin, a potent vasoconstrictor peptide was discovered in 1988 and plasma levels of endothelin-1 are elevated in heart failure. It acts through type A receptors (constrictor) and type B (mediated via generation of nitric oxide and prostacyclin – dilators). Antagonists to the type A receptor, or to both type A and B (e.g. bosentan) have been developed. Preliminary work in heart failure shows an increase in cardiac output and a fall in PVR and SVR.

New sympathetic antagonists
Moxonidine, similar to clonidine, acts centrally on I_1 imidazoline receptors in the medulla reducing sympathetic outflow reducing SVR. Used in hypertension, it may also prove useful in heart failure.

Dopamine beta-hydroxylase antagonists
Acting peripherally, these agents should reduce noradrenaline levels and increase peripheral dopamine levels and hence renal blood flow.

New third-generation calcium antagonists
These drugs are vasodilators with no negative inotropic effect being vascular selective agents.
• *Amlodipine* was shown to be safe in chronic CCF in the PRAISE trial, possibly improving mortality in patients with dilated cardiomyopathy.
• *Mibefradil* is a new T-channel calcium blocker at present being studied in the MACH I trial.
• *Atrial natriuretic peptidase (ANP) inhibitors.* Atrial natriuretic peptide released from stretched myocytes in the left atrial wall causes a diuresis and natriuresis. Levels are elevated in heart failure. Inhibitors of ANP breakdown should have a therapeutic effect and are almost available.

Surgery for cardiac failure
There is increasing interest in surgical options for cardiac failure as the long-term prognosis on medical treatment is so poor. Initially this was a possibility for a few selected patients.

- Mitral valve replacement for mitral regurgitation.
- Left ventricular aneurysmectomy (excision of scar tissue).
- Coronary artery bypass surgery. Reserved for patients who have demonstrable hibernating myocardium on positron emission tomography (PET) scanning, thallium scanning or stress echocardiography.
- Cardiac allograft transplantation. Donor hearts are the rate-limiting factor. Generally patients must be under 60 years old; 1-year survival is approximately 85% and 5-year survival is 50%.

More recently, a variety of other surgical options are being tried but they are all still under assessment and not generally available.

Dynamic cardiomyoplasty

Not suitable for grade IV heart failure patients. The left latissimus dorsi is mobilized keeping its vascular pedicle intact and transposed into the thorax through partial resection of a rib. The muscle flap is wrapped around the ventricles. A specially designed pacemaker/electrical stimulator is implanted in the rectus sheath and attached to the heart via a sensing electrode and stimulating intramuscular electrodes.

After 2 weeks' rest, the latissimus dorsi is gradually transformed from a fast- to a slow-twitch fatigue-resistant muscle by a series of electrical stimuli synchronized with systole.

Operative mortality is approximately 10% and ventricular arrhythmias are the main problem. Intra-aortic balloon pumping is used peri-operatively.

There is still debate how the operation works. Systolic augmentation helps but the main effect is probably the muscle wrap preventing further LV dilatation. Collateral blood flow from the muscle wrap to the LV itself may help.

Left ventricular volume reduction (Batista operation)

This involves resection of a segment of the free wall of the LV. It differs from an aneurysmectomy in that living ventricular muscle is excised to reduce the LV volume and hence wall stress.

Operative mortality is said to be 15%. Results of trials are awaited.

The artificial heart

Major problems with a continuous power source, infection, thrombosis, and haemolysis have so far prevented this being a long-term option.

The Jarvik 7 heart has been used primarily as a bridge to transplantation.

Left ventricular assist device (LVAD)

This has proved a more effective bridge to transplantation than the artificial heart. Some patients have been managed at home with an LVAD waiting for transplantation. The device is implanted in the abdomen with the inflow conduit in the apex of the LV and the outflow conduit in the ascending aorta, incorporating two xenograft valves. Maximum pump output is 11 l/min, and power is supplied by an electrical pack (requiring recharging every 12 h) or bedside console. The LVAD takes all the mitral flow so that the aortic valve does not open significantly and it is thought to be contraindicated in patients with an aortic valve prosthesis with the thrombotic risk. Disadvantages of the system are that it still involves a transcutaneous electric cable. Tunnelling this driveline helps reduce the infection risk. The Heartmate LVAD incorporates a textured titanium surface encouraging neointima formation and reducing the thromboembolism risk. The units are noisy and quite bulky (approximately 800 g).

The LVAD unloads both left and right ventricle and allows some recovery of LV function with regression of LV hypertrophy and myocyte recovery. They have been used in patients unsuitable for transplantation as a 'bridge to recovery' and there have been patients with a dilated cardiomyopathy in whom it has been possible to remove the LVAD after 3–6 months.

Further miniaturization of LVADs is underway and cost will be the limiting factor.

Xenograft transplantation

The theoretical use of a pig heart in man has come a step nearer reality with the development of pigs expressing a human gene for complement regulatory factors. This would prevent acute hyperimmune rejection but not subsequent cellular immune rejection. There is the added worry of transfer of retroviruses from pig to man and to date this operation has not been sanctioned in the UK. Again, cost will be a major problem.

6.4 Cardiogenic shock

A syndrome of inadequate blood supply to vital organs with failure of elimination of metabolites resulting in their functional and structural disturbance. Clinically this amounts to a hypotensive patient with cool pale moist skin, low-volume rapid pulse, oliguria (< 30 ml/hour) and obtunded consciousness.

Causes
It usually results from massive myocardial infarction with > 40% of the myocardium involved. Mortality is approximately 80%. It may result from arrhythmias or valve lesions.

Pathophysiology
Reduction in cardiac output following myocardial infarction results in sympathetic–adrenal discharge and vasoconstriction. Shunting may occur as a result (e.g. lungs) and decreased tissue flow causes tissue hypoxia, anaerobic metabolism and lactic acidosis. Precapillary dilatation and postcapillary constriction may cause fluid extravasation. Stasis, sludging of red cells, further reduces flow. Mitochondrial damage, lysosome release and cell death result. Shunting may result in the wrong organs getting the small output (e.g. splanchnic bed) at the expense of renal, coronary and cerebral vascular beds. Common causes are as follows.

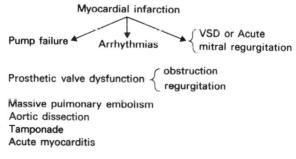

Examination
Should be quick and thorough. Examples of signs to note are as follows.
• General condition: state of consciousness, dyspnoea, peripheral cyanosis, xanthomata. Flows are more important than blood pressure.
• Blood pressure in both arms.
• Pulse: volume, rhythm, ?anacrotic, ?pulsus paradoxus, ?pulsus alternans. Check all peripheral pulses. Auscultate carotids and subclavian arteries.
• Venous pressure: is no guide to LV filling pressure. May be normal in anterior infarction. High in RV infarction or pulmonary embolism.

251

Systolic ('x') descent in tamponade rising with inspiration.

• Apex beat: position and quality, ?high apex beat of anterior infarction, paradoxical of LV aneurysm. ?Hyperdynamic of acute MR. ?Double apex of high LVEDP (prominent 'a' wave). Absent in tamponade. ?RV heave of acute pulmonary embolism.

• Thrills: ?apical with ruptured chordae, retrosternal with VSD or mitral regurgitation, in end-stage aortic stenosis with low flows thrills and murmurs may disappear.

• Auscultation: ?S$_3$ gallop, ?left or right, ?pansystolic murmur of acute VSD or MR.

The murmur of these two conditions may be identical, and both may be heard loudest at the left sternal edge. Consider VSD in anterior infarction with the patient lying fairly flat. Consider mitral regurgitation in inferior or posterior infarction with the patient sitting up in acute pulmonary oedema.

Management

The most important factor in cardiogenic shock is time. If > 2 hours have elapsed from the onset of shock then it is unlikely any intervention will make any difference. Several medical personnel will probably be needed to perform the necessary monitoring requirements.

Stage 1: general measures

Analgesia; oxygen via MC mask or ventilation if necessary; ECG monitoring; 12-lead ECG; urinary catheter; skin (toe) and core (rectal) temperature measurement; bloods for FBC, U and E, LFTs; cardiac enzymes; blood gases; fingertip pulse oximetry.

Insertion of monitoring lines. Swan–Ganz to PA/PAW via subclavian vein; radial artery pressure (acid–base status and arterial gases also); CVP lines × 2 (may be used for drug administration).

Initial CXR. Is performed after insertion of Swan–Ganz catheter to check its position and to exclude a pneumothorax. It is also used to check the following: heart size, lung fields, size of aortic root and upper mediastinum, position of endotracheal tube if patient is ventilated.

Echocardiogram. As soon as possible to exclude pericardial effusion. It provides information about LV size and function, and on two-dimensional machine may show an LV aneurysm. Ruptured chordae will be seen on M-mode as chaotic mitral valve (anterior or posterior leaflet) movement. VSD due to septal perforation can be diagnosed reliably by Doppler echocardiography. A double aortic wall suggestive of dissection may be visualized, but transthoracic echocardiography cannot be relied on. Transoesophageal echocardiography, if available, is much better at visualizing dissection.

Swan–Ganz monitoring

The measurement of left ventricular filling pressure can be performed by right heart catheterization using a balloon flotation catheter introduced by subclavian vein puncture. It can be shown that in the absence of mitral valve stenosis or pulmonary vascular disease then LVEDP = mean PAW pressure.

If a good wedge pressure cannot be obtained, then PAEDP = LVEDP. The catheter can be safely left in PA for > 24–48 hours if necessary. Serial measurements can be made following drug intervention (or exercise testing in fitter patients).

Thermodilution cardiac outputs can be performed. The catheter can be used for:

* cardiac output
* LVFP/PAW/PAEDP measurement
* PA: O_2 content (e.g. for Fick cardiac output)
* right heart saturations (to check for septal perforation in acute myocardial infarction)
* central core temperature (thermistor in PA)
* PA systolic pressure: a useful monitor of ventilation
* $S\dot{V}O_2$ mixed venous (PA) saturation. Normally about 75%. May fall to < 50% in low output state. A useful guide of cardiac output.

Technique. The balloon is tested prior to insertion (usually via subclavian route). Once in RA the balloon is inflated and the catheter gradually advanced until a sudden rise in pressure indicates arrival in RV. The catheter usually easily floats into PA. The balloon is deflated in PA and the pressure recorded. The catheter is advanced until a wedge pressure is achieved. The catheter should not be left in the PAW position for any length of time. The catheter is marked with 10-cm graduation marks to indicate how much has been inserted.

In experienced hands the technique is safe. However, numerous complications have been reported.

* all complications of subclavian puncture (see **7.2**)
* ruptured pulmonary artery (by the balloon)
* damage to pulmonary or tricuspid valves

- pulmonary infarction
- septicaemia
- infective endocarditis
- arrhythmias, often from RV outflow tract
- catheter knotting. This may occur with too vigorous movement of the catheter. The knot should not be pulled out through the subclavian vein. The catheter can be snared from the femoral vein using a Dotter retrieval snare, the catheter is cut at the entry site at the clavicle and the whole catheter pulled out through the femoral vein.

Stage 2: correction of filling pressure

As soon as the Swan–Ganz catheter is *in situ*, attempts are made to get the filling pressure of the left ventricle (mean PAW or PAEDP) to 16–18 mmHg. This is the optimum filling pressure, assuming a normal plasma colloid oncotic pressure. The optimal filling pressure will be lower where the oncotic pressure is lower (e.g. hypoalbuminaemia) or where capillary permeability is greater (e.g. sepsis, myxoedema).

Filling pressure too high.
- With normotension (mean aortic pressure > 90 mmHg) use vasodilators (e.g. nitroprusside), keeping mean aortic pressure > 70 mmHg.
- With hypotension use dopamine 5–10 µg/kg/min.

Filling pressure too low (rare). Give 200 ml plasma and repeat measurement. Vasodilators can always be used if too much plasma is given, and small amounts of plasma may be enough.

Stage 3: improvement of stroke volume

Inotropes are usually required. The choice lies between dobutamine or dopamine (see inotrope section). Note that the skin temperature gradually warms up as peripheral flows improve.

Although set out in stages, the management of cardiogenic shock depends on many of these procedures being performed quickly and more or less simultaneously.

Stage 4: further measures

Percutaneous transluminal coronary angioplasty (see **5.7**).
This should be considered in patients with acute myocardial infarction who are going into cardiogenic shock, whether or not streptokinase

has been given (see thrombolysis, **5.9**). It may still be possible to salvage some myocardium if PTCA is performed early enough and there is little to lose in a condition like this with such high mortality. This can be performed with intra-aortic balloon pumping via the other femoral artery or brachial artery.

Intra-aortic balloon pumping (IABP) (Figure 6.3)
The intra-aortic balloon can now be inserted percutaneously without an arterial cut-down procedure and without X-ray screening. The R wave of the ECG triggers balloon deflation. The sudden 'sump' effect of balloon deflation acts as afterload reduction, reducing systolic work (Figure 6.4).

   The balloon is timed to inflate just after the dicrotic notch of aortic valve closure. Inflation increases coronary and cerebral blood flow. Helium is used as inflation gas.

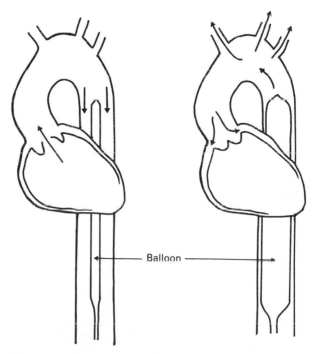

Figure 6.3 Intra-aortic balloon pumping. Inflation of intra-aortic balloon in diastole increases cerebral and coronary blood flow.

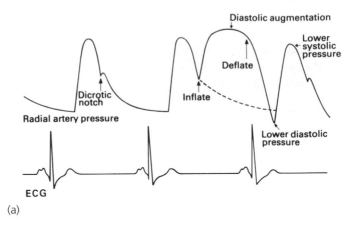

(a)

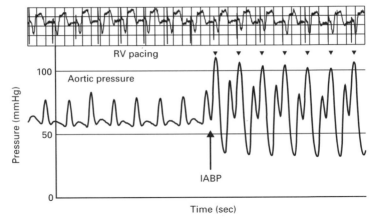

(b)

Figure 6.4 (a) Effect of balloon pumping on arterial pressure. Shows schematic representation of ECG and radial artery pressure during intra-aortic balloon pumping. The balloon is inflated during the second ECG cycle only to show diastolic augmentation of pressure. The balloon is timed to inflate just after the dicrotic notch, and deflation is triggered by the R wave of the ECG. Note also the lower pressure at end diastole prior to the third cycle and the lower systolic pressure of the third cycle. This represents successful afterload reduction by the balloon. (b) Example of intra-aortic balloon pumping (IABP) in cardiogenic shock due to massive inferior infarction. ECG shows RV pacing throughout. Prior to balloon pumping the aortic pressure is 80/57. On starting balloon pumping (large arrow) the peak augmentation pressure is approximately 105 mmHg. Diastolic augmentation is indicated by small arrows. The aortic diastolic pressure is much lower at 32 mmHg with good afterload reduction on balloon deflation. Once IABP had been established this patient went on to successful right coronary artery re-opening and stenting.

Patients are fully heparinized while on the balloon. The balloon can be removed percutaneously after deflation and firm pressure over the femoral artery entry site will secure haemostasis. Surgical removal is advised after prolonged use.

IABP quickly settles unstable angina but is rarely necessary now with drug treatment, followed by coronary angiography and possible PTCA or coronary bypass surgery. Nevertheless it remains a useful tool in severe unstable angina and conventional coronary angiography can be performed with the balloon *in situ* via the other leg. The main indication for IABP remains the low-output state in the preoperative or postoperative cardiac surgical patient. It is also a useful back-up in patients who are at higher risk for coronary angioplasty.

Surgery

In cardiogenic shock this is really reserved for urgent mitral valve replacement (e.g. ruptured papillary muscle), repair of acquired VSD, or for repair of aortic dissection (**10.7**, page 411). Very occasionally repair of sub-acute cardiac rupture is possible (page 205).

6.5 | Cardiac transplantation

About 400 cardiac transplants are performed in the UK annually and about 100 heart–lung transplants. Organ availability is the limiting factor and many patients die on the waiting list. There is no absolute age limit for referral but 55 years for ischaemic heart disease and 60 years for dilated cardiomyopathy is a guide. The 5-year survival is 65% for heart transplants and 50% for heart–lung transplants. The threat in the first year following transplant is infection or rejection and in the long term, the development of allograft coronary disease.

Follow up of cardiac transplant patients

Early follow up will be at the transplant centre. Longer term follow up at the referring centre will be included. There are many potential problems, particularly detecting signs of early rejection, problems secondary to immunosuppresion, prevention of long-term allograft coronary disease, drug interactions and the problem of late malignancy. Close liaison with the transplant centre is essential.

General advice

Smoking is forbidden. Limited alcohol (e.g. 2–3 units daily) is allowed. A low saturated fat diet is encouraged. Weight gain is common (steroids, inactivity and fluid retention), and in patients on longer-term steroids, diabetes should be expected. Patients take their own temperatures and weigh themselves daily contacting the cardiologist if their weight increases by > 2kg over 48 hours. The transplant centre should be consulted by either patient or cardiologist with any problems or queries.

Rejection

Most common in the first year following transplantation. Activated T cells infiltrate the allograft. If suspected, the patient should be referred back to the transplant centre if possible for RV biopsy. Unfortunately early rejection may be asymptomatic with no clinical signs. Suspect it with:

- general malaise, lethargy and fatigue
- dyspnoea and reduction in exercise tolerance
- low-grade fever
- sudden weight gain from fluid retention
- new atrial flutter or fibrillation
- new conduction system abnormalities
- reduction in QRS voltage on ECG.

Many of these are also features of cytomegalovirus (CMV) infection which itself may provoke rejection and early atherosclerosis of the allograft.

Diagnosis is based on RV endomyocardial biopsy via the right internal jugular vein. Initially performed weekly post-transplantation and then at decreasing intervals over the first 6 months. Generally rejection responds well to early treatment (pulsed methylprednisolone 0.5–1.0 g daily over 3 days). Refractory cases may need antithymocyte globulin (ATG) or monoclonal anti-CD3 antibody (OKT3).

Immunosuppression

Initially, patients are on a combination of steroids, cyclosporin and azathioprine, but after about 3 months many can be weaned off their steroids and maintained on cyclosporin and azathioprine. Steroids may need to be continued with poor renal function or continued rejection. Antithymocyte globulin is not used except in acute steroid-resistant rejection as in the long term it predisposes to CMV infection and lymphoma and does not improve long-term prognosis.

Patients must be told to report immediately any symptoms which might be due to oversuppression, e.g. bruising or bleeding, oropharyngeal ulceration or unexplained fever.

Prednisolone

Usual maintenance dose is 10–15 mg daily as a single dose. While patients are on prednisolone they should also take ranitidine for possible peptic ulceration and co-trimoxazole (*Pneumocystis carinii* prophylaxis). Side-effects are inevitable: weight gain from increased appetite and fluid retention, sleep disturbance, redistribution of body fat, fragile skin, acne, hypertension, osteoporosis, muscle wasting and proximal myopathy, exacerbation or development of diabetes, and glaucoma and cataracts. More rarely, aseptic femoral head necrosis, benign intracranial hypertension, psychosis. Growth retardation will occur in children.

Steroids are weaned gradually after a long course. Acute cessation may result in adrenal insufficiency and also a polymyalgia-like syndrome.

Azathioprine

Maintenance dose is 1–2 mg/kg/day It causes a dose-related, usually reversible, depression of all elements of the bone marrow. Aim to keep total white count in the range 4000–6500/mm^3. The total neutrophil count must not fall below 1000/mm^3. Regular blood counts are essential. The drug is generally well tolerated. Hypersensitivity reactions can occur on starting treatment.

The dose of azathioprine must be reduced if allopurinol is started for gout to avoid possible pancytopenia.

Cyclosporin

A cyclic polypeptide originally isolated from fungi now prduced synthetically. It inhibits the resting lymphocyte in G_0 or G_1 phase and prevents the release of interleukin 2 and other lymphokines. Normal maintenance dose is 2–10 mg/kg/day regulated by renal function and drug levels. An oral oily solution (100 mg/ml) is taken once or twice daily in milk or fruit Juice. An i.v. form is available if needed (use one-third oral dose).

Impairment of renal function is the most important side-effect particularly with onset of treatment. It responds to dose reduction. Patients may become hirsute (dark hair), and develop gingival hypertrophy (particularly if on nifedipine). Other side effects are tremor, hypertension (see below), liver dysfunction, gastrointestinal disturbances, migraine and peripheral dysthesiae.

Drug interactions are important with cyclosporin as rises in plasma levels due to other drugs may rapidly cause deterioration in renal function, or increase the infection risk from oversuppression.

Drugs increasing cyclosporin levels	Drugs decreasing cyclosporin levels
Ketoconazole	Phenytoin
Diltiazem	Carbamazepine
Verapamil	Barbiturates
Nicardipine	Rifampicin
Propafenone	Trimethoprim (i.v.)
Erythromycin	
Doxycycline	
Oral contraceptives	
Methylprednisolone (high dose)	

The use of regular ketoconazole or diltiazem with cyclosporin has been used in some centres to cut down the dose (and cost) of cyclosporin, as both drugs inhibit the metabolism of cyclosporin by cytochrome oxidase.

Tacrolimus (FK 506)
A recently introduced immunosuppressive agent with similar side effects to cyclosporin. May cause hypertrophic cardiomyopathy in children, and a long QT interval. Regular echocardiography needed during treatment. Also may cause hyperglycaemia and CNS disturbances.

Hypertension
This is a common problem in heart-transplant recipients, induced by steroids, cyclosporin and renal dysfunction. Long-acting nifedipine is tried first. Avoid verapamil and nicardipine (see above). ACE inhibitors are good but renal function needs watching carefully with patients on cyclosporin. Beta-blockers are unlikely to be tolerated in this group. Avoid thiazides, and care needed with potassium-retaining diuretics.

Hyperlipidaemia
Lipid levels must be measured regularly. The need to lower serum cholesterol in this group of patients is particularly important to try and prevent late onset allograft coronary disease.
• *HMG CoA reductase inhibitors* have been reported as more likely to cause muscle pains and rhabdomyolysis in patients on cyclosporin. Provided the patient is warned to report any unexplained muscle pains and a low dose is prescribed these drugs can be used. One report

suggests that HMG CoA reductase inhibitors might help prevent rejection in addition to their cholesterol lowering properties.
- *Fibrates:* as with HMG CoA reductase inhibitors. Use in low dose and watch for muscle pains.
- *Cholestyramine:* should be avoided as it could interfere with absorption of immunosuppressive drugs.

Contraception

Pregnancy should be strongly discouraged as azathioprine is teratogenic. Oral contraceptives may increase cyclosporin levels unpredictably. This seems to be less of a problem with progesterone-only preparations which are the contraceptive of choice if possible. Cyclosporin levels, renal and liver function should be monitored carefully on starting oral contraceptives, and repeated for the first few months.

The intrauterine contraceptive device should be avoided with the infection risk.

Gout

Hyperuricaemia and gout are common in patients on cyclosporin. Non-steroidal anti-inflammatory agents should be used for as brief a time as possible to avoid deterioration in renal function. If allopurinol is used, the dose should not be > 100 mg/day, the dose of azathioprine should be halved and blood counts performed every 2 weeks for 6–8 weeks.

Infection and antibiotics

It is important to take all cultures pretreatment (nose, throat, urine, sputum and blood).

Bacterial. Amoxycillin, flucloxacillin, cephalosporins and ciprofloxacin are safe. Aminoglycosides should be avoided if possible (combined nephrotoxicity with cyclosporin). Erythromycin increases cyclosporin levels. Antibiotic prophylaxis should be advised for dental procedures, etc. as if the patient had valve disease (see page 392). Single-dose amoxycillin or clindamycin are the drugs of choice. Single-dose erythromycin can be used (see above).

Viral. Cytomegalovirus (CMV) infection is common in the first 6 months and may follow increased immunosuppression given for rejection. Consider if the patient has malaise and pyrexia plus additional symptoms of colitis, retinits, pneumonia or even myocarditis.

Ganciclovir is used for acute CMV infection and its continued use in long-term prophylaxis is increasing.

Acyclovir is given orally for herpes simplex infection, but i.v. for zoster infection initially.

Fungal. Oral nystatin is use for oropharyngeal *Candida* and fluconazole for more severe systemic infection. *Aspergillus* infection commonly involves the lung. Transbronchial or CT-guided lung needle biopsy may be needed to make the diagnosis. Amphotericin use will be limited by renal function. (See section on infective endocarditis, page 384.)

Protozoal. Pneumocystis carinii pneumonia should be prevented with the use of co-trimoxazole. Toxoplasmosis (transmitted with the allograft into non-immune subjects) should be prevented with an initial six week course of pyrimethamine.

Vaccination

Live attenuated viral vaccines must be avoided in immunosuppressed patients. If in doubt consult occupational health centre, professional immunization centre or consultant virologist.

Vaccines to be avoided	Safe vaccines
Oral polio	Polio (killed virus) (i.m.)
Measles	Influenza
Rubella	Tetanus
Yellow fever	Typhoid
Mumps	Hyperimmune gamma-globulin
Hepatitis A or B	Pneumococcal vaccine
BCG	

With the exception of hyperimmune gamma-globulin, the safe vaccines may not generate an immune response and hence be ineffective. Determined energetic patients may require counselling and encouragement to avoid 'at risk' areas.

Allograft coronary disease

This is the commonest cause of late death, and may occur in all age groups. Coronary arteriograms are usually performed at the end of the second year then annually thereafter. The disease process is probably a combination of immune-mediated smooth muscle cell hyperplasia and hypercholesterolaemia. Diffuse coronary disease is common but angina rare (denervated heart), patients presenting with symptoms from deteriorating LV function. The process is diffuse, concentric and may involve the whole length of the artery. It can involve intramyocardial vessels. Coronary angioplasty may occasionally be effective for localized lesions. Retransplantation may be the only possibility.

The search for effective prevention continues. There are already reports of diltiazem and pravastatin reducing the incidence of new coronary disease.

Malignant disease

The incidence of malignant disease increases with long-term immunosuppression, and may occur in 10% of long-term survivors of transplantation. About one-third of these are squamous cell carcinomas. Patients should be advised to avoid strong sunlight or use barrier creams. Any suspicious skin lesions should be excised. Squamous cell carcinomas may recur and plastic surgery may eventually be necessary.

Another one-third of these malignancies are lymphomas (particularly non-Hodgkin's lymphoma). The small tumour mass may respond to high-dose oral acyclovir and a slight decrease in immunosuppression as the non-Hodgkin's lymphoma may be linked to Epstein Barr virus infection. More extensive lymphomas will require chemotherapy and radiotherapy. Close liaison with an oncology team is essential.

Cardiac arrest

Recognition

The recognition of cardiac arrest is based on absent arterial pulsation and an unconscious patient. Spontaneous respiration may continue sporadically for ≤ 1 min after an arrest and the state of the pupils is merely a guide to the time from an arrest.

Ideally, the arrest team should consist of at least three medical personnel (one an anaesthetist) trained in resuscitation, who are called to any hospital arrest. Training non-medical personnel to cope with cardiopulmonary resuscitation is paying dividends in several cities. The training and equipping of ambulance personnel have improved enormously over the last few years. As well as being trained to intubate and give appropriate drugs, the accuracy of emergency ECG diagnosis has been improved with automated external defibrillators.

New concepts

The European resuscitation guidelines published in 1992 have changed

many long-standing traditions in the management of cardiac arrest. These long-held beliefs were not based on firm evidence. In particular, three precautions were emphasized:
• defibrillation at the absolute earliest opportunity with three quick shocks
• lignocaine is not given until several attempts at cardioversion/defibrillation, as this raises defibrillation thresholds
• sodium bicarbonate is not given until late on in the course of the arrest.

Management

Precordial chest thump: check the clock
A few sharp blows to the mid-sternum may revert ventricular tachycardia. It should only be employed if it is possible within a few seconds of the arrest. Occasionally the thumps may start a rhythm in asystolic patients.

External cardiac massage (ECM)
Minimal rate of 70/min in adults, 100/min in infants. When artificial ventilation is under way, pause every 5–6 beats for respiratory cycle. With good cardiac massage, pressure similar to native pressure can be achieved.

In infants the chest is encircled with both hands and the chest compressed with the thumbs. In children ECM is performed with one hand only.

A hard surface beneath the patient is necessary for effective massage. Correct ECM should not fracture ribs, although this occasionally occurs in the elderly. Massage too near the xiphisternum will not be effective and additionally may damage the liver.

Airway and artificial ventilation
The airway should be cleared, dentures removed and vomit aspirated with a sucker. Pillows are removed and the head extended. Initially the patient is ventilated using an oral airway (Guedel), a mask and self-inflating bag connected to an oxygen cylinder. If these are not available a Brooke airway or mouth-to-mouth ventilation is used.

When help arrives:

Establish ECG monitoring
Subsequent action depends on the ECG.
1 *If the monitor shows ventricular fibrillation or ventricular tachycardia*:

....

- Precordial chest thump.
- DC shock 200 J (watt-seconds) in an adult. If performed immediately this should defibrillate 90% of adults. If the patient is very heavy, or if the first shock was delayed, greater energy may be needed. The electrodes should be widely separated. Neither should be directly over the sternum (bone has high impedance to electric current). An electrode paste 'bridge' will short-circuit the shock and prove useless.
- *If this fails* repeat shock at 200 J.
- *If this fails* repeat the shock at 360 J.

If the patient is still in VF after three quick shocks then the resuscitation is unlikely to succeed. Coarse VF is much more likely to be defibrillated successfully than fine VF.

- *Intubation.* This should be attempted after the first three shocks. It should not be attempted by inexperienced personnel, and ventilation using a mask and self-inflating bag should be continued until experienced help is available. Whatever type of ventilation is established, the chest should be auscultated to check that the lungs are being inflated effectively.
- *Establish i.v. access.* Insert a central venous line or preferably two The internal jugular is safest in an emergency. The subclavian vein is an alternative but a pneumothorax will make resuscitation unlikely to succeed. A peripheral vein may be of temporary help only, but several drugs given through a peripheral line will cause tissue necrosis (e.g. dopamine, adrenaline):
  - give adrenaline 1 mg i.v. ⎫
  - 10 CPR sequences ⎬ this sequence is a 'loop'
  - DC shocks 360 J × 3 ⎭
  - repeat the loop twice more
  - consider sodium bicarbonate 50 mmol i.v. 8.4% sodium bicarbonate = 1 mmol/l
  - consider lignocaine 100–200 mg i.v. and then repeat the sequence above: 10 ml 1% lignocaine contains 100 mg, 10 ml 2% lignocaine contains 200 mg
  - if this fails, consider another anti-arrhythmic agent, e.g. bretylium tosylate 100 mg i.v. and repeat the shock.

Continue massage and ventilation between shocks. The value of good massage and ventilation cannot be overemphasized and may ride out arrhythmias (other than VF) that are not being successfully managed with drugs. It is also a safer and a better way of correcting an acidosis than bicarbonate (see below).

2 *If the monitor shows asystole or extreme sinus bradycardia.*

....

- Precordial thump.
- Definitely exclude VF on monitor.
- Intubate and i.v. access as above.
- Adrenaline 1 mg i.v.
- 10 CPR sequences.
- Atropine 3 mg i.v., once only.
- If evidence of electrical activity: emergency pacing; if no evidence of electrical activity: repeat adrenaline i.v. and CPR.

Generally the results of resuscitation in asystole are poor unless the patient has gone into complete AV block (with visible P waves), or asystole has just evolved from extreme sinus bradycardia, or just after VF defibrillation. It is easy to miss fine VF on a monitor and assume it is asystole especially with faulty equipment, artefact or incorrect gain settings.

Calcium chloride 10 ml of 10% i.v. has not been included in the above protocol. There is no evidence that it works and calcium loading has been implicated in myocardial cell injury during ischaemia. It maybe of benefit in occasional cases, but often only transiently.

3 *If there is electromechanical dissociation.* Continuing electrical activity on the monitor with no palpable pulse is a poor prognostic sign unless it occurs transiently during an arrest (e.g. immediately after defibrillation) or is due to a reversible cause such as:

- acute hypovolaemia
- cardiac tamponade
- massive pulmonary embolism
- tension pneumothorax
- hypothermia
- drug intoxication
- electrolyte imbalance, e.g. extreme hyperkalaemia.

Treatment is based on searching for one of these. At the same time resuscitation continues on the lines described under asystole above:

- ECM, intubation, i.v. access
- i.v. adrenaline
- 10 CPR sequences
- consider:
  repeating adrenaline or i.v. calcium
  i.v. bicarbonate
  large dose of adrenaline: 5 mg i.v.

Correction of acidosis and sodium bicarbonate. The use of bicarbonate soon after an arrest is no longer recommended. Effective massage and

....

ventilation should help slow the progression of an acidosis. The measurement of arterial pH and base-deficit bears little relation to the intracellular values, and the inside of the cell may become acidotic (with diffusion of CO_2 into the cell) while the extracellular fluid remains alkalotic. Hyperosmolarity with sodium loading occurs, and an alkalosis may be just as dangerous as an acidosis. A single blood gas measurement provides no indication of the rate of acid production.

If in spite of all this after prolonged resuscitation measures have failed, it is reasonable to give 50 mmol of sodium bicarbonate i.v. and to repeat the blood gas measurements. A separate central line must be used for bicarbonate as it inactivates catecholamines and precipitates out with calcium chloride or gluconate.

Correction of hypotension. If the rhythm is reasonably stable but pulse of low volume:
• check CVP. This is particularly important in inferior (right ventricular) infarctions where a fluid load may improve the cardiac output. Fluid load should not be attempted without Swan–Ganz monitoring (see cardiogenic shock). Generally the CVP should be 5–10 cmH$_2$O from the mid-axillary line.
• start dopamine 5 µg/kg/min increasing to 10 µg/kg/min (for dose regime see **6.3**, page 243) via a central line not used for bicarbonate administration.

Correction of potassium status.
• *Hyperkalaemia* (K$^+$ > 5.0 mmol/l). Give calcium chloride 10 ml 10% and check for possible metabolic acidosis. Correction of metabolic acidosis should reduce serum K$^+$. See also page 233.
• *Hypokalaemia.* Give 20 mmol KCl through central line over 10 min if K$^+$ is < 3.0 mmol/l.

Further measures that may be necessary.
• Insertion of radial artery and Swan–Ganz catheter in pulmonary artery.
• Insertion of urinary catheter.
• Intermittent positive pressure ventilation continued. In the presence of pulmonary oedema and a reasonable arterial pressure (> 100 mmHg) positive end-expiratory pressure (PEEP) may help.
• Insertion of temporary pacing with screening facilities available.
• Echocardiography to exclude pericardial effusion, check LV function, mitral and aortic valve movement and aortic root.

- Aspiration of a pericardial effusion if documented.
- Pass a nasogastric tube and aspirate the stomach.

Procedures that are not recommended.

- *Dexamethasone i.v.* This does not reduce cerebral oedema if given after the event. It should only be used if the arrest was secondary to an anaphylactic reaction.
- *Intracardiac injections.* With a good central line this is unnecessary. It may damage the anterior or inferior surface of the heart.
- *Attempts to assess neurology during resuscitation.* This is very unreliable. Pupils are affected by a wide variety of drugs used in resuscitation. It is preferable to wait and concentrate on resuscitation.

When to discontinue resuscitation attempts
This depends on so many factors such as the precipitating cause for the arrest if known, other medical conditions and the results of resuscitation measures. Usually resuscitation attempts continue for half an hour and longer if the rhythm is still recognizable VF. In younger patients efforts would continue up to an hour or more if there was recognizable electrical activity.

7 Disturbances of Cardiac Rhythm

Contents

7.1 Indications for temporary pacing

AV block in acute myocardial infarction

Complete AV block (Figures 7.1 and 12.4)
In inferior infarction, complete AV block usually results from right coronary artery occlusion. The AV nodal artery is a branch of the right coronary artery. Second-degree AV block (Wenckebach type) does not always represent AV nodal artery occlusion, as vagal hyperactivity may play a part. A localized small inferior infarct may thus cause complete AV block.

In anterior infarction, complete AV block usually represents massive septal necrosis with additional circumflex artery territory damage. The prognosis in complete AV block is dependent on infarct size and site rather than the block itself.

Complete AV block in either type of infarction should be temporarily paced.

Second-degree AV block (Figures 7.1 and 12.4)
1 *Wenckebach (Mobitz Type I).* Incremental increases in PR interval with intermittent complete blocking of the P wave. This is decremental conduction at AV node level. In inferior infarction it does not necessarily require pacing unless the bradycardia is poorly tolerated by the patient. It may respond to atropine. In anterior infarction, Wenckebach AV block should be temporarily paced.
2 *Mobitz Type II AV block.* Fixed PR interval with sudden failure of conduction of atrial impulse (blocking of the P wave). Often occurs in the presence of a wide QRS as this type of block is usually associated with distal fascicular disease. It carries a high risk of developing complete AV block. It usually occurs in association with anterior infarction, but should be prophylactically paced with either type of infarct.

First-degree AV block
Does not require temporary pacing, but approximately 40% will develop higher degrees of AV block, and observation is necessary.

Bundle branch block (Figures 12.6 and 12.7)
This is a more complex group with conflicting evidence from various

Types of 2nd degree AV block

Wenckebach 2nd degree AV block

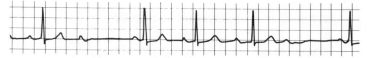

Mobitz type II AV block

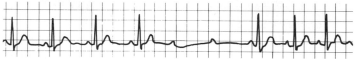

2:1 AV block

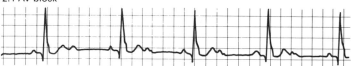

Complete third degree AV block

Congenital: narrow QRS

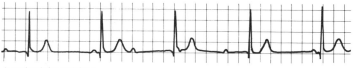

Acquired: broad QRS

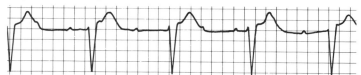

Figure 7.1 Second- and third-degree AV block.

series. Patients with evidence of trifascicular disease or non-adjacent bifascicular disease complicating myocardial infarctions should be prophylactically paced, i.e.

Trifascicular disease
$\begin{cases} \text{Alternating RBBB/LBBB} \\ \text{Long PR interval + new RBBB + LAHB} \\ \text{or new RBBB + LPHB} \\ \text{Long PR + LBBB} \end{cases}$

Non-adjacent bifascicular disease; RBBB + new LPHB (Figure 12.7).

There is no proof that LBBB with a long PR interval is genuine trifascicular disease without measurements from His bundle studies, but if it develops in the presence of septal infarction, LBBB is assumed to be LAHB + LPHB. One of the commonest bundle branch blocks complicating anterior infarction is RBBB and LAHB (usually manifest by RBBB + left axis deviation), as these two fascicles are in the anterior septum. In anterior infarction this combination should only be paced if a long PR interval develops. Measurement of the H–V interval is theoretically useful in acute infarction, but involves insertion of an electrode under fluoroscopy and is not generally practical.

Sino-atrial disease

Profound sinus bradycardia or sinus arrest may occur in acute infarction (typically inferior infarction and right coronary occlusion). The sinus node arterial supply is usually from the right coronary artery. Vagal hyperactivity may contribute and be partially reversed by atropine. However, sinus bradycardia or sinus arrest may need temporary pacing if not reversed by atropine and is poorly tolerated by the patient.

Temporary pacing for general anaesthesia

The same principles apply as those in acute infarction: 24-hour monitoring for those thought to be at risk may provide useful information. Notice should be taken of recent ECG deterioration (e.g. lengthening of PR interval, additional LAHB).

Asymptomatic patients with bifascicular block and a normal PR interval do not need temporary pacing. Patients with sino-atrial disease should have 24 hour ECG monitoring prior to surgery, as vagal influences may produce prolonged sinus arrest.

Temporary pacing during cardiac surgery

Temporary epicardial pacing may be necessary in surgery adjacent to the AV node and bundle of His, e.g.
- aortic valve replacement for calcific aortic stenosis (with calcium extending into the septum)
- tricuspid valve surgery and Ebstein's anomaly
- AV canal defects and ostium primum ASD
- corrected transposition and lesions with AV discordance.

A knowledge of the exact site of the AV node and His bundle can be obtained by endocardial mapping at the time of surgery. Closure of a VSD in corrected transposition or of the ventricular component of a complete AV canal defect may damage the His bundle and permanent epicardial electrodes may be required.

Other indications for temporary pacing

Indications include termination of refractory tachyarrhythmias, during electrophysiological studies, drug overdose (e.g. digoxin, beta-blocking agents, verapamil).

7.2 Pacing difficulties

Failure to pace or sense

Wire displacement

This is the commonest reason for failure to pace and is a common problem with temporary wires that have no tines or screw-in mechanisms. To some extent it can be avoided by stability manoeuvres during wire insertion. Positions just across the tricuspid valve tend not to be very stable.

Positions in the RV apex are usually more stable but sometimes threshold measurements are not ideal here. Wire displacement requires repositioning in either temporary or permanent systems.

Microdisplacement

If not noticed on CXR this may be overcome by increasing pacing output voltage or pulse width. Otherwise repositioning is necessary.

Exit block

This may develop in the first 2 weeks due to a rise in threshold. As the electrode becomes fibrosed into the endocardium the threshold levels off. With temporary units the threshold is checked daily and the voltage increased if necessary. With programmable permanent pacing units the programmer may be used to increase the output.

During temporary wire insertion a threshold of < 1.0 V at 1 ms pulse width is preferable. With permanent pacing the pulse width of the unit to be implanted is used. An acute threshold of < 1.0 V is again preferable. If the wire has been implanted for a few months then a chronic threshold of < 2.0 V is satisfactory as it is unlikely to rise further. Exit block tends to be more of a problem now with epicardial electrodes. Newer endocardial lead design with carbon porous tip and steroid eluting leads should reduce the incidence of exit block.

Wire fracture

This may occur due to kinking of the wire or too severe looping after implantation. Tight silk ligatures may damage the insulation. Complete fracture may be detected on the CXR. Insulation fracture may result in current leakage and pectoral muscle pacing.

Partial fracture results in intermittent pacing, and analysis of the stimulus shows reduced amplitude. A rate drop is not essential with partial wire fracture.

Perforation

This is a rare complication of permanent pacing. It sometimes occurs in patients who are temporarily paced for heart block complicating myocardial infarction. There may be loss of pacing plus signs and symptoms of pericarditis.

The diagnosis can be confirmed by measuring the intracardiac electrogram from the temporary wire. The temporary wire is connected to the V lead of a standard ECG machine. With impaction against the RV wall there should be an endocardial potential of 1.5–8 mV. This is lost with perforation and ST depression and T wave inversion are recorded (Figure 7.2). Repositioning is necessary.

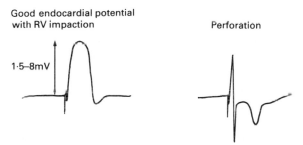

Good endocardial potential with RV impaction

1·5–8mV

Perforation

Figure 7.2 Change in ECG on perforation by pacing wire.

Battery failure

Each permanent pacemaker has its own end-of-life characteristics. Premature battery failure has been a problem with some lithium cell designs. Several factors other than cell design may lead to early battery failure, some of which may be avoided, for example:

- low lead impedance with large electrode tip
- wide pulse width
- constant pacemaker use or fast pacing rate

....

- complex circuitry in automatic pacemakers with two sensing and two pacing circuits (DDD units). Recent units have incorporated microprocessors which drain current.

Thus the choice of electrode is important. If a pacemaker with hysteresis mode is available, the takeover rate may be set lower than the basic pacing rate, conserving battery life. Generally the more complex the pacemaker the shorter the expected battery life.

A pacemaker may have its battery life prolonged by reducing rate, pulse width and output. However, reducing pulse width or output voltage should not be performed until enough time has elapsed from implantation to allow for the establishment of the chronic threshold (e.g. 3 months).

The end-of-life of most pacemaker batteries is indicated by:
- slowing of the basic pacing rate
- increasing pulse width
- decreasing output voltage.

Regular follow up at a pacing clinic is necessary to determine the time for elective pacemaker change. Telemetry may help in some areas.

EMG inhibition (Figure 7.4, page 278)
Electromyographic voltage (e.g. from use of the pectoral muscles) may be of sufficient strength to be sensed by the permanent pacemaker, cause it to be inhibited and hence fail to pace the ventricle. It may exceptionally cause syncope when it is obviously self-limiting. In right-handed patients it is preferable to put the permanent unit on the left side. It is not a problem when a bipolar wire is used and hence does not occur with temporary pacing systems. The problem may be overcome by:
- waiting until any effusion around the unit has resolved
- reprogramming the unit to reduced sensitivity VOO (fixed rate ventricular pacing) mode
- placing a non-conducting 'boot' around the pacemaker
- converting the system to a bipolar system with a new wire.

Sensing failure
The pacemaker fails to notice an intrinsic cardiac impulse and is not inhibited. This may be because the R wave of the intrinsic ECG is too small, the slew rate is too slow or because the pacing unit is too insensitive. In temporary pacing this may be a problem in myocardial infarction (with reduction in or loss of R waves) resulting in stimulus on

T phenomenon. The use of a subcutaneous indifferent electrode as the second pole may help avoid this.

In permanent pacing the sensitivity of the unit may be changed in some programmable units (e.g. R-wave sensitivity increased from 2 mV to 10 mV). A porous tip electrode may offer better sensing capabilities.

False inhibition (oversensing) (Figures 7.3 and 7.4)
Inhibition of the pacemaker by an electrical signal other than by the R wave. EMG inhibition is an example. It may also occur with spurious

Ventricular inhibited pacing

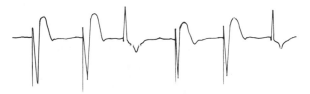

Missing (intermittent failure to pace)

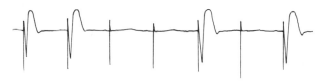

False inhibition (oversensing)

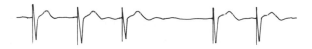

Ventricular triggered pacing

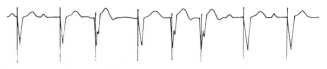

Figure 7.3 Examples of pacing ECGs.

Failure of ventricular capture due to exit block. VVI unipolar system.
Idioventricular rate 36/min

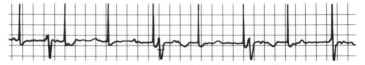

Failure of atrial capture and of atrial sensing with normal ventricular pacing in a
DDD bipolar unit. Unsensed P waves can be seen wandering through the trace

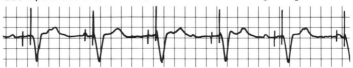

False inhibition (oversensing) in a VVI unit. Lead insulation fracture

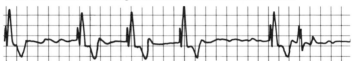

Oversensing and undersensing in a VVI unit programmed to 72/min. Lead
insulation fracture

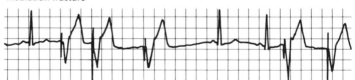

Electromyographic (EMG) inhibition in a unipolar VVI system. Vigorous
pectoral strain produces a signal strong enough to inhibit the unit

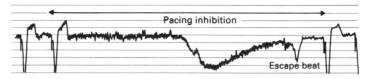

Pacing inhibition

Escape beat

Figure 7.4 Common pacing problems. See also Figure 12.5.

signals from electrode fracture, or inadequate contacts or bad
connections to the internal or external unit. Occasionally, large T-wave
voltage may inhibit the unit. Electromagnetic interference (e.g. leak
from microwave ovens) is another possibility. This used to cause false
inhibition of early permanent pacing units, but is not a problem now.

Complications of wire insertion

Pneumothorax
Following insertion of a pacing wire, the patient should have a chest X-ray to check the wire position and to exclude a pneumothorax.

Infection
Antibiotic prophylaxis is not required for temporary pacing and is only indicated for clinical reasons. After insertion the wire should be anchored with silk sutures to avoid movement and the entry site should be covered with a sterile transparent dressing. If a patient with a temporary wire develops a swinging pyrexia, there is a strong chance that this is due to a staphylococcal septicaemia. Blood cultures should be taken, the patient started on i.v. antibiotics (e.g. flucloxacillin and gentamicin) and the temporary wire removed after a second wire has been put in from the other side (assuming that temporary pacing is still necessary).

Prophylactic antibiotics have been shown to help prevent permanent pacemaker infection. The simplest regime is to give the patient i.v. flucloxacillin 500 mg and ampicillin 500 mg i.v. just prior to the procedure itself. No further antibiotics are necessary.

Once a permanent unit is infected (e.g. extrusion of a corner of a box through ulcerated skin) it should be removed, together with the wire (if possible). There is no point in trying to rescue the situation with antibiotics and resuturing. A new system should be implanted on the other side.

Haemorrhage
This uncommon complication may result from puncture of the subclavian artery with a haemothorax or widening mediastinum features appearing on the chest X-ray. The subclavian artery lies posterior to the vein, and arterial puncture occurs if the entry site is too posterior (supraclavicular approach) or if the needle is directed too posteriorly (supra- and infraclavicular approach). Usually needle puncture of the subclavian artery does not result in complications if the clotting screen is normal. In elective permanent pacing, if the patient is on anticoagulants, these should be discontinued where possible to allow the INR/prothrombin time ratio to fall to $\leq 1.5 : 1$. Aspirin should also be stopped if possible 3–4 days prior to implantation.

Thrombophlebitis
This is usually only a problem with median cubital vein entry site, which

should be avoided where at all possible. Temporary pacing from the femoral vein (other than at formal cardiac catheterization) should be avoided because of the risk of infection and deep vein thrombosis.

Brachial plexus injury

This is rare and also occurs with entry site being too posterior. If the needle track is kept strictly subclavicular this will be avoided.

Thoracic duct injury

This is rare. The main thoracic duct drains into the junction of the left subclavian and left internal jugular vein. Temporary pacing via the right subclavian vein should therefore be attempted first.

Arrhythmias

Manipulation of the wire in the RA may produce atrial ectopics, atrial tachycardia or atrial fibrillation. Manipulation in the RV (especially postinfarction) may produce ventricular tachycardia or VF. If the RV is very irritable, a lignocaine infusion should be set up (starting with 100 mg i.v. stat and 4 mg/min). Atrial arrhythmias are usually transient and of less serious consequence, especially if the wire is being inserted for complete AV block.

7.3 Glossary of pacing terms in common use

Automatic interval (basic interval)

The stimulus–stimulus interval during regular pacing.

Bipolar pacing system

Most temporary wires use a bipolar pacing wire with two ring electrodes. The proximal ring electrode (approximately 1 cm from electrode tip) is the anode, and the distal (tip) electrode the cathode. Sometimes the position of the anode may be higher up the wire (e.g. in the SVC). The pacing spike is small on the surface ECG. Bipolar wires are also available for permanent pacing. A permanent polar system is immune to external signals. See **7.9**, page 311.

Blanking period

The time interval after a pacing impulse during which the pacemaker is insensitive to signals from the heart or from the other channel (avoiding cross-talk).

Chronotropic incompetence

The inability of the heart to increase its rate in response to exercise or metabolic demand.

Committed

A dual-chamber pacing system in which the delivery of an atrial stimulus forces the delivery of a ventricular stimulus after a programmed AV delay.

Cross-talk

In DDD units sensing of electronic events from one channel by the other channel, e.g. an atrial stimulus sensed by the ventricular channel resulting in dangerous inhibition of the ventricular impulse. This is avoided by the blanking period (see Figure 7.10, pages 305–306.

Demand pacing (inhibited)

Unlike the fixed-rate mode, spontaneous cardiac activity is sensed and inhibits the pacemaker, which fires a stimulus only after a pre-set interval if no further impulse is sensed. Thus pacing is inhibited by sensed impulses (atrial or ventricular, see codes, page 296).

Entrance block

The failure of a pacemaker to sense cardiac events because the sensitivity of the pacemaker is too low, the signals are of too low an amplitude or the lead is fractured.

Epicardial system

Pacing wires attached to the epicardium either at thoracotomy or by subxiphoid route. The permanent unit is usually intra-abdominal (beneath the rectus muscle and extraperitoneal). It is used in:
- recurrent failure of endocardial systems (infection, exit block, etc.)
- small children where rapid growth makes transvenous pacing difficult
- heart block developing during cardiac surgery
- tricuspid mechanical valve prosthesis.

Epicardial systems tend to be less reliable in the long term. Wire displacement and fracture may occur due to kinking and vigorous movement.

Escape interval

The interval between a spontaneous cardiac impulse which is sensed and the next pacing stimulus. This is usually the same as the automatic pacing interval unless the pacemaker is programmed to hysteresis mode, in which case the escape interval is longer than the automatic interval.

Fixed-rate pacing
Constant stimulation of the heart at a fixed rate not influenced by spontaneous cardiac activity.

Hysteresis
The takeover rate of the pacemaker is lower than the pacing rate, e.g. a pacemaker with a pacing rate of 72 bpm and hysteresis mode set at 60 bpm will not start pacing until the patient's heart rate falls to < 60 bpm, then the pacing rate jumps to 72 bpm. Patients may notice the abrupt change in rate, but it conserves battery life.

Lead impedance
This is a vital factor in battery life. It includes the electrical resistance of the electrode itself plus the impedance of the electrode tip–tissue interface. The size of the electrode tip influences impedance of the wire. (The larger the tip, the lower the impedance.) Low-impedance wires result in early battery depletion. Average lead impedance is 510 Ω. Development of newer electrodes has resulted in smaller electrode tips (from standard 12 or 14 mm^2 down to 6 mm^2).

Magnet rate
Application of a magnet over some VVI units converts them to a faster (fixed) pacing rate. This is used to test battery life and satisfactory pacing if there is competition at a slower demand rate.

Missing
The term used to denote failure of a pacing stimulus to capture and depolarize atrial or ventricular myocardium. It may be due to incorrect lead positioning, too low an output voltage or too high a myocardial threshold. Initial management is to increase pacing voltage if a temporary system, and then reposition the wire if this is not successful. Missing with a permanent system cannot be ignored. The unit must be removed, the wire threshold tested and either repositioned or changed.

Mode-switching
The ability of a dual chamber pacemaker to switch between DDDR and VVIR modes. Thus when a patient with paroxysmal AF or atrial

tachycardia goes into AF or SVT the pacemaker will switch to VVIR mode, thus avoiding atrial tracking with fast ventricular rates: e.g. rates of > 175 for 5–10 cycles or even less in some units will trigger the mode-switch. The unit switches back to DDDR mode when sinus rhythm reappears or the atrial rate falls. In patients with regular atrial arrhythmias, some units can mode switch to DDIR mode thus avoiding atrial tracking.

Myopotential (EMG) inhibition (Figure 7.4)
Electrical signal from skeletal muscle (usually pectoral) which is sensed by the pacemaker, incorrectly interpreted as cardiac in origin and falsely inhibits the pacemaker impulse.

Non-committed
A dual-chamber pacemaker in which the sensing of ventricular activity during the AV interval can inhibit the delivery of a ventricular impulse.

Oversensing (false inhibition) (Figures 7.3 and 7.4)
Inhibition of the pacemaker by non-physiological electromagnetic interference or by physiological myopotential signals. In this instance pacemaker sensitivity must be reprogrammed to a lower setting.

Paired pacing
A double impulse fired in rapid succession to the ventricle results in an increased force of contraction, but a much greater MVO_2 and a risk of inducing VT. It is not used in clinical pacing.

Pulse width/pulse duration
The duration of the pacing stimulus (usually between 0.5 ms and 1.0 ms). The broader pulse width may capture the ventricle and pace it when narrower pulse widths fail, but this will drain more current and shorten battery life of permanent units. The same applies to atrial pacing.

Relative threshold
Some pacing units have an analysable threshold once implanted permanently. The relative threshold is the minimum percentage of total available voltage required to pace the heart. Thus a relative threshold of 25% with maximum unit voltage of say 5.2 V is 1.3 V.

Rate-responsive pacing (adaptive rate pacing)
A permanent pacing system in which the pacemaker speeds up and

slows down in response to certain physiological stimuli. May be single-chamber (AAIR or VVIR) or dual-chamber (DDDR), see page 306.

Sequential pacing
Pacing of the atrium followed at a pre-set interval by pacing of the ventricle. This allows physiological atrial transport (see physiological pacing, page 300).

Slew rate
The rate of rise of the endocardial potential (dV/dt). Potentials with a low slew rate may not be sensed.

Telemetry
A pacemaker facility to transmit a radiofrequency signal containing information about battery life, programmable functions, frequency of pacemaker use, etc.

Tilt testing
Used to provoke syncope in patients with possible cardioneurogenic syncope. Patients lie flat for 20–30 min and are then tilted head up to 60° for 45 min. Continuous ECG and blood pressure recordings (ideally from a radial artery line) are needed.

Triggered pacing (see Figure 7.3)
A sensed spontaneous R wave results in immediate pacing stimulus fired into the R wave (the heart obviously refractory and not paced). Triggered pacing units have a built-in refractory period to protect against fast electrical interference inducing ventricular tachycardia. Ventricular triggered pacing may be used:
• to avoid EMG inhibition
• when a temporary wire is inserted to cover a failing permanent unit. Stimuli from the failing implanted unit trigger the external unit to fire an impulse. This falls in the absolute refractory period (if the internal unit's impulse depolarized the heart) or alternatively paces the heart if the internal/permanent unit impulse fails to depolarize the heart. It is thus a fail-safe mechanism.

Unipolar pacing system
Most permanent units are unipolar: using the pacing box as the anode (+) and the pacing wire as the cathode (−). The pacing spike is large on the surface ECG.

Voltage threshold
Minimum voltage which will pace the heart.

7.4) Permanent pacing for bradyarrhythmias

There has been an enormous increase in pacemaker technology since the first pacemaker was implanted by the Karolinska Hospital team in 1958. Permanent pacing is one of the most cost-effective forms of treatment in the whole of medicine. Numbers of implants are increasing, but the implant rate in the UK is amongst the lowest in Europe, due in part to the lack of pacing centres and in part to the low referral rate for pacing. Data from BPEG registry (see appendix) shows a gradual increase in number of pacemakers implanted in the UK over the last 6 years with an increase in dual chamber systems:

Parameter	1989	1995
Pacing centres (n)	106	140
Patients paced (n)	10 500	17 800
Implants/million population (n)	175	258
VVI units (%)	79	47
VVIR units (%)	2.5	9.5
DDD units (%)	16	34
DDDR units (%)	1	6

Indications for permanent pacing
These vary from country to country, but certain definite categories are recognized.

Chronic complete AV block with Stokes–Adams episodes
This is usually due to central bundle branch fibrosis (Lenegre's disease), often with normal coronary arteries in the older group. QRS complex is wide. Pacing should abolish symptoms and prolong life (1-year mortality: 35–50% unpaced, 5% paced). Symptoms other than frank syncope, which may be due to AV block, include giddiness, transient amnesia and misdiagnosed epilepsy.

In the younger age group coronary artery disease may be an additional prognostic factor.

Chronic complete AV block with no symptoms
This is a smaller group of patients who should also be paced because life expectancy is increased, and the first Stokes–Adams episode may be fatal: ECG monitoring for 24 hours usually reveals very slow idioventricular rhythm at night (e.g. < 20 bpm).

Congenital complete AV block (Figure 7.1)

In this condition the level of block is higher up in the His bundle or AV node. The QRS complex is narrow, the idioventricular rhythm faster and it may respond slightly to exercise or to other autonomic stimuli. Asymptomatic children may survive into adult life, when a permanent transvenous system is easier to insert. Indications for pacing in congenital complete AV block are:

• development of any rate-related symptoms

• wide QRS

• other cardiac lesions and cardiac surgery

• early presentation

• failure of AV node to respond to exercise, etc. ('lazy junction')

• 24-hour monitoring evidence of junctional exit block or paroxysmal tachyarrhythmias

• a daytime mean junctional rate < 50/min: as this carries a higher long-term risk of syncope and sudden death.

Mobitz Type II AV block (Figures 7.1 and 12.4)

This type of AV block is characterized by a constant PR interval and the sudden failure of conduction of an atrial impulse through the AV node. There is a high incidence of complete AV block developing and patients with this type of AV block should be paced permanently.

It should be noted that Wenckebach Type I AV block is not an indication for permanent pacing. It may be due to high vagal tone in athletes or children, and may be a transient phenomenon in acute inferior infarction (involving the AV nodal artery). It may result from drug toxicity (digoxin, beta-blockade, verapamil). Generally it is a benign, transient rhythm disturbance.

Postmyocardial infarction

Following inferior ipfarction second or third-degree AV block is normally transient, and permanent pacing does not need to be considered for 2–3 weeks postinfarct.

Following anterior infarction, complete AV block usually represents massive septal necrosis, and mortality from LV failure is high. Persistent complete AV block is permanently paced. More difficult is an AV block that regresses during hospital stay. This is still a subject for debate, but 24-hour Holter monitoring may help identify subjects at risk who need permanent pacing. The ventricular myocardium is often very irritable in the postinfarct period and if possible permanent pacing should be avoided in the first 3–4 weeks.

Chronic bundle branch block

Early work which suggested that His bundle electrograms would identify patients at risk has not been substantiated. Theoretically a prolonged H–V interval in the presence of bifascicular block would indicate the third fascicle at risk. However, this does not seem to be prognostically useful. The incidence of chronic asymptomatic patients with bifascicular block developing complete AV block is low. It does not seem to be precipitated by general anaesthesia. Again 24-hour Holter monitoring may be helpful. Generally, asymptomatic patients with bifascicular block do not merit permanent pacing. Pacing is indicated for patients with symptoms plus bifascicular block, e.g. symptoms plus:

- RBBB ı LAHB   } bifascicular disease
- RBBB ı LPHB   } (Figure 12.7)
- RBBB with alternating LAHB/LPHB
- LBBB with alternating RBBB   } 'trifascicular' disease
- LBBB + long PR interval

Sick sinus syndrome (SSS)

SSS is also known as sino-atrial disease, tachycardia–bradycardia syndrome or generalized conduction system disease. Although primarily involving the sinus node and atrial myocardium it may develop into a condition including AV node disease, or even be associated with a cardiomyopathy. Systemic emboli are a recognized complication (possibly related to prolonged periods of sinus arrest).

Common ECG abnormalities include (often switching from one to another) (Figure 7.5)

- sinus arrest: chronic or paroxysmal
- sinus bradycardia: not necessarily responding to effort or atropine
- sinus exit block
- paroxysmal { atrial tachycardia / atrial flutter / atrial fibrillation
- carotid sinus hypersensitivity
- AV block – usually in the older age group, who may have AF with complete AV block and a slow idioventricular rhythm.

Permanent pacing in SSS does not prolong life. The indications for permanent pacing are
- symptoms with a documented bradycardia.
- symptoms due to drug-induced bradycardia (used to control the

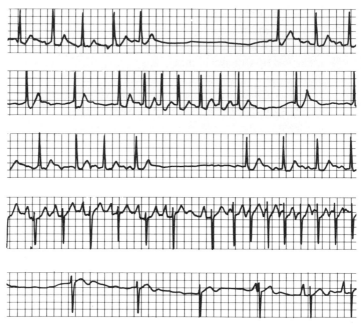

Figure 7.5 Sino-atrial disease. Segments of a single 24-hour monitored ECG in a patient with this condition (also known as sick sinus syndrome). The ECG shows episodes of wandering atrial pacemaker and sinus arrest (first line), junctional escape rhythm and AF (second line), sinus arrest (third line), sinus rhythm and supraventricular tachycardia (fourth line) and junctional bradycardia moving into sinus rhythm (fifth line).

tachyarrhythmias). AAI pacing will maintain atrial transport while AV nodal concluction is still normal. However, the development of AV block may require a change to DDDR pacing (see page 307).

7.5 Pacing for tachyarrhythmias

Implantation of a designated antitachycardia pacing device is now rarely needed. Catheter radiofrequency ablation has replaced antitachycardia pacemakers as treatment for supraventricular arrhythmias. Antitachycardia pacing is still useful in certain situations:
• as part of tiered therapy in the implantable cardioverter defibrillator (ICD) in the management of VT (see pages 291–296 and Figure 7.6)
• as an emergency in the catheter laboratory when SVT or VT may occur during cardiac catheterization

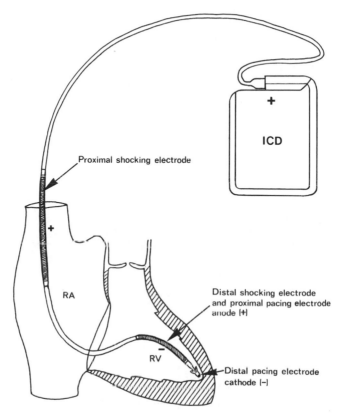

Figure 7.6 Example of a single lead implantable cardioverter defibrillator (ICD). The distal shocking electrode is positioned against the RV septum. For shock delivery, the proximal shocking electrode and the ICD unit itself (hot can) act together as the anode (+) and the distal shocking electrode as the cathode ( ). For pacing, the distal shocking electrode acts as the anode and the distal pacing electrode as the cathode.

- in the CCU or ITU setting where drug therapy has failed or is inappropriate.
- very occasionally in patients with permanent pacemakers by programming the rate up and AV delay down. Permanent overdrive pacing at a higher rate my help prevent VT.

Antitachycardia pacing in the ICD for VT has several advantages:

- automatic: no patient cooperation required
- less drug therapy
- no drug effects on LV function
- less battery requirements than for DC shocks
- rapid termination prevents deterioration of the rhythm, hypotension or cerebral hypoperfusion
- no drug side-effects
- possible method of arrhythmia control in pregnancy
- no negative inotropic effect on LV function
- may work when drugs fail
- rapid termination preventing hypotension or cerebral hypoperfusion
- patient normal between attacks
- easily reversible (explantation or reprogramming).

Methods of antitachycardia pacing

Overdrive suppression

1 Permanent overdrive pacing: single chamber. Suppression of ectopics by overdrive pacing may prevent SVT or VT. Prevention of bradycardia may abolish episodes of bradycardia-dependent VT although this is not very effective in the long term.

2 Permanent overdrive pacing: dual chamber. AV pacing with a short programmed AV delay (e.g. 50–150 ms) can prevent recurrent re-entry tachycardia using the AV node as part of the circuit. It may also help reduce episodes of VT.

Tachycardia termination/version

Bursts of tachycardia can be terminated using overdrive or underdrive pacing or bursts of extrastimuli. Underdrive pacing (VOO mode) is the least effective relying on random competition and rarely effective at faster rates (> 160/min).

In VT termination using the ICD careful electrophysiological studies are needed to select the best algorithm. The number and timing of extrastimuli need to be programmed. Ramp or autodecremental pacing may be needed if standard extrastimuli at fixed intervals fail (see Figure 7.7).

Implantable cardioverter defibrillator (ICD)

Following the pioneering work of Mirowski implanting a device in a dog in 1969, the first unit was implanted in 1980 in a human. The box was 200 cc in volume. Initially the box was implanted in the abdomen with a thoracotomy also required for an epicardial patch plus two i.v. wires. The units have become much smaller now (down to 60 cc), a thoracotomy is rarely required and one transvenous wire provides both shocking, sensing and pacing electrodes. Advances in technology now provide greater control.

• Tiered pacing therapy for VT with programmed initial antitachycardia pacing followed by a DC shock if attempts at pacing overdrive are unsuccessful. An example of successful overdrive pacing by an ICD is shown in Figure 7.7 and a 15 J shock defibrillating the patient on another occasion (Figure 7.8).

• Tiered shock therapy: initial shock is about 15 J with further shocks of 29–34 J if the initial shock is unsuccessful. Biphasic shock waveform (with the polarity of the shock reversing half way through the shock) allows for a lower defibrillation threshold (DFT).

• Back-up VVI pacing for bradycardia. Dual-chamber pacing back-up is available now.

• Full telemetry and programming facitilities. This can store information such as battery status, number of previous shocks, stored electrograms, etc.

• Improved sensitivity with automatic gain control allowing better differentiation of fast AF from VF.

• The hot can (active can). The ICD itself acts as an anode in conjunction with the proximal shocking electrode (see Figure 7.6). This lowers defibrillation thresholds.

This technology does not come cheap: units with wire(s) are over £22 000 each. The UK implant rate for ICDs is 5 per million population and 79 per million in the USA.

Indications for ICD therapy

• Recurrent sustained (> 30 s) preferably monomorphic VT.
• Recurrent proven VF.
• VT inducible at EP study and refractory to drug therapy .
• Prognosis > 1 year on other cardiac and non-cardiac grounds.
• Psychologically suitable.

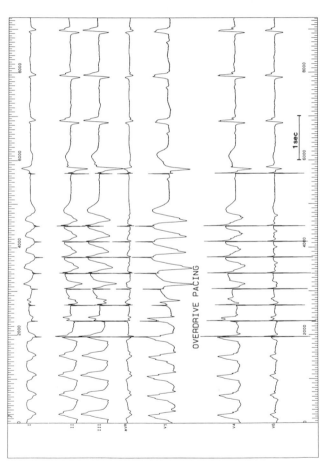

Figure 7.7 Successful overdrive pacing of ventricular tachycardia by the ICD. The VT is relatively slow (135/min) and is overdriven by a train of eight paced beats at 166/min. The first beat after the pacing train is back-up paced and then sinus rhythm resumes.

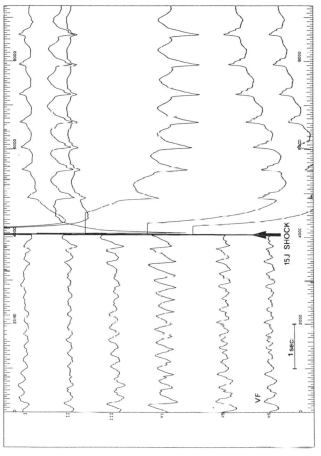

Figure 7.8 Defibrillation of VF by the ICD with a single 15-J shock to a LBBB tachycardia.

Most ICDs can now be implanted in a similar fashion to permanent pacemakers but general anaesthesia is required. The device is very little bigger than a DDD pacing unit (60–100 cc only). The ICD is implanted beneath the pectoralis major with the wire(s) introduced via the cephalic or subclavian veins. The left side is preferable. Newer leads are smaller (11 Fr). In very thin patients the box can be implanted in the abdomen beneath the rectus sheath.

The defibrillation threshold is checked at implantation and should be < 20 J. The wire position is the most crucial factor with the tip lying up against the septum. The use of the hot can and a subcutaneous array electrode helps. In a very few patients in whom satisfactory DFTs are unobtainable using a single transvenous wire with a subcutaneous array a thoracotomy as a separate procedure is needed to implant an epicardial patch. Following successful implantation, the patient should have a second general anaesthetic a few days later to programme the antitachycardia facilities.

The antitachycardia pacing facility has greatly improved battery life which should be good for > 100 shocks. It takes 5–15 s for the capacitors to charge once antitachycardia pacing has been unsuccessful. Some units incorporate an audible bleeping tone to warn the patient that a shock is imminent (useful if he/she is cooking for instance). The patient if still conscious may describe a sensation of being suddenly kicked in the back. Anyone touching the patient at the time of the shock will not be harmed. Initial shocks can be programmed to 15 J. This should be 10 J more than the lowest successful shock strength at the EP study at implantation. Further shocks of 29–34 J are then delivered if the 15 J shock was unsuccessful.

Operative mortality is now 1% but the slightly more bulky unit and wire results in a higher morbidity than conventional pacing with problems such as wire or box extrusion, pocket infection and sensing malfunction resulting in inappropriate shocks. Extensive psychological support is also needed both before and following implantation.

Contraindications to ICD therapy
- VT secondary to drugs or metabolic disturbance.
- VT in acute myocardial ischaemia or infarction.
- Acute myocarditis.
- Unsustained VT (< 30 s)
- Incessant or very frequent VT.
- The arrhythmia is supraventricular (see atrioversion, below).

- There is a unipolar pacing system *in situ*. It must be removed and converted to a dedicated bipolar system only.
- Symptomatic patients with spontaneous episodes suspected of having VT but without ECG evidence.

Follow up of patients with ICDs

Driving is not allowed. There are no problems with X-rays, microwave ovens, bathing, sex, etc.

Patients should be told to avoid:

- big electrical transformers
- large loudspeakers with strong magnets
- digital portable telephones. An analogue phone may be used but should not be put in the breast pocket over the ICD, see also page 313
- magnetic resonance imaging (MRI)
- electrocautery. If surgery with diathermy is needed the ICD must be deactivated. If no programmer is available, a magnet should be taped over the unit. The magnet will not affect back-up pacing
- transcutaneous electrical nerve stimulation (TENS) device. This may be possible, but with the ICD on monitor only the sensed electrogram should be recorded with the TENS machine switched on to check there is no oversensing. If there is, the TENS electrodes must be moved
- additional anti-arrhythmic therapy is allowed but drugs like amiodarone may increase the DFTs and shock impedance which will have to be checked once the patient is loaded on the drug.

ICD device with additional permanent pacing

With earlier ICDs it may be necessary to implant an additional DDD pacemaker when simple VVI back-up pacing is inadequate or producing the pacemaker syndrome. It is essential that a dedicated pacemaker is used which can only pace in bipolar mode. If a unipolar unit is already *in situ* at the time of ICD implantation it must be removed. Finally it is important that during implantation of the additional pacing unit that the ICD is only sensing one event (i.e. not both the pacing spike and the evoked potential). The bipolar pacing spike is small and should not be sensed by the ICD. The additional pacing electrode should be positioned as far from the ICD electrode as possible.

Long-term results

These vary from series to series but mortality of about 10% per year may be expected chiefly dependant on LV function. About 30% patients who have an ICD implanted do not use it in the first year after implantation. Once an ICD has been implanted the physician is committed to replacing it when necessary.

Patients with better prognosis include the following.
• Patients whose arrhythmia is well tolerated.
• Patients whose VT cannot be induced at EP study.
• Patients with VT inducible and suppressible at EP study by drug therapy.
• Patients whose tachycardia is slowed by drug therapy even if not suppressed
• LV ejection fraction > 0.4.

Although much criticized the MADIT trial compared ICD therapy with conventional drug therapy in a randomized trial over 5 years in patients with inducible non-suppressible VT postinfarction and a LVEF of < 35%. Patients receiving an ICD had a better prognosis with no evidence that drug therapy influenced survival. The results of further trials are awaited.

 ## Pacemaker codes

With increasing complexity of permanent pacemakers, codes have been developed to enable operators to identify the capabilities of individual units.

The initial three-letter code was introduced by Parsonnet in 1974 and is currently in use on the European Pacemaker card. This has been agreed by the International Association of Pacemaker Manufacturers. The three-letter code is now in general use, but already likely to be superseded by a five-letter code, to cope with facilities available on newer programmable units. A sixth letter may one day be included to cope with telemetric capabilities.

As will be seen in the pacemaker code table, the first letter of the code always relates to the chamber paced, the second to the chamber sensed. The third letter indicates the pacemaker response to the sensed impulse. Formerly this third letter was replaced by a 'fraction', e.g. T/I or T/I/I, since the more complex pacemaker responded in different ways to stimuli from atrium and ventricle.

The most frequently used pacemaker in the UK has the code VVI (47% of UK implants in 1995. See page 285).

Individual pacing codes explained
These are shown diagrammatically with a schematic ECG alongside each.

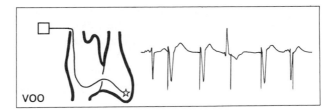

VOO This is fixed-rate ventricular pacing only, and is now rarely used, i.e. ventricular pacing, no sensing and no response. The pacemaker is not inhibited by spontaneous ventricular impulses, and there is a risk of stimulus on T phenomenon causing ventricular tachycardia.

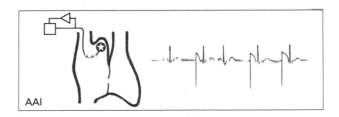

VVI Ventricular pacing that is inhibited by sensed ventricular impulses. It is the unit of choice in patients with AV block and atrial fibrillation, and sick sinus syndrome with atrial paralysis.

However, patients with AV block and persistent sinus node function will lose atrial contribution to ventricular filling as often the atria contract against closed AV valves. There will be cannon waves in the JVP, and intermittent reversal of atrial flow. Retrograde AV conduction compounds the problem.

Programmable VVI units may partly overcome this by being programmed to a lower rate, or with hysteresis.

AAI   This is atrial pacing only that is inhibited by sensed P waves. This type of pacemaker is used in patients with sick sinus syndrome who have normal AV node function. (It does not matter if they have retrograde AV conduction.) It may be used in patients with profound sinus bradycardia or in drug-induced sinus bradycardia (in the sick sinus syndrome) (Figure 12.5). Atrial transport is preserved.

However, this pacing relies on normal AV node function, and patients with SSS may develop abnormalities in AV conduction after the unit has been implanted (≤ 30% in one series). Also it is obviously unsuitable for patients with SSS and intermittent AF, which may also develop after the unit has been implanted.

Contraindications to AAI pacing are:
- AV block or Wenckebach block with atrial pacing up to 150/min
- bifascicular block on 12-lead ECG
- atrial flutter, fibrillation or atrial paralysis
- carotid sinus syndrome
- H–V interval > 55 ms or prolonging with high atrial rates.

Thus His bundle electrograms and atrial pacing studies are necessary before choosing to implant an AAI unit.

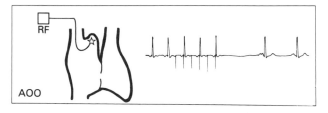

AOO   Asynchronous atrial pacing. Rarely used except in patient-activated bursts to overdrive atrial tachycardias. In using rapid atrial stimulation bursts it is important to be certain there is no preexcitation pathway to the ventricle.

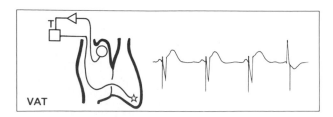

VAT   Ventricular pacing triggered by a sensed atrial impulse. Two
       leads are required. This is P-wave synchronous pacing with
       normal sinus node function. It cannot be used in patients with
       atrial dysrhythmias, AF or atrial flutter.
           Its major disadvantage is that it does not sense ventricular
       impulses, and hence will compete with spontaneous ventricular
       activity. If the patient has frequent ventricular ectopics there is
       the risk of stimulus on T phenomenon.
           It is the simplest way of perserving atrial transport in patients
       with AV block (Figure 12.5) but rarely used now.

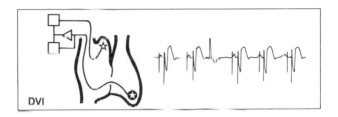

DVI   Atrial and ventricular pacing, but only spontaneous ventricular
       activity is sensed. Spontaneous atrial activity is ignored. Two
       leads are required. After a spontaneous ventricular impulse is
       sensed the pacemaker resets to one V–A interval and fires an
       atrial impulse followed by a ventricular impulse. Spontaneous P
       waves occurring within this V–A interval are not sensed.
           It can be used in complete AV block or sinus bradycardia.
       It cannot be used in AF. Although atrial synchrony is maintained
       at a basal rate it will not follow an increase in sinus rate with
       exercise, and competes with atrial rates faster than the
       pacemaker rate. It is useful in patients with retrograde VA
       conduction.

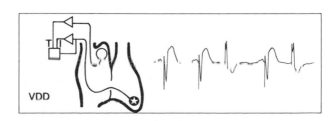

VDD   Also known as ASVIP, atrially sensed ventricular inhibited pacing. Both chambers are sensed (once two leads were required, but a new single pass lead with atrial electrodes is now available) and the spontaneous impulse triggers the pacemaker to stimulate the ventricle. Spontaneous ventricular impulses inhibit the pacemaker, which is reset to fire after one standby period.

It is suitable for simple AV block without any evidence of sino-atrial disease. Sinus node function should be normal. If AF develops, the pacemaker reverts to VVI mode. This also occurs if the spontaneous atrial rate falls below the escape rate of the pacemaker.

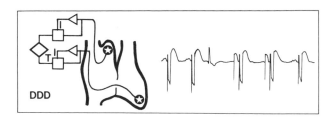

DDD   This is the only fully automatic unit that paces and senses both chambers (two leads required). This unit will either sense the atrial impulse and then pace the ventricle, or pace the atrium and then pace the ventricle if no spontaneous atrial impulse is sensed. It is the necessary advance on the VDD unit as it can be used in the sick sinus syndrome with additional AV nodal disease. If AF develops it also reverts to the VVI mode (mode switching).

KEY TO SYMBOLS

☆ Pacing only ◯ Sensing only ◇ Logic function
✪ Pacing and Sensing   I   Inhibited
▢ Pacing output circuit   T   Triggered
◁ Sensing circuit   RF Radio frequency signal

7.7 Physiological pacing

The VVI unit involves a single ventricular pacing lead only, and ignores atrial contribution to cardiac output. Atrial systole may contribute ≤ 25% of cardiac output in some patients by increasing LVEDV and stroke volume. Utilization of atrial systole by either sensing and/or

Pacemaker code table

	Code letter position				
	1st	2nd	3rd	4th	5th
Category	Chamber(s) paced	Chamber(s) sensed	Mode of pacemaker response	Programmable functions	Tachyarrhythmia functions
Letters used	V = ventricle A = atrium D = dual *S = single	V = ventricle A = atrium D = dual O = none *S = single	T = triggered I = inhibited D = dual R = reverse T/I = atrially triggered and ventricular inhibited T/I = fully automatic	P = programmable (rate and/or output only) M = multipro-grammable O = none R = rate responsive	B = burst N = normal rate competition S = scanning E = controlled external (magnet or AF)

*i.e. either atrium or ventricle.

pacing in synchrony with ventricular pacing has been called 'physiological pacing'. It has many limitations and cannot be strictly physiological at high heart rates. Nevertheless it may improve cardiac output in patients with borderline left ventricular function. It may also help to avoid systemic emboli in patients with sick sinus syndrome by avoiding stagnation in a flaccid left atrium, and may help prevent the development of AF.

A few patients with AV block may actually do worse with VVI pacing. The AV node may still conduct retrogradely and atrial stimulation may cause atrial contraction against closed AV valves. This has been shown to put up pulmonary wedge pressure: the pacemaker syndrome.

Ideally the choice of a physiological pacing unit should involve knowledge of certain facts, but time rarely allows this degree of investigation:

• The cardiac output should be measured with ventricular pacing and AV synchronous pacing to ensure that the more expensive and sophisticated physiological unit will confer extra benefit to the patient.
• A knowledge of sinus node function. ECG monitoring for 24 hours will provide some information. Tests of sinus node function (sinus node recovery time, sino-atrial conduction time) unfortunately do not reliably predict sinus node function if normal.
• A knowledge of AV conduction, both anterograde and retrograde.
• Does the patient develop SVT or other atrial tachyarrhythmias? ECG monitoring for 24 hours and provocation with atrial extrastimulus testing may help here.

Sino-atrial disease with normal AV-node function
Single-lead AAI pacing is adequate. The addition of rate response (AAIR) is a theoretical attempt to improve cardiac output on effort in the presence of chronotropic incompetence (inability to increase heart rate with exercise). However, it seems to carry little benefit over AAI pacing. Atrial pacing helps prevent systemic emboli and the development of AF.

The development of AV block in sino-atrial disease is low. About 2–4% of patients will require upgrading to a dual-chamber unit (DDD or DDDR) with the development of AV block. This is a small number and most patients can be managed on atrial pacing alone.

Complete AV block with normal sinus-node function
Ideally all patients should have DDD units. Owing to the expense of the

units, and the elderly and frail nature of many of the patients presenting with Stokes–Adams attacks, many individuals have been managed and cured with VVI pacing. With these economic problems a reasonable compromise is the provision of DDD units for:

- patients with poor LV function ⎫ both have high LVEDP
   and need atrial
- patients with LV hypertrophy ⎭ transport to maintain cardiac output
- the younger or mobile elderly patient
- patients with documented retrograde VA conduction
- the development of a pacemaker syndrome with VVI pacing.

The older patient with limited mobility can be managed with a VVI unit in most cases.

Complete AV block with additional sino-atrial disease

The theoretical ideal is a DDDR system (see above). If the patient exercises, and the sinus node does not follow, there is rate-responsive back-up. A simpler DDD unit will not allow an exercise-induced increase in heart rate if there is background chronotropic incompetence of the sinus node. It has, however, yet to be proved that a DDDR system is superior to DDD in this situation.

Chronic AF with complete AV block

A single-chamber rate-responsive system is best (VVIR) allowing some increase in cardiac output on exercise. VVI unit is a second-best alternative.

Carotid sinus syndrome

This is a rare condition with a minimal stimulus to the carotid sinus causing AV block or ventricular standstill (see Figure 7.9). Stimuli which may provoke syncope include head turning, shaving, coughing, heavy

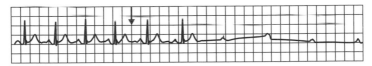

Figure 7.9 Carotid sinus hypersensitivity. Normal sinus rhythm is converted to ventricular standstill by the lightest touch on the carotid sinus (arrowed). The sinus node is slowed but there is complete AV block with no ventricular escape. Atropine and a brief period of cardiac massage were required to restore sinus rhythm.

lifting, or a Valsalva manoeuvre. If a sufferer has a sore throat, even swallowing may provoke syncope. Tight collars must be avoided. Carotid sinus stimulation affects both the sinus node and AV node (see Figure 7.9). DDD or DDDR pacing is necessary.

Neurocardiogenic syncope (malignant vasovagal syndrome)

This syndrome is incompletely understood. Increased parasympathetic and inhibited sympathetic outflow result in peripheral vasodilatation (vasodepressor response). The diagnosis can be made on head up tilt testing. Hypotension and bradycardia occur but the problem is only partly relieved by pacing. Treatment involves DDD pacing and drug therapy. Drugs tried have included adenosine blockade (e.g. theophylline) anticholinergics agents (e.g. transdermal scopolamine or oral disopyramide), beta-blockade, serotonin re-uptake inhibitors (sertraline, fluoxetine) and fludrocortisone. Alpha-agonists may help, e.g. ephedrine, and more recently a new drug, midodrine. Support stockings may help.

Advances in pacing algorithms have allowed some units implanted for this condition to pace at 120/min for 2 min as soon as a sudden rate drop is sensed. This helps abolish an episode before it has time to develop.

Problems with physiological pacing units

Against the obvious advantages of greater cardiac output and higher blood pressure with physiological pacing there are several disadvantages compared with VVI pacing:
• Two leads generally required except in AAI pacing. The atrial wire positioning can be difflcult with both stability and threshold problems especially in patients who have had cardiac surgery, with no right atrial appendage and often a fibrotic or flabby right atrium. Single-pass leads are available for VDD and DDD pacing with both atrial and ventricular electrodes. Atrial capture may not always be reliable. Temporary pacing with single pass leads can be useful in the ITU.
• Units more expensive.
• Shorter battery life.
• Problems with reliability of complex units and their programming equipment.
• Angina (e.g. SVT developing in VDD pacing causing high ventricular rate).
• Uncertainty at high atrial rates: e.g. episodes of SVT in DDD pacing causing ventricular tachycardia. This is dealt with by programming in an

....

upper rate limit (e.g. 140/min), beyond which 2 : 1 AV block occurs. This rate should be set lower in patients with angina.

• Retrograde VA conduction with reciprocating tachycardia (pacemaker-mediated tachycardia). Retrograde conduction occurs in about 70% of patients with normal AV node function and 40% in first degree AV block. Retrograde conduction of a P wave is sensed by the atrial electrode. It starts an AV interval which is followed by a paced ventricular impulse and a re-entry tachycardia using the pacemaker. This can be prevented by increasing the postventricular atrial refractory period or PVARP (see section on basic intervals below). This technique limits the maximum physiological pacing rate, but 150/min is usually considered fast enough. If increasing the PVARP fails to stop the pacemaker-mediated tachycardia, the pacemaker unit should be programmed to DVI (no atrial sensing or tracking) or DDI mode (no atrial tracking).

• Disease progression that limits the pacemaker's potential, e.g. development of AV block in AAI pacing, development of sick sinus syndrome in VDD pacing, development of AF in any DDD system.

Many physiological pacing systems are vulnerable to progression of conduction system disease. DDD units are vulnerable to the development of AF and have to be programmed to VVI mode unless they have an automatic mode switching facility (page 282).

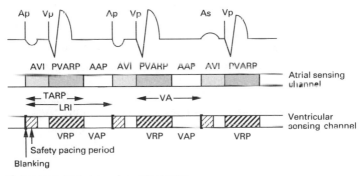

Figure 7.10 Basic intervals in DDD pacing.

Basic intervals in DDD pacing

AVI   The AV interval starts after the initial atrial pacing stimulus (Ap) The atrial sensing channel is refractory during the AVI.

PVARP   The post ventricular atrial refractory period starts after the ventricular pacing stimulus (Vp) during which the atrial sensing channel remains refractory. This helps prevent pacemaker mediated tachycardia due to retrograde VA conduction (see page 305). Both the AVI and PVARP can be programmed. It is rarely necessary to programme the PVARP beyond 400 ms.

TARP The total atrial refractory period = AVI + PVARP. This interval determines at what heart rate 2:1 AV block will occur (upper tracking limit), e.g. AVI of 170 ms, and PVARP of 350 ms = TARP of 520 ms and an upper tracking limit of 115/min. Above this, 2:1 block will occur.

AAP Atrial alert period. The atrial channel will sense spontaneous P waves.

LRI Lower rate interval or pulse interval. LRI = AVI + VA interval.

VA Starts after ventricular stimulus or ventricular sensed beat and ends with either an atrial simulus or an atrial sensed beat.

Blanking In the ventricular sensing channel there are two periods when the circuit is closed to external signals. The first is 5–15 ms after the atrial pacing spike and prevents the ventricular channel sensing the atrial pacing output (crosstalk). The second is VRP.

VRP Ventricular refractory period. Unresponsive to any signal. Programmable. Begins after a paced or sensed ventricular event.

Safety pacing period This occurs in the AVI just after the blanking period in the ventricular sensing channel. If a ventricular extrasystole falls in this period it is interpreted as noise and commits the pacemaker to fire in a safety ventricular pacing spike 100–110 ms after the atrial spike. This prevents inappropriate inhibition of ventricular output. A normal VA interval then follows.

VAP Ventricular alert period. The ventricular channel will sense spontaneous ventricular events.

Rate-responsive pacing (adaptive rate pacing): VVIR

This is a form of physiological pacing that is a useful alternative to dual-chamber pacing. Only one chamber (the ventricle) is paced (as in VVI units), but the pacemaker increases its pacing rate during exercise and slows down physiologically to its basal rate at rest.

A variety of biological sensors have been developed that detect a physiological change and signal for an increased (or decreased) heart rate. These must imitate the atrium in physiological terms, and many sensors are still in development. The two most commonly used are:

1 *QT interval.* This shortens during exercise due to catecholamine release, the pacemaker senses the stimulus to T interval (the evoked QT interval). This is the most physiological of all forms of rate-responsive pacing. Early problems resulted from a misconception that the QT interval and heart rate were linearly related. This produced a slow rise in heart rate with effort. The new algorithms have solved this problem.

2 *Body activity.* A piezo-electric crystal is mounted inside the pacemaker can. Vibrations from increased body activity are sensed. However, on some occasions there is little increase in heart rate: e.g. mental activity, isometric exercise and swimming, as there is little body vibration.

Other sensors detect changes in:
- mixed venous oxygen saturation
- RV dP/dt
- stroke volume
- temperature
- pH of right atrial blood
- changes in thoracic impedance
- minute volume
- respiratory activity.

Added to all this technology is the fact that some units contain more than one physiological sensor for optimal rate response (e.g. minute volume and thoracic impedance). At lower levels the body activity or thoracic impedance acts as the sensor, with the minute volume taking over as the sensor at higher work loads.

The minute volume sensor pacemaker should be avoided in patients with chronic lung disease. Pacemakers using thoracic impedance as a sensor probably have a shorter battery life. Rate-responsive pacemakers are rapidly increasing in popularity. They allow an increased cardiac output on exercise denied to the patient with a single VVI unit. Their advantages over DDD pacing and their drawbacks are summarized below.

Advantages of VVIR rate-responsive pacing compared with DDD pacing
- Single ventricular wire only. Easier and quicker to implant. No problem with unstable atrial wire.
- Units cheaper than DDD units.
- Possible use in sino-atrial disease or AF.

Advantages of DDD pacing compared with VVIR
- The only system to incorporate atrial contribution to cardiac output.
- Avoids the pacemaker syndrome.
- Of greater benefit in patients with poor LV function and high LVEDP.

DDDR pacing

Pacemakers are now available which incorporate the best of both systems: i.e. a dual chamber pacing system with rate responsive back up should the patient develop sino-atrial disease (DDDR pacing) or atrial fibrillation (VVIR) pacing. The pacing unit can mode switch between these if paroxysmal AF occurs and telemetry will indicate how many times mode switching has been employed.

Summary of optimum pacing modes

Condition	Best	Second best	Comments
Sino-atrial disease	AAIR	AAI	AAI may be as good
Sino-atrial disease plus AV block	DDDR	DDD	DDD may be as good
Atrio-ventricular block	DDD	VVI	See text for choice
Chronic AF plus AV block	VVIR	VVI	
Carotid sinus syndrome	DDD	VVI	
Malignant vasovagal syndrome	DDD	VVI	

7.8 Electrophysiological measurements and pacing

Sinus node recovery time (SNRT)

The right atrium is paced at a rate faster than the intrinsic sinus rate for ≤ 5 min and then pacing is switched off. Rates up to 160 bpm are used. The SNRT is the longest interval between the last paced beat and first sinus beat. Maximum SNRT is < 1.4 s. Corrected SNRT = SNRT − (spontaneous cycle length before pacing) = < 400 ms.

Sino-atrial conduction time (SACT)

This is calculated by firing an atrial premature stimulus late in the spontaneous cycle. The atrial premature beat collides with and extinguishes the next sinus impulse. A pause follows as the sinus node is reset. The atrial premature stimulus has to enter the sinus node and the subsequent reset sinus impulse has to leave it to the atrium. Thus:

$$SACT = \frac{(A_2 - A_3) - (A_1 - A_1)}{2} = < 100 \text{ ms (see Figure 7.11)}$$

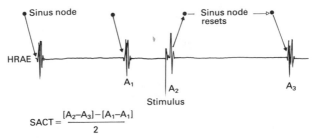

$$SACT = \frac{[A_2-A_3]-[A_1-A_1]}{2}$$

Figure 7.11 Calculation of sino-atrial conduction time.

where $(A_1 - A_1)$ = spontaneous cycle length
$(A_2 - A_3)$ = premature atrial stimulus to next spontaneous cycle

The distance of the catheter from the sinus node is important. The SNRT and SACT are only useful if abnormal. Normal results are unhelpful and cannot be relied upon to predict normal sinus node function.

His bundle intervals (Figure 7.12)
Prolongation of the PR interval may be due to electrical delay in any part of the atrio-ventricular conducting system. His bundle studies divide the PR interval into A–H interval (AV node conduction) and H–V interval (His–Purkinje conduction) (Figure 7.12).

PA interval (20–40 ms)
Lengthening of this is uncommon, usually associated with atrial dilatation or large atrial septal defects. The delay is prior to the P wave.

A–H interval (50–120 ms)
This represents AV node conduction time. The AV node normally shows decremental conduction (increasing delay in conduction with increased frequency of impulses). With graded atrial pacing the A–H time is gradually prolonged to the 'Wenckebach point'. This depends on vagal tone and may be altered by drugs.
   Long A–H time is intra-AV-nodal delay. It occurs in:
- first degree heart block; vagal overactivity; athletes
- Wenckebach second-degree AV block
- inferior infarction
- congenital heart block
- drugs, i.e. digoxin, verapamil, beta-blocking agents, amiodarone.
   Shortening of the A–H time is usually due to accessory pathways or

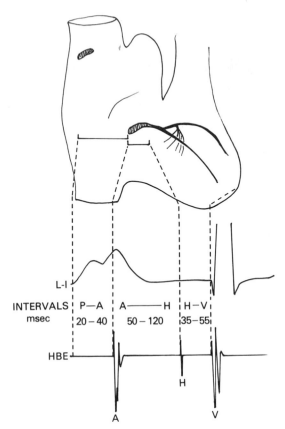

Figure 7.12 Normal HBE intervals. L–I standard lead I of ECG. HBE = His bundle electrogram.

sympathetic overactivity. It occurs in:

- sympathetic overactivity
- drugs: atropine, catecholamines
- accessory atrio-nodal or atrio-His pathways (James pathways)
- junctional ectopics

In Wolff–Parkinson–White syndrome the accessory pathway (Kent pathway) is not part of the AV node and does not affect the A–H time.

H–V interval (35–55 ms)

This represents His–Purkinje system conduction. Rarely, two His spikes may be seen (split His potential), suggesting conduction delay within the His bundle. Lengthening of the H–V time indicates delay in conduction within the His bundle or intra-ventricular conduction system. It occurs in:

- acquired heart block in the elderly (Lev's Lenegre's disease)
- Mobitz Type II AV block
- anterior infarction
- surgical trauma
- drugs (quinidine, disopyramide, ajmaline, flecainide).

Measurement of the H–V interval in patients with bifascicular block will not predict the small number who will develop complete AV block (approximately 6% patients with RBBB and LAHB).

Shortening of the H–V interval usually is due to accessory pathways arising from the normal AV node or His bundle (Mahaim pathways) or direct atrioventricular pathways (Kent pathway). Shortening occurs in:

- sympathetic overactivity
- drugs; catecholamines
- nodoventricular or His–ventricular pathways (Mahaim)
- atrioventricular pathways (Kent)
- idioventricular rhythm arising from one of the fascicles.

Spurious short H–V intervals may be produced by recording right bundle branch activity. Delivery of increasingly premature atrial stimuli until RBBB develops should help differentiate this. If the so-called His spike disappears with the development of RBBB, then the spike was not a true His spike but arose from the right bundle branch.

7.9 Advice to the pacemaker patient before going home

Pacemaker interference from environmental factors

Before a patient with a permanent pacemaker goes home he or she should be warned that external signals may rarely interfere with the pacemaker and alter its function. The pacemaker wire acts as an aerial for the signal and it is usually only a problem with a unipolar system. The typical response of the pacemaker to an external signal is to switch to fixed-rate pacing (magnet rate, page 282). This increase in heart rate is noticed by the patient, who can then walk away from the source of interference and negate the problem.

Bursts of interference may cause inhibition of the pacemaker and pulsed electromagnetic fields are particular culprits (e.g. airport weapon detectors). The inhibition is quickly noticed by the patient.

As long as the patient is aware of the possibility of pacemaker interference he or she can check his or her own pulse if near a possible signal source. Particular warning should be given about getting too close to the following situations.

• Mains-driven electric motors, especially if sparking or with faulty suppression (e.g. electrical kitchen equipment, vacuum cleaners, electric razors, electric power drills, motor cycles, lawn mowers, outboard motors, old car engines).

• Airport weapon detectors. Hand-held detectors are safe.

• Microwave ovens if faulty with inadequate door seal.

• High-power radar stations. Hand-held police radar guns are safe.

• CB radio transmitting systems.

• Some dental drills (e.g. ultrasonic cleaner).

• Some equipment used by physiotherapists (e.g. short-wave heat therapy, faradism, etc.).

• Shop anti-theft equipment. The pacemaker may trigger the alarm system as the patient walks out of the shop, and he or she should warn the shopkeeper.

• Public libraries have a system that can inhibit the pacemaker.

• Vibration. Hovercraft, helicopters and other sources of vibration may increase the rate of activity-sensing pacemakers. Patients should be warned that this effect may occur.

If a patient is at frequent risk from external interference he or she can use a magnet to switch the pacemaker to fixed-rate mode, during which it is immune to external signals. If this is inconvenient the unipolar system may have to be explanted and changed to a bipolar system (as in EMG inhibition, page 283). Generally the risks are very small and are chiefly related to faulty electric motors.

Pacemakers and sport
Vigorous contact sports are best avoided by patients with permanent pacemakers, to avoid injury to the unit (e.g. rugby football, soccer, boxing, judo or karate). Squash should be discouraged if possible. A full golf swing may be uncomfortable with a pacemaker in the supramammary pouch, often more so if it is implanted on the left side.

Pacemakers and radiotherapy
Ionizing radiation may damage pacemaker circuitry. If possible the pacemaker should be shielded during courses of irradiation. Close monitoring of pacemaker function is necessary after each dose of irradiation. A typical sign of pacemaker damage is a noticeable drift in the automatic pacing interval to a slower rate.

Pacemakers and surgery

Should a patient with a permanent pacemaker require surgery there is usually no problem provided the anaesthetist is aware of the hazards. A common problem is prostatic surgery with permanent pacemakers *in situ* and a few precautions are necessary.

• The patient should have ECG monitoring throughout.

• Full DC cardioverting equipment should be available.

• The diathermy plate should be as far from the pacemaker as possible (i.e. not on the chest or back). Diathermy should not be performed near the pacemaker box.

• Short bursts of diathermy may inhibit the pacemaker temporarily. This can be avoided by placing a magnet over the unit converting it to fixed-rate mode (VOO). Alternatively the pacemaker can be programmed to VOO mode at the start of the operation and reprogrammed immediately after the operation.

• There is a remote risk of VT or VF induced by diathermy with the pacing electrode acting as an aerial. This will not be prevented by magnet override.

Pacemakers and driving (see Appendix 6)

Patients with permanent pacemakers may not hold LGV or PCV licences. They should not drive a car for 3 months after the unit's implantation. Provided they are under regular pacemaker follow up they may hold a driving licence and should not have to pay an extra insurance premium.

Pacemakers and mobile telephones

Close proximity of a mobile telephone to a pacemaker may cause pacemaker inhibition. This is most likely to occur with a high-power output from the phone, maximum sensitivity of the pacemaker and unipolar pacing. It is much more likely with digital phones than analogue phones. The commonest interference is inappropriate atrial tracking up to the upper tracking limit of the pacemaker. Ventricular inhibition may also occur.

   Patients wishing to use digital phones must be programmed to bipolar pacing with sensing thresholds programmed as high as possible and be tested in the pacing clinic using the phone. Patients should not carry the phone close to the pacemaker. They should hold the phone away from the body when dialling, and to use the ear remote from the pacemaker. If interference from digital phone still occurs in spite of these caveats patients should revert to an analogue system.

7.10 Principles of paroxysmal tachycardia diagnosis

In patients with intermittent (paroxysmal) tachycardias diagnosis may be difficult. It is useful to know if the arrhythmia starts and stops suddenly, whether it is regular or irregular, and if there are any factors that start it or stop it. 'Catching' the arrhythmia may not always be possible with the limited services of 24-hour ECG monitoring, and the patient may not be able to get to a hospital to have the arrhythmia recorded when it occurs. A patient-activated recorder may help.

Diagnosis of paroxysmal tachycardia involves:

• recognition of likely associated cardiac lesions. AF: alcohol, mitral valve disease, thyrotoxicosis, coronary artery disease, pericarditis, postcardiac surgery, etc. VT: LV aneurysm, recent myocardial infarct

• recognition of resting 12-lead ECG abnormalities, e.g. pre-excitation with short PR interval:

without delta-wave: Lown–Ganong–Levine syndrome

with delta-wave: Wolff–Parkinson–White (WPW) syndrome

apparent long QT interval due to prominent 'u' wave: hypokalaemia

long QT interval: may be caused by metabolic abnormalities, drugs or rare genetic defects; torsades de pointes may result (see pages 337–339)

• Recognition of other cardiotoxic drugs: e.g. sympathomimetic agents: beta-2 agonists (SVT or VT), digoxin (paroxysmal SVT with varying block), L-dopa, tricyclic antidepressants (VT), Adriamycin, doxorubicin (SVT or VT).

• Recognition of other precipitating factors: caffeine (tea or coffee excess), smoking, alcohol, emotional stress, fatigue.

• Metabolic upsets: K^+ or Ca^{2+} high or low, hypoxia, hypercapnia, metabolic acidosis, hypomagnesaemia, phaeochromocytoma, febrile illnesses, pneumonia, etc.

• ECG monitoring for 24 hours. Several recordings are often needed in a single patient. Telemetry is an alternative, and is useful for ambulant patients during hospital admission.

• Provocation of the arrhythmia. This is sometimes necessary to establish a diagnosis, to assess provocation factors and to assess treatment. The commonest provocation test is the exercise test. Unifocal ectopic beats in the normal heart are common and usually decrease in number during exercise, recurring with rest. The abnormal heart may develop multifocal frequent ectopics, or even ventricular tachycardia on effort. A few patients with WPW may develop tachycardia on effort, but this is uncommon.

Other provocative tests in patients with paroxysmal tachycardia include the use of the tilt table (orthostatic tachycardia), isoprenaline infusion (WPW syndrome), electrophysiological stimulation or cardiac catheterization with LV and coronary angiography. A more detailed protocol for provocation studies of ventricular tachycardia is discussed on page 335.

Most intermittent tachycardias can usually be diagnosed without provocation tests. Electrophysiological studies may be needed to assess the effect of drug therapy.

7.11 Classification of anti-arrhythmic drugs

The table on page 319 shows the Vaughan-Williams classification Some drugs fit into more than one class and some drugs fit into none of them. The table on page 321 also shows a classification based on the clinical effects of the drugs and their sites of action. It does not contain any electrophysiological data but is probably more useful at the bedside.

7.12 Management of specific tachyarrhythmias

Atrial fibrillation (AF)

Established AF

In established AF, drug therapy is used to control the rate of ventricular response by increasing AV node refractoriness. Vagal manoeuvres will do this temporarily and may be useful in the diagnosis of fast AF.

Digoxin is still the drug of choice in AF (see Inotropes section, page 236). If the ventricular response is still too fast in a well-digitalized patient, a small dose of a beta-blocking agent is added (e.g. metoprolol 50 mg tds) and the dose gradually increased if necessary. Before adding a beta-blocking agent it is important to be sure that LV function is adequate and the patient is not thyrotoxic. If the LV function is poor, verapamil is added to digoxin, starting at 40 mg tds and increasing the dose if necessary up to 120 mg tds. If this fails to control the response, amiodarone can be tried. Usually, however, digoxin plus beta-blockade controls the ventricular response.

Very occasionally in AF the conduction pathway to the ventricles is anomalous (e.g. Kent accessory pathway in WPW). In this situation digoxin, beta-blockade and verapamil are not effective. Digoxin and verapamil may even increase anterograde condition in the accessory pathway and are contra-indicated. If an ECG in AF shows intermittent or constant delta-waves or if the ventricular response in AF is very fast (e.g. RR intervals of 200–250 ms), then WPW is a strong possibility (see Figure 7.17). Intravenous disopyramide 50–150 mg or flecainide 50–150 mg i.v. are the drugs of choice. Other agents that can be effective are quinidine, procainamide, amiodarone. Do not use more than one drug i.v.; if your choice fails then proceed to DC cardioversion.

Paroxysmal AF

In the euthyroid patient, alcohol is the commonest precipitating factor. Caffeine, nicotine and emotional stress have been implicated but with little evidence. Attacks are not usually effort related except in the younger patient (see below). Therapy is aimed at reducing the number and duration of attacks but is unlikely to suppress them completely. It is likely over the years that in spite of treatment attacks will become more frequent and eventually AF become fully established.

Drugs of value are amiodarone, flecainide, propafenone, disopyramide and beta-blockade. Quinidine is also of proven value but rarely used in the UK because of side-effects (page 352). Class 1b agents should be avoided. Flecainide is the initial drug of choice provided LV function is good and there is no known coronary disease. The same cautions hold for propafenone. Amiodarone (probably the most effective drug) is reserved for patients with LV dysfunction, coronary disease, or failed treatment with flecainide or propafenone. Beta-blockade is useful adjunctive therapy. Possible pro-arrhythmias induced particularly by Class 1 agents must be considered.

A few younger patients with normal hearts will have episodes of AF induced by autonomic factors. Those where AF is induced by exercise, or on waking or with emotional stress should be beta-blocked. Others where AF occurs, while asleep, or after meals (vagal activity) should be tried on disopyramide or flecainide.

Digoxin is not in this list and merely controls ventricular response if AF occurs. Amiodarone is very useful, but photosensitivity is its most limiting side-effect. Anticoagulation should be considered as there is an embolic risk.

Classification of anti-arrhythmic drugs (Vaughan–Williams)

	Class 1	Class 2	Class 3	Class 4
Method of action	Block fast sodium channel	Beta-sympathetic blockade	Potassium channel blockade	Slow calcium channel blockade
Effect on cardiac action potential	Slow Phase 0 rate of rise. Depress Phase 4 rate of rise. Also effect on APD varies: 1a ↑ APD, 1b ↓ APD, 1c No effect APD	Depress Phase 4 rate of rise	Increase APD	Depress Phases 2 and 3
Primary site of action	Atrium, Ventricle, Bypass / Ventricle / His–Purkinje, Ventricle, Bypass	Sinus and AV nodes	Atrium, AV node, His–Purkinje, Ventricle, Accessory pathway	AV node
Examples of drugs	Quinidine, Procainamide, Disopyramide, Ajmaline / Lignocaine, Phenytoin, Mexiletine, Aprindine, Tocainide, Moricizine / Flecainide, Encainide, Lorcainide, Propafenone	Beta-blocking agent, Bretylium, Guanethidine	Dofetilide, Amiodarone, Disopyramide, Sotalol, Several other beta-blocking agents, Bethanidine, Bretylium	Verapamil, Diltiazem, Adenosine
Effect on AV nodes and His–Purkinje system	Variable or AV node ↑ His–Purkinje refractory period / Variable on AV node ↑ His–Purkinje refractory period / ↑ A–H ↑ H–V time ↑ His–Purkinje refractory period	↑ A–H time ↑ AV node refractory period No effect on His–Purkinje refractory period	↑ A–H time Little effect on H–V time ↑ Refractory periods of both AV node and His–Purkinje system	↑ A–H time ↑ AV node refractory period

Anticoagulation and AF

This should be considered in patients with frequent episodes of uncontrolled AF, in patients needing DC cardioversion (see below) and in the long-term management of established AF. The annual CVA risk for patients in their sixties with lone AF is between 3 and 8%. There are now seven major trials comparing warfarin with placebo and four comparing warfarin with aspirin in AF. It is now clear that warfarin is superior to aspirin in the prevention of thromboembolic events. These trials have identified patients at particular risk of thromboembolism.

- Hypertension. Systolic blood pressure > 160 mmHg.
- Poor LV function. LVEF < 25%.
- Age > 75 years.
- Diabetics.
- Previous emboli, CVA or transient ischaemic attack.

In these high-risk patients, warfarin is important controlling the INR beween 2.0 and 3.0. A regime of low dose warfarin plus aspirin is not an alternative and is ineffective.

Drug cardioversion

This is most likely to succeed with recent onset AF. Flecainide 2 mg/kg i.v. over 10 min is the drug of choice but should be avoided in patients with poor LV function as it has a negative inotropic effect. Disopyramide 50–150 mg i.v. slowly over 5 min is an alternative. Fibrillatory waves may coarsen and the ventricular response increase before sinus rhythm is achieved. Amiodarone given orally (200 mg tds up to 400 mg tds for 1 week) may also result in version to sinus rhythm. The dose is reduced after 1 week. Amiodarone is also very useful given i.v.: 5 mg/kg over 4 hours in 5% dextrose. The maximum i.v. dose over 24 hours in an adult is 1200 mg. An immediate result should not be expected: it may take 24–48 hours to convert the patient back to sinus rhythm. The patient can be converted to oral amiodarone when practical.

DC cardioversion

This is not used for established or paroxysmal AF. Its role is chiefly in two types of situation.

1 As an elective procedure following a first attack of AF with an identifiable cause, e.g. attack of pneumonia, a thoracotomy, pulmonary embolus, controlled thyrotoxicosis following thyroidectomy, following coronary artery surgery, ASD closure, mitral valve surgery, etc. If no known cause the patient is labelled 'lone AF' and one attempt at cardioversion is certainly worth trying.

2 As an emergency procedure where atrial transport is vital to the maintenance of a reasonable cardiac output. The patient is usually very sick and the chances of success are not great. Examples are in HCM, aortic valve stenosis and acute myocardial infarction.

Cardioversion and the need for anticoagulation

If the left atrium is small and AF has only been present for 24–48 hours, prior anticoagulation is unnecessary. If the LA is dilated, there is mitral valve disease or AF has been prolonged, then the patient is anticoagulated with warfarin for 4 weeks prior to DC cardioversion. The risk of systemic emboli is about 5–7% without anticoagulation and < 1.6% with it. Recent experience with transoesophageal echocardiography (TOE) has shown that thrombi in the atrial appendage occur in about 13% of patients with AF. If no thrombi are seen on TOE then DC cardioversion may be performed safely without prior anticoagulation. If bi- or multiplane TOE is not available then patients should be anticoagulated beforehand. Patients with spontaneous echo contrast in the LA (thought to be a prelude to thrombi) should also be anticoagulated (see Figure 12.31).

A dilated LA and prolonged AF make it less likely that DC cardioversion will succeed. Anticoagulation should be continued for 1 month after successful cardioversion. Reversion to AF is common and about 30% stay in sinus rhythm. Disopyramide, beta-blockade or amiodarone help maintain sinus rhythm.

Suggested protocol for DC cardioversion

- Serum potassium between 4.5 and 5.5 mmol/l if possible.
- There is no need to stop digoxin beforehand but DC cardioversion is not performed if there is any suspicion of digoxin toxicity (page 239).
- Fast for 6 h. Consent should include explanation of remote risk of cerebral emboli.
- General anaesthesia with short-acting i.v. agent (e.g. propofol).
- Start with 200-J shock (100 J if in atrial flutter). If failure to cardiovert: second shock, 300 J. If failure: give disopyramide 100 mg i.v or flecainide 50–100 mg slowly over 5–10 min.
Third shock 360 J with paddles in anteroposterior position. If still failure: consider treatment with amiodarone for 1 month and a further attempt or just accept AF as definitive rhythm and treat with digoxin and long-term warfarin.

Atrial flutter (see Figures 7.13 and 12.2)
The atrial rate in atrial flutter is 280–320/min and 2 : 1 ventricular

Atrial flutter with 2:1 AV block. Flutter rate is 270/min. Ventricular rate is 135/min

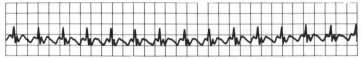

Carotid sinus massage (CSM) in atrial flutter produces transient complete AV block revealing the atrial flutter waves. Lead III

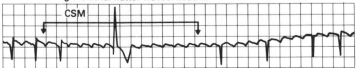

Chronic atrial flutter. Effect of digoxin. Atrial flutter rate 280/min. 4:1 AV block reduces ventricular rate to 70/min

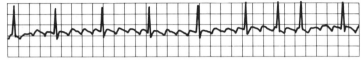

Chronic atrial flutter. Effect of amiodarone. Slows intrinsic flutter rate to 190/min. 3:1 AV block results in ventricular rate of 63/min. Lead II

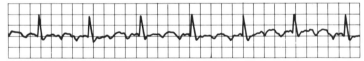

Figure 7.13 Atrial flutter.

response results in a ventricular rate of 150/min. With a 4 : 1 response, the ventricular rate is 75/min; however, it is unusual to be able to keep the response at a regular 4 : 1.

Carotid sinus massage will increase the degree of AV block temporarily and this can be useful in diagnosis of the rhythm, as the typical saw-tooth pattern of flutter becomes obvious (especially in leads II and V1 in the ECG). An isolated event of atrial flutter is best treated by DC cardioversion. It is the most likely arrhythmia to convert to SR and only small energy shocks are needed (50–100 J in the adult). If AF is produced the patient is shocked again into sinus rhythm.

Paroxysmal atrial flutter has to be controlled by drug therapy. Digoxin may produce atrial fibrillation, which tends to be easier to manage. In difficult cases of paroxysmal atrial flutter the atrium can be fibrillated using a right atrial endocardial pacing lead.

Amiodarone is also useful as it reduces the atrial flutter rate, making

Drugs available for specific tachycardias

Sinus tachycardia	Atrial fibrillation / Atrial flutter / Supraventricular tachycardia	Junctional tachycardia	WPW bypass tachycardia	Ventricular tachycardia
More initially	*Version to SR*	(Vagal manoeuvres)	*At AV node*	*Prevention and termination*
Look for cause:	Disopyramide	Verapamil	Beta-blockade	Lignocaine
Pain	Amiodarone	Beta-blockade		Mexiletine
Anxiety	Flecainide	Digoxin	*At accessory pathway*	Tocainide
Fever, sepsis		Flecainide	Disopyramide	Procainamide
Hypovolaemia	*Rate control at AV node*		Quinidine	Quinidine
Low-output state	Adenosine		Amiodarone	Phenytoin
Shock	Digoxin		Procainamide	Beta-blockade
Thyrotoxicosis	Verapamil		Flecainide	Amiodarone
	Beta-blockade		Sotalol	Disopyramide
			Propafenone	Propafenone
	Prevention		Ajmaline	
	Disopyramide			*Version only*
	Amiodarone			Bretylium tosylate
	Flecainide			Ajmaline
	Propafenone			
	Procainamide			
	Quinidine			

even 2 : 1 ventricular response more acceptable (e.g. down to 130–140/min). It probably also reduces the number of bursts of flutter. RF ablation is possible for chronic atrial flutter (see page 346).

Atrial tachycardia (see Figures 7.14 and 12.2)
• Ectopic atrial tachycardia (supraventricular tachycardia – SVT, primary atrial tachycardia – PAT). Atrial rate is 150–250/min. Often atrial rate is about 160–170/min, and ventricular response is 1 : 1 (P waves may not be visible on the ECG but appear with carotid sinus massage). Figure 7.14 shows an ectopic atrial tachycardia with a faster atrial rate of 260/min and 2 : 1 AV block.
• Paroxysmal atrial tachycardia with varying block secondary to digoxin toxicity (PATB). Ventricular response is less likely to be a 1 : 1 response. P waves are usually visible (Figure 7.14).

Adenosine
The purine nucleoside adenosine has taken over from verapamil as the drug of choice in an acute episode of atrial tachycardia. It is given as 3 mg i.v. followed by a saline flush. If necessary a second dose of 6 mg and a third of 12 mg may be given at 2-min intervals (dose for children 0.0375–0.25 mg/kg). The very short half-life of the drug (5–10 s) makes it safe even in wide complex tachycardias, but means that the SVT may recur. If it does then verapamil is used (see below).

Ectopic atrial tachycardia with 2:1 AV block. Atrial rate 260/min. P waves arrowed. Ventricular rate 130/min

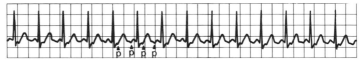

Atrial tachycardia with varying block. P waves arrowed. Atrial rate 214/min. PATB. Could be digoxin toxicity

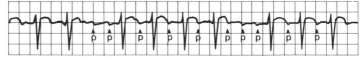

Atrial flutter with 4:1 AV block. Flutter rate 288/min. Ventricular rate 72/min

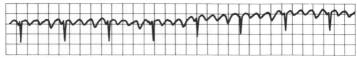

Figure 7.14 Atrial tachycardias.

Side-effects of adenosine: transient chest pain, flushing, nausea, headache and dyspnoea. If troublesome, these can be reversed with i.v. aminophylline. Dose reduction needed in patients on dipyridamole (inhibits breakdown). Dose increase needed in patients on aminophylline (blocks adenosine receptor).

Verapamil

Almost as effective in SVT as adenosine but has a negative inotropic effect and is contra-indicated in wide complex tachycardias in case these are ventricular in origin. It can be used in recurrent SVT following initial success with adenosine. It is given as 5–10 mg as a fast i.v. bolus. The dose can be repeated in 20 min if still necessary. It is more hazardous in patients already on beta-blockade but can still be used with careful monitoring (risk of complete AV block) in an emergency DC shock may be needed.

Paroxysmal atrial tachycardia in the long term can be managed on oral verapamil, beta-blockade or even digoxin. Disopyramide, flecainide, propafenone and amiodarone are also very useful. Long-acting quinidine preparations are still used, but gastrointestinal side-effects may prove a problem.

In atrial tachycardia with block (digoxin toxicity) the drug is stopped, and the K^+ checked. The potassium should be > 4.5 mmol/l and oral or i.v. KCl may be necessary. Verapamil or beta-blockade is used to slow ventricular response if necessary. DC cardioversion is avoided if possible, and if used low-energy shock is given (25–50 J) under lignocaine cover. Rapid atrial pacing can be used to extinguish the atrial focus.

The use of disopyramide in atrial tachycardia may slow the atrial rate, but quicken the ventricular response before version to sinus rhythm. Disopyramide prolongs atrial effective refractory period, slowing atrial rate, but its anticholinergic effect on the AV node may increase ventricular response. The net effect depends on vagal tone. It is a more useful drug for long-term prophylaxis than for acute i.v. administration in atrial tachycardia.

Junctional tachycardias (AV nodal tachycardias) (Figure 7.15)

These are commonly divided into:

- AVNRT: atrioventricular nodal re-entry tachycardia
- AVRT: atrioventricular re-entry tachycardia
- His bundle tachycardia.

Atrioventricular re-entry tachycardia (AVRT). Common type. Inverted P waves seen just after QRS complexes. PR > RP, i.e. a short RP tachycardia

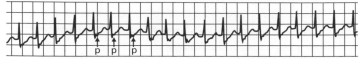

Atrioventricular re-entry tachycardia (AVRT) at 160/min reverting spontaneously to sinus rhythm. Although no P waves can be seen following the QRS complex as in the trace above, this ECG shows QRS alternans. If the narrow complex tachycardia is < 210/min QRS alternans is diagnostic of AVRT

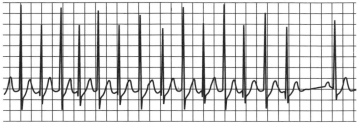

AV nodal re-entry tachycardia (AVNRT). Rate 214/min. Common type. P waves buried in QRS complexes as ventricle and atrium depolarize simultaneously

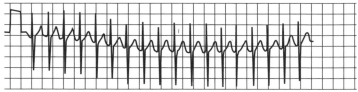

Figure 7.15 Junctional tachycardias.

AVNRT (common slow–fast type) (Figures 7.15 and 7.16)

A re-entry circuit in or very close to the AV node. There is usually a slow anterograde limb and a fast retrograde limb to the circuit. Atrium and ventricles are depolarized simultaneously so that the P wave is typically buried in the QRS complex. If visible it occurs as a positive blip just at the end of the QRS and may be mistaken for incomplete RBBB.

AVNRT (uncommon fast–slow type – a long RP tachycardia)

As above but the anterograde limb is fast and the retrograde limb slow. Atrial depolarization is thus late and there are inverted P waves in inferior leads half-way between the QRS complexes. PR interval less than RP'. A long RP tachycardia.

....

AVRT (common type: a short RP' tachycardia)

(Figures 7.15 and 7.16)

These tachycardias involve accessory pathways remote from the AV node such as WPW syndrome. During tachycardia there is slow anterograde conduction through the AV node and fast retrograde conduction through the accessory pathway (see Figure 7.23). The delta-waves are lost (no anterograde conduction through the accessory pathway) and the P waves which may be difficult to see are between the QRS complexes with PR > RP'. QRS alternans may occur at fast rates (Figure 7.15). QRS alternans below rates of 210/min is virtually diagnostic of AVRT. At rates higher than this it may occur in AVNRT.

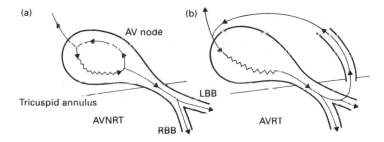

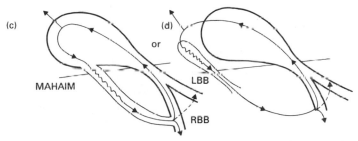

Figure 7.16 Examples of re-entry pathways involving the AV node: junctional tachycardias. Each circuit has a slow pathway (the zig-zag line representing decremental conduction) and a fast pathway. (a) AV nodal re-entry tachycardia (AVNRT). The re-entry circuit is entirely within the AV node. Atria and ventricles are depolarized together. The P waves are buried within the QRS complexes. See also Figure 7.15. (b) Atrio-ventricular re-entry tachycardia (AVRT). The re-entry fast pathway is remote from the AV node (as in WPW tachycardia). Atrial depolarization occurs after ventricular and P waves follow QRS complexes. PR is thus greater than RP'. A short RP' tachycardia. Common type. See also Figures 7.15 and 12.2. (c) Mahaim nodofascicular pathway. Late depolarization of the left bundle branch (LBB) results in the tachycardia having an LBBB morphology. (d) Mahaim free-wall pathway. The slow limb of the circuit is often in the anterior tricuspid annulus.

AVRT (uncommon type – a long RP' tachycardia)

Usually occurring in children, this incessant tachycardia has a fast limb through the AV node and a slow retrograde limb close to the AV node – similar to the uncommon form of AVNRT with the P wave late in the cycle so that PR < RP'. The accessory pathway is usually concealed and the resting ECG normal.

His bundle tachycardia (junctional ectopic tachycardia)

Rare. Again seen in children sometimes postcardiac surgery. The QRS complexes look normal but there is AV dissociation with dissociated (slower) sinus P waves. This is best managed with Class 1 anti-arrhythmic agents not verapamil.

Management

Where anterograde conduction through the AV node is involved in the tachycardia circuit then vagal manoeuvres are worth trying initially and the patient should be taught these (eyeball massage is dangerous and so is excluded).

• Ice-cold water splashed on the face. Ice-cubes in a polythene bag placed on the face. The 'duck-diving' reflex.
• Carotid sinus massage. One side at a time with the patient lying flat.
• Stimulation of the soft palate (gag reflex).
• Valsalva or Müller manoeuvres.
• Straining, lifting heavy weights, changes in posture.

If the AV node is involved, anterograde conduction will be blocked by adenosine or by beta-blockade. Verapamil should be avoided (page 343). In the long term, beta-blockade and amiodarone are very useful, but RF ablation is playing an increasing role in both AVRT and in some cases of AVNRT where the slow pathway is very close to the AV node.

Wolff–Parkinson–White syndrome is discussed separately (page 339).

Wide complex tachycardia: differentiation of SVT from VT

QRS complexes > 120 ms are classified as wide. The table on page 329 gives a general guide. See also Figures 7.17, 12.2 and 12.3.

It is important to remember that the haemodynamic state of the patient is no guide at all to the source of the tachycardia, as this depends on heart rate and LV function, irrespective of the origin of the tachycardia. It is safer to assume that wide complex tachycardia is ventricular in origin unless the patient has had a firm diagnosis made before. Vagal manoeuvres are worth trying as is a test dose of i.v. adenosine. If this fails to influence the tachycardia and the patient is in

Ventricular tachycardia.

Wide complex tachycardia with RBBB pattern in a man with an inferior infarct (see first complex in standard leads). Rsr' in V1 and V2. QRS duration > 140 msec. No p wave preceding first bizarre QRS. Extreme left axis > –30 degrees. RS ratio in V6 < 1.

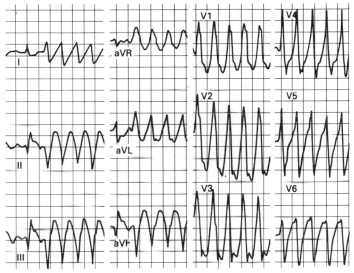

Atrial fibrillation with pre-excitation. WPW Type A.

Bizarre wide QRS with delta waves. Negative delta waves in I aVL and V6 suggest left lateral pathway. Note irregular tachycardia (sustained VT is regular as above).

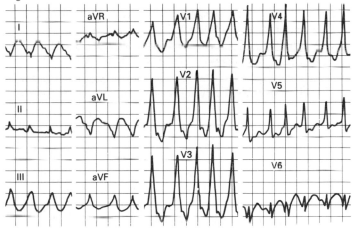

Figure 7.17 Wide complex tachycardias.

a reasonable haemodynamic state then lignocaine is the drug of choice (see **7.14**). It may be impossible to decide on the origin of tachycardia, especially with paroxysmal wide complex tachycardia picked up on a 24-hour ECG. An oesophageal electrode (easily swallowed as a 'pill on a wire') may help in identifying atrial activity from the left atrium. Electrophysiological studies with provocation may be necessary to decide between the two.

7.13 Ventricular premature beats (VPBs)

Ventricular ectopics on routine 24-hour monitoring

Routine 24-hour ECG monitoring in an apparently healthy population will reveal ectopic beats in more than half, and in about 10% these will be multifocal. They do not necessarily imply underlying heart disease. They probably occur with increasing frequency in the older population. Important points in the decision to treat them are:

• are the ectopics producing troublesome symptoms?
• is there an excessive consumption of alcohol, tea, coffee, cola, tobacco?
• any recent febrile or influenza-type illness?
• any associated drug therapy that might be implicated?
e.g. digoxin, sympathomimetics, tricyclic anti-depressants, diuretics inducing hypokalaemia
• is there any underlying cardiac condition?
e.g. mitral leaflet prolapse, recent myocardial infarction, sino-atrial disease, cardiomyopathy, aortic valve disease, etc.

Clearing up these points will require echocardiography and probably exercise testing. Innocent ectopics tend to disappear with increasing heart rate. More pathological ones may increase in frequency with possible short salvos of ventricular tachycardia on effort (Figure 12.3).

If full clinical examination is normal echocardiography is normal and an exercise test is negative (page 451), then the patient should be reassured. Treatment will only be necessary if in spite of reassurance and avoidance of possible precipitating factors, symptoms are still troublesome. Usually a small dose of a beta-blocking agent or disopyramide is effective, but should rarely be necessary.

Excessive zeal in trying to quench ectopic beats may result in drug side-effects being worse than the condition itself.

Differentiation of SVT with aberrant conduction from ventricular tachycardia

Sign	SVT with aberrancy	Ventricular tachycardia
Vagal manoeuvres or adenosine i.v.	May slow ventricular response to reveal atrial activity	Ineffective
Signs of AV dissociation		
Cannon waves	Absent	Present
First heart sound	Normal	Variable
Fusion beats	Absent	May be present
Capture beats (narrow QRS)	Absent	May be present
Independent P waves	Absent	May be seen
ECG pattern		
Onset of tachycardia	Usually RBBB	Bizarre wide QRS, RBBB or LBBB
	P wave preceding first wide QRS	No P wave preceding first bizarre QRS
QRS duration	< 140 ms	> 140 ms
QRS axis	Normal	More negative than −30°
V leads polarity	Discordant (some positive some negative)	Concordant (all negative or all positive)
If in RBBB		
Features in V1	rSR' in V1	Rsr' in V1
RS ratio in V6	> 1	< 1
Tip of S wave in V1	Down to or below isoelectric line	Well above isoelectric line
If in LBBB		
Initial R wave in V1	< 30 ms	> 30 ms
S wave in V1	No notch on S wave	Notch on S wave
Onset r to nadir S in V1	< 60 ms	> 60 ms
Onset to nadir S in other chest leads	< 100 ms	> 100 ms
Q in V6	Absent	Present
rS complexes in V leads	Present	May be absent

Ventricular premature beats following myocardial infarction

The treatment of ventricular premature beats following myocardial infarction is still controversial. Lown (1967) proposed certain types of premature beads were more likely to lead to VF and should be suppressed. These warning arrhythmias were:

- frequent VPBs
- multi-focal VPBs
- R-on-T phenomenon
- salvos of VPBs (two or more).

Since then it has been established that as many as 50% of cases of VF postinfarction occur with no warning arrhythmias at all. It has also been established that there is no case for routine use of anti-arrhythmic drugs in all patients entering a coronary care unit. There is no justification for a single-drug policy for all patients.

Ventricular premature beats are possibly just a marker of the extent of myocardial damage and do not necessarily cause sudden death. In an uncomplicated myocardial infarct, suppression of simple unifocal ectopic beats is not justified.

This has been shown to be dangerous in the cardiac arrhythmia suppression trial (CAST study) in which patients receiving flecainide or encainide had a higher mortality (7.7%) than if just taking a placebo (3%) and the trial was stopped early. The drugs were presumed to have a pro-arrhythmic effect.

Suppression of ventricular premature beats following myocardial infarction:

- check K^+, other drugs (e.g. digoxin), acid–base state and blood bases (hypoxia, hypercapnia), and correct them if possible. K^+ should be 4.5–5.5 mmol/l.
- consider prophylactic anti-arrhythmic drug if: poor haemodynamic state, frequent multi-focal VPBs, R-on-T or salvos of VPBs. Lignocaine is given as an infusion, switching to an oral agent after 48 hours. If LV function is good, consider beta-blockade or disopyramide. If LV function is poor, use amiodarone. Two big trials, the European and the Canadian myocardial infarct amiodarone trials (EMIAT and CAMIAT) have shown a reduction in arrhythmic deaths (but not overall mortality) in patients treated with amiodarone post myocardial infarction. Amiodarone should be particularly considered in patients with > 10–20 ventricular premature beats/hour on Holter monitoring postinfarction plus poor LV function (LV ejection fraction < 40%).
- Consider temporary pacing if ectopics are related to atropine-resistant bradycardia.

7.14 Ventricular tachycardia (VT) (Figures 7.17, 7.19 and 12.3)

Available drugs

Commonly used drugs in the management of VT are shown in the table on pages 332–334. Many of the Class 1 agents (lignocaine, mexiletine, tocainide) have similar side-effects predominantly affecting the CNS (tremor, dizziness, confusion, cerebellar ataxia, fits) and the gastrointestinal tract (nausea, anorexia, vomiting). The large number of drugs testify to the failure of a single drug to work in all cases of VT, and sometimes several drugs need to be used in prophylaxis.

Treatment of ventricular tachycardia

Treatment of ventricular tachycardia depends on the patient's condition. If present right at the onset of ventricular tachycardia in a monitored patient, a chest thump or getting the patient to give a vigorous cough may succeed in re-establishing sinus rhythm. In the very sick patient DC cardioversion is necessary. If VT is well tolerated, lignocaine 100–200 mg i.v. is given followed by an infusion (4 mg/min for 30 min, 2 mg/min for 2 hours, then 1 mg/min is normally satisfactory). If lignocaine fails to control the tachycardia a second drug can be tried provided that the patient's condition is still good. Disopyramide, amiodarone and procainamide have all been shown to be valuable in this situation, with amiodarone having the least negative inotropic effect. If two drugs fail to work:

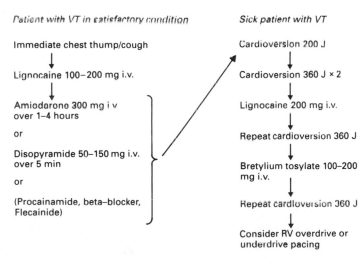

Patient with VT in satisfactory condition

Immediate chest thump/cough
↓
Lignocaine 100–200 mg i.v.
↓
Amiodarone 300 mg i v
over 1–4 hours

or

Disopyramide 50–150 mg i.v.
over 5 min

or

(Procainamide, beta–blocker, Flecainide)

Sick patient with VT

Cardioversion 200 J
↓
Cardioversion 360 J × 2
↓
Lignocaine 200 mg i.v.
↓
Repeat cardioversion 360 J
↓
Bretylium tosylate 100–200 mg i.v.
↓
Repeat cardioversion 360 J
↓
Consider RV overdrive or underdrive pacing

331

Drugs commonly used in ventricular arrhythmias

Drug (proprietary name's)	Oral dose	Intravenous dose	Half-life (approx.)	Therapeutic plasma level	Side-effects
Lignocaine (Xylocard)	—	100–200 mg i.v. bolus 4 mg/min for 30 min 2 mg/min for 2 hours then 1 mg/min	30 min	1.5–6.0 µg/ml	Drowsiness + confusion, paraesthesiae and numbness, dysarthria, fits
Quinidine (Kinidin, Kiditard, Quinicardine)	200 mg test dose 200–400 mg tds or qds long-acting preparation bd	Rarely used 6–10 mg/kg over 0.5 hour (quinidine gluconate)	7 hours	2–5 µg/ml	Visual disturbances, tinnitus, vertigo, thrombocytopenia, agranulocytosis, diarrhoea, paroxysmal VT or VF, half-dose digoxin, warfarin, etc.
Procainamide (Pronestyl)	375 mg 4 hourly	100 mg over 5 min repeat up to max. 1 g over 1 hour 2–5 mg/ min infusion	3 hours	5–10 µg/ml	Hypotension, AV block, insomnia, fever, rash, arthralgia, arteritis (lupus syndrome), agranulocytosis
Disopyramide (Rhythmodan, Norpace)	100–200 mg (max.) 6 hourly	50 mg i.v. over 5 min repeat to max. 150 mg, and to 300 mg in 1 hour	6 hours	2–6 µg/ml	Dry mouth, blurred vision, urinary retention, constipation, hypotension, VT

Drug	Dose (oral)	Dose (IV)	Half-life	Therapeutic level	Side effects
Propafenone (Arythmol, Rythmonorm)	150 mg tds up to 300 mg tds	2 mg/kg then 2 mg/min	6 hours	0.2–3.0 µg/ml	Dizziness, headache, anti-cholinergic
Phenytoin (Epanutin)	100 mg tds to 200 mg bd	50 mg over 5 min, repeating to 500 mg	22 hours	10–18 µg/ml	Cerebellar signs, gum hypertrophy, megaloblastic anaemia (folate), lupus syndrome, bradycardia, hypotension
Mexiletine (Mexitil)	Loading dose 400 mg then 200 mg tds	100–250 mg over 10 min; 4 mg/min for 1 hour, 2 mg/min for 1 hour, then 0.5 mg/min	16 hours	1–2 µg/ml	Anorexia, nausea, vomiting, tremor, cerebellar signs, bradycardia, hypotension
Aprindine (Fiboran, Fibocil)	Loading dose 200 mg then 100–200 mg od	25 mg over 5 min repeated to 150 mg	12–66 hours 28 hours	1–3 µg/ml	Tremor, giddiness, diplopia, hallucinations, ataxia, agranulocytosis, jaundice (rare)
Tocainide (Tonocard)	400 mg tds to 800 mg tds	0.5–0.75 mg/kg/min over 15 min	14 hours	5–10 µg/ml	Nausea, vomiting, CNS disturbance, giddiness, cerebellar signs, blood dyscrasias

Continued on page 334

Drugs commonly used in ventricular arrhythmias (Contd).

Drug (proprietary name's)	Oral dose	Intravenous dose	Half-life Therapeutic (approx.)	plasma level	Side-effects
Flecainide (Tambocor)	100–200 mg bd	1.5–2 mg/kg over 10 min	12–27 hours mean 20 hours	200–800 ng/ml	Avoid in paced patients. Giddiness, blurred vision
Propranolol (Inderal)	40 mg tds (range 10–240 mg tds)	0.1–0.2 mg/kg over 5 min	3 hours	30–50 ng/ml oral 50–100 µg/ml i.v.	Hypotension, AV block, depression, LV failure, cold peripheries, bronchospasm
Amiodarone (Cordarone X)	200 mg tds for 1 week reducing to ≤ 200 mg od	5 mg/kg over 2–4 hours 10–20 mg/kg/day infusion	28 days	0.1 µg/ml	Photosensitivity, corneal microdeposits, thyroid dysfunction, sleep disturbance, etc., alveolitis, half-dose digoxin, warfarin
Bretylium tosylate (Bretylate, Bretylol)	Poorly absorbed	5 mg/kg over 10 min then 1–2 mg/min bolus dose if in VF	8 hours	0.5–1 µg/ml	Hypotension, dizziness, avoid in digoxin toxicity
Ajmaline (Cardiorhythmine)	Not suitable as very short half-life	5 mg over 2 min Repeated after 10 min	1–2 min	1–3 µg/ml	Caution if also on digoxin as may induce AV block

- check K$^+$, acid–base state and blood gases
- proceed to DC cardioversion
- in the sick patient cardiac massage may help correct the arrhythmia.

Management and long-term prophylaxis

Check blood for K$^+$, acid–base balance and blood gases in all patients and correct if necessary (including artificial ventilation). In the sick patient with low-output state, cardiac massage may help correct the arrhythmia.

Once successfully cardioverted, prophylactic therapy is started orally. The effect of the chosen drug is monitored with 24-hour Holter taping and/or VT provocation study (see below). It is important to keep the serum K$^+$ between 4.5 and 5.5 mmol/l. If VT was secondary to myocardial infarction or acute myocarditis it is probably wise to continue drug therapy for 3 months in the first instance, and then repeat 24-hour monitoring both on the drug and after its withdrawal. In some cases more than one drug will be necessary and indefinite oral therapy may be required. Cardiac catheterization is indicated to delineate an LV aneurysm if this is a suspected cause of recurrent VT

Regimes of choice are one or more of these drugs:

Disopyramide 100 mg tds or qds

Mexiletine 200 mg tds

Amiodarone 200 mg tds for 1 week then reducing

Propafenone 150–300 mg tds

Beta-blocking agent

Flecainide 100–200 mg bd.

Drugs of second choice may be added or tried separately:

Procainamide 375 mg 4 hourly

Quinidine durules, two twice daily

Phenytoin 100 mg tds to 200 mg bd.

The best combinations of the first group are those from different Vaughan-Williams classes (e.g. disopyramide and amiodarone). There is evidence that amiodarone may be more effective than long-term beta-blockade in prevention of recurrent VT in patients with HCM. The implantable cardioverter defibrillator (ICD) is now important in the long-term management of recurrent VT (page 291).

Provocation of ventricular tachycardia

It is important to check that the ventricular tachycardia is being successfully suppressed by drug treatment. Patients who have VT still provokable at catheter studies are at much greater risk than those whose rhythm is successfully suppressed. A provocation study and Holter monitoring are the two equally important methods for identifying those at risk (the ESVEM trial).

Figure 7.18 shows the simple form of a provocation study. An anaesthetist should be present in the laboratory in case DC cardioversion is needed.

Ventricular pacing is established at 100/min (R–R interval 600 ms). After at least 8 paced beats a ventricular extrastimulus (E1) is interposed at an interval of 300 ms. If VT is not provoked then the extrastimulus is brought in 10 ms (R–ectopic interval 290 ms) and the cycle repeated. The cycle is repeated each time with the R–extrastimulus interval 10 ms less until the extrastimulus no longer captures: the effective refractory period (ERP). The extrastimulus is then moved to an interval of ERP plus 50 ms. A second extrastimulus (E2) is then added at 300 ms and E2 moved in each time with an E1–E2

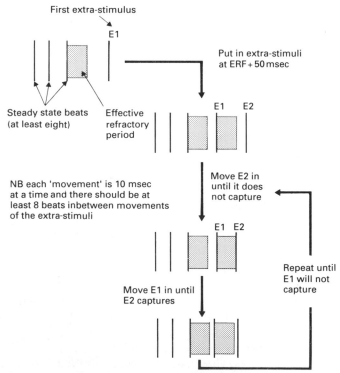

Figure 7.18 A simplified approach to ventricular provocation.

interval 10 ms less than the previous cycle. When E2 fails to capture then E1 is moved in 10 ms until E2 captures. The sequence is then repeated moving in E2.

The protocol is repeated with three extrastimuli, and then at a ventricular paced rhythm of 120/min (R–R interval 500 ms) and if necessary at 150/min (R–R interval 400 ms). If VT is still not provoked, a different pacing site can be chosen in the RV, and then isoprenaline infused if a really rigorous protocol is wanted.

Long QT syndromes (LQTS)

The normal QTc is 0.38–0.46 s (see page 437). A long QT interval may predispose to ventricular tachycardia often of the polymorphic torsades de pointes type (see Figures 7.19 and 12.3, pages 340 and 442).

QT dispersion

This is the difference between the maximum and minimum QT interval on the surface 12 lead ECG. In ischaemic patients QT dispersion will be increased by pacing. It is possible wide QT dispersion may be a marker for ventricular arrhythmias and sudden death as it indicates wide differences in repolarization times in the myocardium.

A long QT interval may be congenital (inherited gene defects) or acquired (drug or electrolyte effects) resulting from abnormalities of the ion channels controlling the duration of repolarization.

Congenital long QT syndrome genetic defects

These are rare syndromes. Only 500 families worldwide were on a registry by 1995. Two clinical syndromes were originally recognized.
• Jervell and Lange Nielsen (1957), a family with long QT interval, congenital deaf mutism and sudden death. Autosomal recessive.
• Romano-Ward (1963–64): QT prolongation and risk of sudden death. Normal hearing. Autosomal dominant transmission. Genetic heterogeneity present as commoner in females.
Both syndromes are characterized by:
• genetically prolonged QT interval. ECG could also show T-wave alternans, notched or biphasic T waves, sinus pauses, or even AV block
• frequent syncopal attacks provoked by emotional or physical stress. Symptoms still may occur during rest or sleep
• high mortality in untreated cases: 21% dying in 1 year from first syncope. 50% at 10 years.
Dominance of the left sympathetic nerves appears to be

pathogenetic and therapy is aimed at this. Beta-blockade is 80% effective. If this fails left sympathetic nerve denervation is considered (cardiac sympathectomy), or a combination of pacing plus beta-blockade. Higher rate pacing (e.g. 100/min) keeps the QT interval short. Implantable cardioverter defibrillators (ICDs) have been used but these patients are usually children. An ICD shock may induce pain or fear regenerating the original VT. There are also all the problems of child growth, marriage prospects, etc. Fortunately most children can be managed without an ICD.

Particularly bad prognostic features are:
- family history of syncope and sudden death
- QTc > 0.54 s
- congenital deafness
- AV block
- documented ventricular arrhythmias.

Schwarz and his colleagues have now identified three different genetic types with different ion channel defects, and in time this will make therapy more specific, e.g.

LQT1: Mutation on chromosome 11. The most common type. *KVLQT1* gene. A novel voltage gated K⁺-channel abnormality. High risk with effort/emotion, low risk in sleep. Unlikely to benefit from pacing. Treat with beta-blockade or left cardiac sympathectomy.

LQT2: Mutation on chromosome 7 (1995). *HERG* gene. Defect in inward K⁺ rectifier. High risk with exercise or arousal. Low risk in sleep. Unlikely to benefit from pacing as they do not shorten the QT interval with increasing heart rate. Beta-blockade first choice.

LQT3: Mutation on chromosome 3 *SCN5A* gene. Na⁺-channel dysfunction. Rarest. Highest risk during bradycardia (sleep). Should benefit from pacing but less from beta-blockade. Mexiletene may be helpful abolishing the persistent current in the defective Na⁺ channel.

Acquired long QT interval

This is most commonly drug induced or secondary to hypocalcaemia or hypomagnesaemia. May occur in anorexia nervosa. Prolongation of the QT interval is part of the therapeutic benefit of drugs like amiodarone and sotalol and the finding of a long QT interval is not necessarily an indication to stop the drug unless the QT interval is > 500 ms. Torsades de pointes is unlikely to occur unless the QT interval exceeds this. Patients should not receive two of the drugs from this list at the same time with the increased risk of inducing polymorphic VT. Hypokalaemia must be avoided. Two commoner examples of a long QT interval are shown in Figure 7.19 due to amiodarone therapy and hypocalcaemia. Although amiodarone commonly prolongs the QT interval polymorphic ventricular tachycardia due to the drug is rare.

Drugs prolonging the QT interval

Anti-arrhythmics	Psychiatric drugs	Antimalarials/ antibiotics	Serotonin antagonists	Others
Quinidine	Thioridazine	Erythromycin	Ketanserin	Probucol
Procainamide	Pimozide	Pentamidine	Cisapride	Vasopressin
Disopyramide	Chlorpromazine	Halofantrine		Terfenadine
Amiodarone	Haloperidol	Amantidine		Astemizole
Sotalol	Tricyclics	Quinine		Tacrolimus
d-Sotalol	Lithium	Chloroquine		
Bretylium	Sertindole			
Bepridil				

Measurement of the QT interval before and shortly after starting treatment is needed. Several drugs have been withdrawn because of their effect on the QT interval (prenylamine, terodiline) and terfenadine, originally an over the counter drug is now only available on prescription in the UK.

Management of torsades de pointes

Torsades respond poorly to conventional drugs and may be made worse by class 1a agents, e.g. lignocaine or class III agents. The likely culprit drug is stopped. Increasing the heart rate will help prevent torsades and shortens the QT interval. Consider isoprenaline infusion, i.v. magnesium (even if magnesium level is normal) or overdrive atrial pacing to rates of 90–110/min.

7.15 Wolff–Parkinson–White (WPW) syndrome

A variety of eponyms have become attached to accessory pathways that cause paroxysmal tachycardia using the pathway as a re-entry circuit. The three most well known are:

1 *Kent bundle* (1893). Atrioventricular accessory pathway separate from AV node. Short PR interval on ECG and delta-wave. Wolff–Parkinson–White syndrome. The great majority of accessory pathway tachycardias (Figure 7.23).

2 *Mahaim pathway.* Often young patients with LBBB pattern tachycardia. Nodoventricular pathway including fasciculo-ventricular

Salvos of monomorphic VT. Lead V1. RBBB pattern

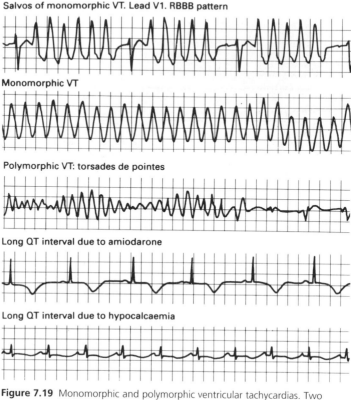

Monomorphic VT

Polymorphic VT: torsades de pointes

Long QT interval due to amiodarone

Long QT interval due to hypocalcaemia

Figure 7.19 Monomorphic and polymorphic ventricular tachycardias. Two common causes of long QT on ECG.

and His–ventricular pathways. Most Mahaim paths seem to be in the anterior tricuspid annulus separate from the AV node. Rare (Figure 7.16).

3 *James pathway.* Atrionodal or atriofascicular/atrio-Hisian tracts. Short PR interval on ECG but no delta-wave. Lown–Ganong–Levine syndrome. Uncommon.

WPW syndrome occurs in 1–3/1000 of the population but less than a quarter have episodes of sustained tachycardia. This may be partly due to the fact that the accessory pathway can lose its ability to conduct anterogradely over the years. The delta-wave is due to premature activation of part of the ventricular myocardium by the accessory pathway. There may in addition be repolarization abnormalities resembling ischaemia and a false positive exercise test is common. The accessory pathway may be in the anterior or posterior septum or in either the right or left atrial free wall. Two broad types are recognized. Type A (positive delta-wave in V1 – left ventricular pathway; Figure 7.20) and Type B (negative delta-wave in V1 – right ventricular pathway; Figure 7.21). A guide to localization of WPW accessory pathways is shown in Figure 7.22. More detailed localization is possible, analysing the initial delta-wave polarity.

Type	Site of accessory pathway	ECG appearances
Type A	Posterior left atrial wall to left ventricle or paraseptal	Positive delta-wave in leads V1–V6. Negative delta-wave in lead I
Type B	Lateral right atrial wall to right ventricle	Biphasic or negative delta-wave in leads V1–V3. Positive delta-wave in lead I

The ECG complex in WPW syndrome is thus a fusion complex of abnormally activated and normally activated myocardium. The ECG

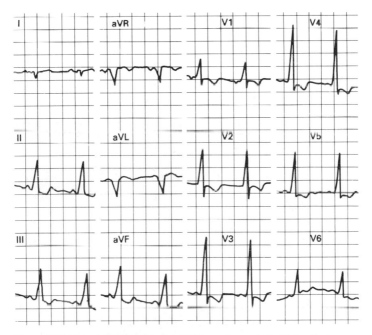

Figure 7.20 Type A Wolff–Parkinson–White syndrome. Left-sided pathway. Using the algorithm in Figure 7.22 it is shown to be a left lateral pathway.

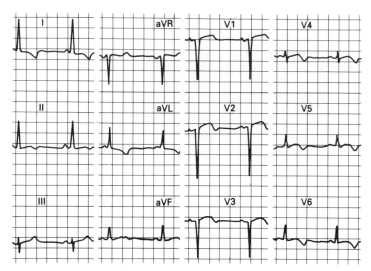

Figure 7.21 Type B Wolff–Parkinson–White syndrome. Right-sided anteroseptal pathway. Note repolarization abnormalities mimicking myocardial ischaemia.

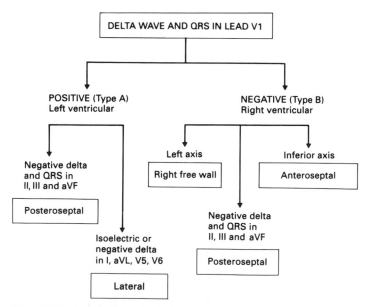

Figure 7.22 Accessory pathway localization in WPW.

appearances may mimic other conditions:
- LBBB (Type B)
- true posterior infarction, RV hypertrophy or RBBB (Type A).

Associated lesions
WPW syndrome may occur as an isolated condition or in association with other cardiac lesions (e.g. Ebstein's anomaly, hypertrophic obstructive cardiomyopathy, mitral valve prolapse), and paroxysmal tachycardia is a common problem in these conditions. WPW syndrome may be concealed and not obvious on the surface ECG. In this situation the accessory pathway only conducts retrogradely.

WPW tachycardia
The development of tachycaxrdia results from unidirectional block in the accessory pathway (Figure 7.23). A circus movement is set up with anterograde conduction down the AV node, and retrograde conduction in the Kent bundle (due to prolonged anterograde refractoriness of the Kent bundle). During tachycardia the delta-wave is lost, as ventricular activation occurs only via the AV node, and the ECG and its axis may appear very different from the ECG in normal sinus rhythm. Very occasionally, in small children the circuit is established the wrong way round (i.e. anterogradely via the accessory pathway) and the QRS complexes are wide.

Drug treatment
Drugs can act at three sites in WPW tachycardia (see Figure 7.23). Vagal manoeuvres may help in some cases.

WPW tachycardia can be treated by i.v. disopyramide (50–150 mg), i.v. flecainide (50–150 mg), i.v. propranolol (1–10 mg) or i.v. ajmaline (50–100 mg). Intravenous amiodarone is dangerous unless given very slowly (over 1–4 hours). Long-term prophylaxis may require a combination of drugs (e.g. disopyramide + beta-blockade, amiodarone + beta-blockade). DC cardioversion should be used early if the tachycardia is poorly tolerated.

Digoxin and verapamil should be avoided in WPW tachycardia, as the drugs may accelerate anterograde conduction down the Kent bundle.

Electrophysiological studies and RF ablation
Patients who are unresponsive to medical treatment, who dislike their treatment or have frequent or disabling attacks are candidates for RF

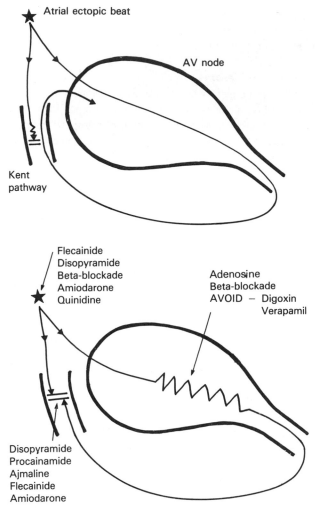

Figure 7.23 Mechanisms and treatment of re-entry tachycardia in WPW syndrome. The upper panel shows the re-entry circuit. A premature atrial beat (star) is blocked at the Kent bundle anterogradely and conducted normally through the AV node. The Kent bundle is not refractory to retrograde conduction and the circus movement is set up. The lower panel shows the sites of drug action. The atrial premature beat can be abolished by disopyramide, beta-blockade, amiodarone, flecainide or quinidine. Anterograde conduction down the AV node is delayed by adenosine or beta-blockade. Retrograde conduction up the Kent pathway is blocked by disopyramide, amiodarone, flecainide, ajmaline, procainamide, sotalol and propafenone. Verapamil and digoxin are contraindicated.

....

ablation, which is curative and avoids the need for any further drug treatment. The EP study and the RF ablation can be done as one procedure.

So successful is RF ablation now that patients rarely require surgical ablation of the bypass. Epicardial mapping is necessary prior to surgical ablation as the pathway is usually invisible. Septal tracts are difficult with a risk of complete AV block, and posteroseptal pathways difficult with the proximity of the coronary sinus. Patients who are absolutely asymptomatic and found to have WPW on a routine ECG do not need EP study unless they plan high-rise activities, such as rock-climbing, etc.

Catheter ablation

DC ablation
In 1982 Gallagher described the use of high energy DC shocks delivered to the His bundle by a standard tripolar recording catheter in the catheter laboratory in eight patients with refractory supraventricular tachycardia. It was described as a 'tactic of last resort'. Shocks of up to 300 J were used, and a general anaesthetic was required. Although the shocks were subsequently modified, it became clear that high-energy catheter ablation produced explosive barotrauma in the heart sometimes resulting in:
- hypotension requiring volume loading
- coronary spasm
- cardiac perforation
- transient electromechanical dissociation
- permanent RV dysfunction
- ventricular arrhythmias at follow up.

AV nodal ablation with the development of complete AV block was possible with the implantation of a permanent pacemaker. It proved very valuable for patients with fast intractable AF or SVT. However, complete AV block was sometimes induced inadvertently in an attempt to ablate accessory pathways near the AV node, and the technique was imprecise.

RF ablation
Radiofrequency current uses energy similar to surgical diathermy. The use of this form of energy is a huge advance and at last has brought a permanent non-surgical cure to many patients with disabling tachycardias whose lives were a misery on drug treatment. Particular advantages of the technique are:

- low voltages only required 40–60 V, no cardiac barotrauma
- no neuromuscular stimulation so no general anaesthetic required; sedation only
- discrete precise lesions with minimal cardiac damage
- possible to perform electrophysiological study and ablation in one procedure
- high success rate and low recurrence rate with very few complications.

The disadvantage with the technique is that it is time consuming with a long learning curve and often a long screening time. Average length of the procedure is 1–3 hours, but occasionally > 6 hrs with screening times of 2 hours. Two to five catheters are introduced via the femoral vein. A femoral artery catheter to the left heart is needed for left-sided accessory pathways, and possibly a subclavian puncture or arm vein catheter for coronary sinus catheterization. The ablating catheter tip must be negotiated gradually to within < 1 mm of the accessory pathway. The use of orthogonal and steerable catheters has helped. The technique can be used for WPW tachycardias of any type even if the pathway is close to the AV node. Sometimes multiple accessory pathways have to be dealt with. Ablation can if necessary be performed in the coronary sinus but there is a small risk of pericarditis or perforation here. Shocks lasting for a few seconds are delivered once the accessory pathway action potential has been recorded and the device switches off automatically if the impedance rises due to blood coagulum. Recurrence rate is small (5%) and complications few. Patients are sedated and heparinized throughout the procedure.

Atrio-ventricular nodal re-entrant tachycardia (AVNRT) has also been successfully dealt with by RF ablation. The slow component of the pathway in the posterior septum can be safely ablated without damaging the AV node. There is a 2% risk of complete AV block requiring permanent pacing, and this must be discussed with the patient prior to the procedure, especially the younger patient with infrequent attacks.

Fast atrial fibrillation can be dealt with by a direct AV node ablation 'modifying conduction' but permanent pacing will be needed. Some cases of atrial flutter can be managed by delivering several shocks to the triangle of Koch between the His bundle and the ostium of the coronary sinus. This destroys the area of slow conduction and may obviate the need for permanent pacing. RF ablation is possible for VT in either ventricle but the success rate is lower than for accessory pathway ablation. VT arising from the RV outflow tract (LBBB pattern with inferior axis) is the VT which is most likely to be successfully ablated. It may also be useful in idiopathic VT in otherwise normal hearts, and in very frequent or incessant VT following myocardial infarction (where an ICD is inappropriate).

Following RF ablation the patient is kept in overnight and echocardiography is performed the following morning before discharge to exclude a possible pericardial collection.

Surgical techniques for the management of arrhythmias

The management of arrhythmias that are refractory to drug treatment may include:

- anti-tachycardia pacing (temporary or permanent) (page 288)
- catheter ablation of AV node, bypass tract or arrhythmogenic focus (page 343)
- implantation of automatic cardioverter defibrillator (page 291)
- other surgical procedures.

RF ablation for WPW tachycardia has largely removed this condition from the sphere of the surgeon. Frequent ventricular tachycardia refractory to drug treatment may still need surgery. The best surgical case is that of the patient with well-tolerated inducible monomorphic VT with a localized infarct or aneurysm and good residual LV function. Results for polymorphic VT are not so good and patients with additional poor LV function are probably best managed with an ICD.

Direct division or ablation of an accessory pathway or arrhythmogenic focus can be performed during open heart surgery. Careful epicardial and occasionally endocardial electrographic mapping are required to detect the activation sequence over the atrial and ventricular myocardium. Detection of the earliest activation site on the myocardium helps establish the site of the accessory pathway (e.g. in WPW syndrome) or the arrhythmogenic focus (e.g. in ventricular tachycardia).

Surgical techniques may involve the following approaches.

- Cryotherapy: a cryoprobe can produce temporary ablation at $-10°C$, or permanent at $-65°C$, e.g. of accessory pathway or His bundle.
- Ventriculotomy. Encircling ventriculotomy is performed during VT.
- Endocardial resection. Performed during cardiopulmonary bypass.
- Ventricular aneurysmectomy. Performed alone may miss the site of origin of the VT, as this is often at the junction of scar tissue and more normal myocardium.
- Mitral valve replacement (for arrhythmias with mitral valve prolapse).

- Cardiac transplantation. For the extreme case where drugs and other ablative techniques have failed.

Combinations of these techniques may be necessary, e.g. mapping-directed endocardial resection plus the implantation of a cardioverter defibrillator (ICD).

7.16 Problems with individual anti-arrhythmic drugs

Amiodarone

This iodine-containing compound has a very long half-life and is strongly bound to plasma proteins. It is highly fat soluble and probably binds with phospholipids on the cell membrane and modifies adenyl cyclase activity.

Given orally it takes 5–10 days to saturate the tissues. It is of great value in both atrial and ventricular arrhythmias, as well as WPW syndrome where it acts by increasing the bypass anterograde effective refractory period (ERP).

Electrophysiological effects

It increases action potential duration (APD) in both sinus and AV nodes, but more so in the His–Purkinje system and ventricular muscle. It increases the AH interval without changing the H–V time. It slightly reduces the sinus node discharge rate and sinus node recovery time. It reduces conduction in the WPW accessory pathway, and reduces the anterograde ERP more than the retrograde ERP. It reduces excitability of all cardiac tissues, and the automaticity of SA and AV nodes is reduced. There is probably no chronic effect on contractility, although acute i.v. administration produces vasodilatation with afterload reduction, which affects acute contractility measurements.

Drug interactions

The doses of digoxin and warfarin should be halved in patients starting amiodarone (displacement of digoxin from myocardial receptors increases plasma digoxin, but reduces the direct cardiac effect). Amiodarone can be used with verapamil or beta-blockers, but care is needed (effects on AV node).

Side-effects

These are common and sometimes require stopping the drug. Patients should be warned about possible photosensitivity. They should shield themselves from the sun and use barrier creams if necessary.

Thyroid function is checked before starting the drug, especially in patients with AF. It is best avoided in patients with known thyroid dysfunction.

Amiodarone side-effects

Common side-effects	Rarer side-effects
Photosensitivity (> 50% patients)	Peripheral neuropathy
Skin rash	Pulmonary fibrosis (fibrosing alveolitis)
Headache	Thyroid dysfunction (hypothyroidism
Tremor	more than hyperthyroidism)
Sleep disturbance, insomnia	Slate-grey skin and melanosis
and nightmares	Hepatic dysfunction (raised enzymes)
Gut effects: nausea, constipation	Visual symptoms
Corneal microdeposits	Epididymitis
Increased prothrombin time	

Thyroid dysfunction (hypothyroidism) is due to inhibition of T_3 production and enhancement of reversed T_3 production (inactive). Corneal microdeposits are very common, but only visible on the slit lamp. They are reversible if the drug is stopped and regular eye checks are no longer needed. Only about 6% of patients on the drug develop visual disturbance.

The drug is safe in moderate renal dysfunction.

Pulmonary fibrosis occurs in about 5% of patients taking amiodarone. It is commoner in the older patient, in those with low pre-treatment pulmonary diffusion capacity (DLCO) and with high maintenance doses of amiodarone. It is rare with a maintenance dose of < 300 mg/day. It may be reversible if the drug is stopped soon enough. Steroid therapy needed for six months.

Cardioversion on amiodarone
If the patient has sino-atrial disease care is needed (effect on reducing sinus node automaticity), but it is usually safe.

Dosage
• Oral therapy: 200 mg tds for 1 week, reducing to 200 mg daily or less. It is very important to follow up patients taking amiodarone closely and to ensure that they are taking the smallest possible maintenance dose.
• Intravenous administration can be dangerous if given quickly (alpha-blocking effect). It is avoided if possible in the elderly and patients with

large hearts. In AF or VT it may restore sinus rhythm without the need for DC cardioversion in about 50% of patients. Infusion dose is 5 mg/kg in 100 ml 5% dextrose (not N-saline) over 1–4 hours. Maximum dose is 1200 mg in 24 hours. Abnormal rhythm may not be abolished immediately, sometimes reverting several hours after the infusion has stopped.

Drug levels
In chronic therapy it may be helpful to assay plasma amiodarone levels, and the level of its principal metabolite desethyl amiodarone. Normal range for both is 0.6–2.5 mg/l; both are anti-arrhythmic.

Disopyramide
A drug with both class 1a and class 3 actions, disopyramide also has an anticholinergic effect. The anticholinergic effect on the heart depends on the vagal tone present (in the normal heart, disopyramide may occasionally increase heart rate slightly by this 'vagolytic' action).

About 90% is bioavailable taken orally, and with normal serum levels (2–6 μg/ml) about 30–50% is free in serum. Half is excreted unchanged in urine.

Electrophysiological effects
It prolongs atrial effective refractory period, it has a variable effect on AV node refractory period, and prolongs ventricular refractory period. Conduction times in AV node and His–Purkinje system are little affected (unless there is pronounced vagal tone). It slows accessory pathway conduction.

It is a useful drug in atrial ectopics, prevention of AF or paroxysmal SVT because it causes a rise in atrial ERP; in WPW tachycardia because it causes a rise in accessory pathway conduction time; and in ventricular ectopics or tachycardia because it causes a rise in ventricular ERP.

Dosage
Oral. Loading dose is 300 mg in the adult (200 mg if < 50 kg) followed by 150 mg 6 hourly (100 mg if < 50 kg).
Increase dose interval if renal dysfunction (e.g. once daily for creatinine clearance ≤ 15 ml/min).
Intravenous. Dose of 50 mg is given slowly over 5 min, and may be carefully repeated up to 150 mg if necessary and contraindications have not appeared (see below).

Relative contraindications to disopyramide (where the drug has to be used with great care)

- Congestive cardiac failure with a large heart, poor LV function or cardiogenic shock.
- Sino-atrial disease (prolongs atrial ERP).
- 2° or 3° AV block.
- Prostatic hypertrophy.
- Glaucoma.
- Hypokalaemia: rarely it may precipitate VT (torsades de pointes) as with quinidine.

Disopyramide toxicity on ECG: watch for lengthening QT interval, widening of QRS complex, bradycardia or conduction defects. Also watch for hypotension. More likely with too rapid i.v. administration, especially if the patient is also on beta-blockade or other antihypertensive medication.

Common (anticholinergic) side-effects	Less common
Dry mouth, eyes, nose	Urinary retention
Blurred vision	Acute psychosis
Hesitancy in men with prostatic hypertrophy	Cholestatic jaundice
Constipation	Hypoglycaemia
Nausea	Agranulocytosis

Other points to note

- A dry mouth is an expected side-effect and is neither a guide to plasma level nor drug toxicity.
- Occasionally the drug may potentiate warfarin.
- It does not interact with lignocaine and can be used where lignocaine fails. It has only a weak negative inotropic effect.

Procainamide

A class 1a anti-arrhythmic with electrophysiological properties similar to quinidine. Up to 90% is absorbed orally and 15% only is protein bound. The drug is acetylated in the liver (first-pass metabolism), and acetylator status is important in determining plasma levels and toxic side-effects. About 50% of the drug is excreted in the urine. The acetyl metabolite is also anti-arrhythmic, and has a longer half-life.

Dosage

- In the adult the drug is given 4 hourly, in some difficult cases this means waking the patient at night to maintain plasma levels (5–10 μg/ml).

....

- Average adult dose is 375 mg, 4 hourly (250–500 mg 4 hourly).
- Slow-release preparation: procainamide durules can be taken 8 hourly (dose 1–1.5 g, 8 hourly).
- Acetylator status.

fast acetylators: may not reach necessary plasma levels of procainamide, but acetyl metabolite is anti-arrhythmic and less toxic
slow acetylators: may have high plasma levels and risk toxicity.

- Intravenous dose is 100 mg slowly over 5 min up to a maximum of 1 g in 1 hour.

Electrophysiological effects of procainamide

Little effect on AV node conduction (A–H time), dose-dependent increase in His–Purkinje conduction (H–V time). Increase in refractory period of Kent pathway making it useful in WPW tachycardia.

Side-effects

Make it a more useful drug in acute management of ventricular arrhythmias than in chronic suppression.

Intravenously it is a little safer than quinidine and can be tried if lignocaine fails. Side-effects following intravenous administration are:
- hypotension due to vasodilatation (reversed by phenylephrine)
- complete AV block. The drug should not be given in complete AV block as it may slow or extinguish the idioventricular rhythm
- in atrial flutter or fibrillation a vagolytic effect on the AV node may increase ventricular response (as with disopyramide). Procainamide is not usually used for atrial dysrhythmias although it may extinguish atrial ectopics.

Long-term side-effects

- The lupus syndrome: rash, arthralgia, fever, arteritis, pleurisy and pericarditis, but not renal involvement. The effects resolve on stopping the drug. Antinuclear antibodies occur in half the patients receiving the drug.
- Agranulocytosis.

Unless absolutely essential, procainamide should be restricted to 3–6 months oral therapy.

Quinidine

The original anti-arrhythmic drug with class 1a activity. The drug is completely absorbed orally and intravenous administration can be dangerous and is rarely used.

Unlike procainamide, 80% is protein bound, causing resulting drug interactions. The drug is hydroxylated in the liver, and in CCF, liver congestion results in high plasma quinidine levels. Alkaline urine may result in toxic metabolic accumulation.

Quinidine may be tried in paroxysmal AF or other atrial arrhythmias, and may help keep a patient in SR after cardioversion. Atrial arrhythmias are the main indication for its use; it is rarely used for ventricular arrhythmias now, as less toxic drugs are available. It is contraindicated in sino-atrial disease, digoxin toxicity and complete AV block.

Dosage

A test dose of quinidine sulphate of 200 mg is given to check for drug idiosyncrasy (anaphylaxis).

Quinidine durules are then started, initially two twice daily (= 500 mg quinidine bisulphate bd) to three times daily maximum. When starting treatment, quinidine displacement of other drugs from plasma proteins necessitates reducing the doses of other drugs, so the dose of concomitant warfarin or digoxin should be halved.

Electrophysiological effects

As in procainamide: no change in A–H time (or even slight shortening due to vagolytic effect), plus lengthening of H–V time.
Surface ECG shows:
- widening QRS
- prolonged QT interval } these are useful guides to toxicity
- T-wave changes

QRS widening > 120 ms is an indication to stop the drug.
With increasing toxicity the following may occur:
- atrial standstill
- ventricular tachycardia (torsades de pointes) (Figures 7.19 and 12.3)
- VF.

Side-effects

These are commonly gastrointestinal. Any others are indications to stop the drug.
- gastrointestinal: diarrhoea is expected, with nausea and vomiting.
- cinchonism: tinnitus, vertigo, deafness, visual disturbances, blindness.
- haematological: thrombocytopenia, purpura, agranulocytosis
- neuromuscular blocking effect: this may potentiate muscle relaxants. Its vagolytic action inhibits anticholinesterase activity in myasthenia

- quinidine syncope. This may be due to AV block, VT or VF.
  A prolonged QT interval plus an early ectopic (R on T) may be the cause.

Lignocaine
A class 1b anti-arrhythmic that shortens the action potential duration. It differs from procainamide and quinidine in several respects (see table).

	Class 1a: Procainamide Quinidine	Class 1b: Lignocaine
APD	Lengthened	Shortened
Peripheral vessels	Vasodilator	Vasoconstrictor
Oral preparation	Yes	No
Useful in atrial arrhythmias	Yes	No
Conduction of His–Purkinje system	Prolongs H–V time	Little effect
CNS toxicity	Uncommon	Common
Myocardial depression	In toxic doses	Minimal
Use in sino-atrial disease	No	Safe

It is the standard drug in use for ventricular arrhythmias in the CCU. It is rapidly metabolized in the liver, allowing flexible control and has to be given intravenously. Liver dysfunction or congestion (as in heart failure) requires dose reduction. It is not protein bound.

Lignocaine metabolites are excreted in the urine and contribute to CNS toxicity. It is safer than i.v. procainamide in low-output states or in patients with degrees of AV block.

Dosage
There are numerous suggested schedules. One of the easiest is:

200 mg i.v. bolus over 5 min, followed by infusion of 4 mg/min for 30 min, then 2 mg/min for 2 hours, then 1 mg/min.

In low-output states the initial 4 mg/min infusion period is omitted and the infusion is started at 2 mg/min. Plasma levels should be 1.5–6 µg/ml. Significant plasma levels can be obtained after i.m. lignocaine (300 mg in the adult) after about 15 min. Lignocaine infiltration used for minor surgery, pacemaker insertion, etc. can also produce significant plasma levels.

Side-effects

These are primarily neurological, especially in the elderly, and include: numbness, drowsiness, confusion, nausea, vomiting, dizziness, dysarthria and eventually convulsions. Convulsions are managed with i.v. diazepam.

Lignocaine is safer in cardiac failure or cardiogenic shock than procainamide, provided lower infusion rates are used.

What to do if lignocaine fails:

- check adequate infusion rate and drip still functional
- check plasma K^+: lignocaine is less effective in hypokalaemia
- check for additional drug therapy, possibly causing arrhythmias: digitalis, other inotropes, etc.
- gradually increase lignocaine infusion rate until early toxic signs appear
- if still ineffective switch to alternative drug, e.g. disopyramide, flecainide, amiodarone or bretylium tosylate.

Mexiletine

A class 1b agent similar to lignocaine, but available for oral administration. Hepatic metabolism is slower than with lignocaine, and renal excretion is reduced if the urine is alkaline.

Electrophysiological effects are variable; the H–V time has been reported to increase or decrease. Generally it has little effect on AV conduction.

Dosage

Orally: 200–400 mg 8 hourly in the adult. Dosage i.v. is complicated as with lignocaine, since there is a small margin between therapeutic effect and side-effects. Suggested i.v. regime: 100–250 mg i.v. over 10 min, 4 mg/min for 1 hour, 2 mg/min for 1 hour, then 0.5 mg/min.

Close attention is needed with i.v. mexiletine as the long half-life (16 hours) compared with lignocaine means that fine tuning of the regime is much more difficult. Neurological side-effects are common with i.v. therapy. Chronic oral therapy is much easier, and side-effects are less likely.

Side-effects

As with lignocaine: dizziness, numbness, paraesthesiae, tremor, dysarthria, tinnitus myoclonus, convulsions, nausea and vomiting, hiccoughs, bradycardia and hypotension. The bradycardia usually responds to atropine.

On oral therapy common complaints are nausea, anorexia and a continuous unpleasant taste in the mouth.

Tocainide
Also similar to lignocaine in structure and anti-arrhythmic effect but is available orally and has a longer half-life (11–14 hours). Fifty per cent is protein bound. About 40% is excreted unchanged in the urine. Electrophysiological effects are similar to those of lignocaine.

As with lignocaine, it is safe in low-output states, but dosage should be reduced in patients with heart failure, renal disease or post-myocardial infarction as the half-life is prolonged (e.g. 17–19 hours) and twice-daily dosage is sufficient in these patients.

Dosage
Oral. 400-800 mg 8 hourly, 400–600 mg 12 hourly in hepatic, disease or CCF.
Intravenous. 0.5–0.75 mg/kg/min over 15–30 min, followed by oral therapy.

Side-effects are similar to lignocaine and mexiletine and, unfortunately, as common. The main adverse effects are nausea, vomiting, dizziness and light headedness, tremors and paraesthesiae.

Recently, neutropenia, agranulocytosis, thrombocytopenia and aplastic anaemia have been reported. The drug should only be used for life-threatening arrhythmias and weekly blood counts are necessary while patients are on the drug.

Flecainide
A class 1c anti-arrhythmic agent that has recently received bad coverage in the CAST study. This study showed that patients taking flecainide or encainide for ectopic beats following a myocardial infarction had a higher mortality than those taking a placebo. This was thought to be due to a pro-arrhythmic effect of these drugs. The CAST trial results led to the drug being largely abandoned for a wide variety of arrhythmias unrelated to myocardial infarction. Flecainide is still of great value in refractory arrhythmias not responding to other drugs:
• life-threatening VT
• paroxysmal atrial arrhythmias, AF or atrial flutter
• reciprocating tachycardias involving accessory pathways (either intra- or extranodal).

Like tocainide it has a long half-life (approximately 20 hours) and twice-daily dosage is adequate. In common with other class 1c drugs, it does not prolong the action potential duration, but prolongs the refractory period in His–Purkinje and accessory bypass tracts.

Dosage

Oral. 100–200 mg 12 hourly. Maximum daily dose 400 mg. The long-term dose should be reduced if possible, especially in the elderly.

Intravenous. 0.5–2.0 mg/kg slowly i.v. up to a maximum of 150 mg. Careful ECG monitoring needed if the patient is in VT. In patients with poor LV function it is safer to give the drug as a mini-infusion over 30 min.

Side-effects are not common and generally the drug is well tolerated. Giddiness, light headedness and blurred vision are the commonest complaints. The pro-arrhythmic effect occurs in a small number of patients (probably < 10%). It has a mild negative inotropic effect.

Flecainide should be avoided in:

• patients in cardiac failure
• patients with permanent pacing who do not have a programmable unit. The pacing threshold may rise and the pacemaker may need programming to a higher output voltage or pulse width. A similar increase in pacing voltage may be needed with temporary wires
• second or third-degree AV block
• sino-atrial disease
• post-myocardial infarction ectopic beats

Propafenone

This is another class 1c agent recently available in the UK. It is valuable in the management of both supraventricular and ventricular arrhythmias as well as those re-entrant arrhythmias involving accessory pathway conduction. It blocks retrograde conduction in the accessory pathway.

Bioavailability is 50% and protein binding 90%. Half-life is approximately 6 hours. The drug is given 8 hourly. Dose: 150–300 mg tds. Side effects are dizziness, unusual taste and headache. It is mildly negatively inotropic. It has anticholinergic effects. Care is needed in patients with airway obstruction as it has mild beta-blocking activity. It should be avoided in patients with myasthenia gravis.

Bretylium tosylate

A drug that tends to be used as a last resort in patients with VT or VF resistant to other anti-arrhythmic therapy. It is only available i.v. or i.m.

Its mode of action is not well understood, but it has both class 2 and 3 effects. Eighty per cent is excreted unchanged in the urine. Half-life is about 8 hours.

Dosage

Intramuscularly: 5 mg/kg 8 hourly or 200 mg 2 hourly until the drug works (up to a maximum 2 g).

Intravenously: single bolus of 5 mg/kg for VF.

Side-effects

Hypotension, nausea, nasal stuffiness (sympathetic blockade); parotid pain with prolonged use; patients receiving bretylium should be lying flat, and hypotension (the commonest side-effect) can be reversed by volume loading and a pressor agent if necessary (e.g. phenylephrine).

8 Pericardial Disease

8.1) Acute pericarditis

Inflammation of the parietal and visceral layers of the pericardium may be a primary condition or secondary to systemic disease.

Causes

- Acute rheumatic fever.
- Other bacterial infections.
- Viruses, e.g. Coxsackie group, Epstein–Barr virus.
- Fungi infections: patients on immunosuppressive agents.
- Uraemia.
- Trauma, e.g. road traffic accident with steering wheel injury.
- Collagen vascular disease, particularly systemic lupus erythematosus, rheumatoid arthritis.
- Postmyocardial infarction (page 204) acute.
- Postcardiotomy syndrome, Dressler's syndrome (page 208).
- Malignant disease.
- Radiotherapy.
- Hypothyroidism.
- Many cases are idiopathic.

Pericardial pain and other symptoms

Pain is variable in intensity and site. It is usually retrosternal, radiating to the neck, left shoulder, back and around the left scapula. It may be epigastric only. It is often quite sharp in quality, unlike the heavy sensation of angina. Its most important characteristics are its:
- relation to position. It is relieved by sitting forward and made worse by lying flat, twisting the thorax or lying on the left side.
- relation to respiration. It is frequently worsened by deep inspiration, coughing, etc.

The pain does not necessarily improve as a pericardial effusion develops. Dyspnoea is a common symptom. The patient frequently takes small rapid breaths, as any major respiratory movement causes pain.

An enlarging effusion increases dyspnoea. Other symptoms include and depend on associated conditions, e.g. fever, dry cough, sweating, arthralgia, rash, pruritus, etc.

Physical signs

Venous pressure may be normal initially, rising as and if an effusion develops. Prominent `x` descent suggests tamponade (page 363) may be developing.

The pericardial rub is best heard at the left sternal edge with the patient leaning forward. It is variable with respiration and often transient, coming and going over a few hours. It may be confused with and sound very similar to true cardiac murmurs (e.g. the to-and-fro murmur of aortic regurgitation). The heart sounds are soft with a pericardial effusion.

Bronchial breathing at the left base with large effusions compressing the left lower lobe (Ewart's sign).

Signs of tamponade (page 363).

Investigations
Obviously depend on the suspected aetiology but the list below is an example of the possible difficulties in making a diagnosis:

FBC and ESR, U and E, creatinine

ASO titre, anti-DNAse B titre, etc. throat swabs

Blood cultures x 3

Viral titres: acutely and 2 weeks later, urine + faecal samples

Paul Bunnell screen

Cold agglutinins (*Mycoplasma*)

LE cells, ANF, anti-DNA antibodies, immune complex titres, complement levels

T_4, T_3, TSH

Sputum culture and cytology

Mantoux test

Fungal precipitins

CXR, heart shape and size, lung pathology

ECG

Echocardiogram

Pericardial fluid for culture, Ziehl–Neelsen staining, guinea-pig inoculation, cytology and fungal culture

ECG changes (Figure 12.9, page 447)
Are often non-specific showing T-wave inversion only. 'Saddle-shaped' ST-segment elevation may occur, and be confused with myocardial infarction, but in pericarditis the ST segment is concave upwards (convex upwards in infarction).

With the development of a pericardial effusion the voltage falls, and with very large effusions electrical alternans may occur (Figure 8.2).

Echocardiography (Figure 12.24, page 475)
Is most valuable in confirming the presence of an effusion, its site and

size. Left ventricular function is assessed regularly for possible deterioration, e.g. associated myocarditis.

Cardiac catheterization

Is rarely necessary now. RA cineangiography prior to pericardial aspiration will confirm the diagnosis with an obviously thickened pericardium.

Management

Analgesia and bed rest are the main forms of therapy. Soluble aspirin or non-steroidal anti-inflammatory agents are very successful in relieving pain in most cases. A short course of steroids (e.g. 2 weeks) will also work, but care must be taken to follow the patient carefully after cessation of treatment, as the symptoms may recur. Idiopathic benign recurrent pericarditis is treated symptomatically. Colchicine may be helpful in preventing relapses.

Aspiration of the effusion is indicated for diagnosis and/or the relief of symptoms or tamponade. Patients with recurrent effusions not settling on medical treatment should have surgical drainage with a pericardial window and direct histology may be helpful. Specific therapy is necessary for the possible associated condition.

Recurrent loculated effusions may require extensive pericardectomy.

8.2) Tamponade

An acute situation that requires quick diagnosis and pericardial aspiration. Patients, if conscious, complain of dyspnoea, a dull central chest pain, facial engorgement, abdominal and ankle swelling. A chronic form of tamponade does occur.

Acute causes

- Myocardial infarction with rupture of ventricular wall.
- Aortic dissection into the pericardial space.
- Following cardiac surgery.
- Chest trauma.
- Following transseptal puncture at cardiac catheter.
- Uraemic patients undergoing haemodialysis (and heparinization).
- Malignant disease and/or radiotherapy.
- Patients on anticoagulants.
- Associated with acute pericarditis.

  Chronic pericardial effusion may in addition occur with collagen

....

diseases, Dressler's syndrome, viral, bacterial or tuberculous pericarditis. Chylous effusions can occur with lymphatic obstruction.

Diagnosis of tamponade should be considered in any patient with a low-output state, high venous pressure, oliguria or anuria who is not responding to inotropes.

Physical signs

JVP. Raised, prominent 'x' descent (systolic). Forward flow from cavae only occurs during ventricular systole. No 'y' descent (Figure 1.1). Inspiratory filling of the neck veins is not common.

BP. Low. May be undetectable on inspiration.

Pulse. Low volume. Pulsus paradoxus. An abnormally excessive reduction in pulse volume on inspiration. The exact mechanism is still debated, but increased venous return on inspiration fills the right heart, and left heart filling is less possible with increased RV volume occupying more space in the 'rigid box'. Other factors also contribute (e.g. the normal inspiratory reduction of intra-thoracic pressure transmitted to the aorta, and a relative failure of intra-pericardial pressure to fall much on inspiration). Diaphragmatic traction on the pericardium is now thought irrelevant.

Normally there is a slight reduction of systolic pressure on inspiration (e.g. about 5 mmHg). Reduction of systolic pressure of > 10 mmHg is suggestive of pulsus paradoxus (Figure 8.1).

Other causes of pulsus paradoxus are:

• constrictive pericarditis (less commonly)
• status asthmaticus (exaggerated pressure swings within the thorax transmitted to the aorta)

Heart sounds are soft. There may be a pericardial rub in tamponade.

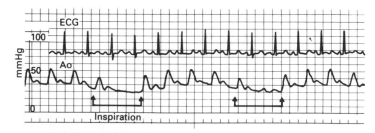

Figure 8.1 Pulsus paradoxus in tamponade. Simultaneous arterial pressure (Ao) and ECG in a man with subacute cardiac rupture. The patient was in shock and hypotensive. On inspiration the pulse pressure disappears, and returns immediately on the onset of expiration.

Oliguria or anuria rapidly develops with tamponade, and a brisk diuresis occurs when tamponade is relieved.

Other help in diagnosis

ECG: shows progressive reduction in voltage, and sometimes electrical alternans (Figure 8.2). This may be due to the heart moving around within the fluid-filled pericardium.

CXR: shows a symmetrical globular enlargement of the heart.

Echocardiography: confirms a large pericardial fluid collection with right atrial and/or right ventricular diastolic collapse. The size of the collection is a better predictor of tamponade than right heart collapse (Figure 12.24, page 475).

Right atrial cineangiogram: confirms diagnosis but is not necessary now with two-dimensional echocardiography.

Management

Pericardial needle aspiration may be life saving, but usually is only of temporary benefit. Insertion of a surgical drain or creation of a pericardial window is frequently necessary.

Needle aspiration is best performed via the xiphisternal route with the patient supine, using ECG control if screening is not available. The V lead of a standard ECG is attached to the aspiration needle with a crocodile clip. The needle is inserted 0.5 inch below the xiphisternum and, keeping it horizontal, the tip is rotated 45° to the left (towards the left shoulder tip). The cardiac pulsation can usually be felt at the end of the needle, but if the needle penetrates the myocardium itself, ST-segment elevation occurs ('injury potential').

Pericardial fluid should be sent for cytology if no obvious diagnosis is apparent. Creation of a pericardial window allows a pericardial biopsy to be taken. Removal of even a small amount of fluid from the

Pre

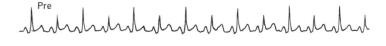

Post

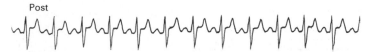

Figure 8.2 ECG lead II in tamponade pre and postpericardiocentesis. The ECG prior to aspiration shows electrical alternans. Following pericardiocentesis, this disappears, the voltage has increased and the axis has changed.

pericardial sac (e.g. only 50–100 ml) can produce a considerable improvement in haemodynamics as the intrapericardial pressure falls sharply.

Instillation of chemotherapeutic agents is possible in confirmed malignant disease with reaccumulation of fluid (e.g. 5-fluorouracil, nitrogen mustard or ^{32}P). Instilling tetracycline in patients with recurrent malignant pericardial effusions may help obliterate the pericardial space.

8.3 Chronic constrictive pericarditis

Constrictive pericarditis and restrictive cardiomyopathy usually present in a similar way with signs and symptoms of both right- and left-sided heart failure. However, there is no history of hypertension, angina is rare and the heart is not grossly enlarged (as in dilated cardiomyopathy). Clinically, right-sided signs are prominent with marked elevation of venous pressure, hepatomegaly and often ankle oedema or ascites. The cause is often not identified. It is probably the result of haemorrhagic pericarditis producing fibrosis with organization of the exudate.

Possible causes
- Viral.
- Mediastinal radiotherapy and/or malignancy.
- Tuberculosis.
- Collagen/autoimmune disease, rheumatoid arthritis.
- Other bacterial infections.
- Rarely, uraemia, drugs (procainamide, hydralazine), trauma.

Physical signs
JVP. The most important sign is appearance of prominent 'x' and 'y' descents (Figure 8.3) in the venous pressure. This is an important differential diagnostic point from tamponade. These two prominent descents can be seen even if the patient is in AF. Forward flow occurs during ventricular systole and on tricuspid valve opening. Inspiratory filling of the neck veins may occur (Kussmaul's sign) but it is not a particularly reliable sign.

Pulsus paradoxus is uncommon in constrictive pericarditis.

Ankle oedema and ascites are common, as is hepatosplenomegaly.

Heart sounds are soft. There may be an early third sound associated

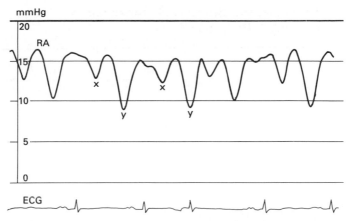

Figure 8.3 Right atrial pressure in pericardial constriction. The mean RA pressure is high and the 'x' and 'y' descents are prominent.

with rapid early ventricular filling (pericardial knock).

AF is common.

Although the condition is chronic, the development of oedema and ascites may be acute and sudden.

Conditions clinically similar to chronic pericardial constriction

• Chronic pericardial effusion (see table on page 368).

• Restrictive cardiomyopathy: amyloidosis, endomyocardial fibrosis, Loeffler's eosinophilic endocarditis.

• Dilated cardiomyopathy (DCM).

• Mitral stenosis with pulmonary hypertension and tricuspid regurgitation.

• HCM involving RV and LV.

• Thromboembolic pulmonary hypertension.

• Ischaemic CCF.

The heart is large in DCM and ischaemic CCF but tends to be smaller or normal in constrictive pericarditis and restrictive cardiomyopathy.

Left ventricular systolic function is usually normal in restrictive cardiomyopathy and often normal in constrictive pericarditis. It is grossly reduced in DCM and ischaemic CCF.

Severe pulmonary hypertension is not a feature of constriction or restriction, but is frequently found in the other conditions listed above.

Cardiac catheterization may be the only way to reach a definitive diagnosis.

Similarities and differences between tamponade and pericardial constriction

	Tamponade	Constrictive pericarditis
JVP/RA pressure	Prominent 'x' descent	Prominent 'x' and 'y' descents
Kussmaul's sign	Usually absent	May be present
Pulsus paradoxus	Invariable	Not common
Atrial pressures	Equal	Equal
LVEDP/RVEDP	Equal	Equal
Diastolic dip and plateau waveform	Absent	Present

Investigations

Are usually unrewarding. There is little point in viral titres in such a chronic disease. The important feature is a vigorous search for tuberculosis, e.g.

- Mantoux, early morning sputum and urine.
- ANF, DNA antibodies, rheumatoid factor.
- CXR, calcification of the pericardium strongly suggests a tuberculous aetiology.
- Echocardiography shows normal LV size with rapid early filling and diastasis (best seen on posterior wall movement).

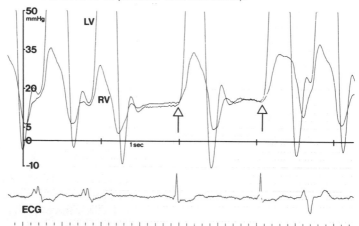

Figure 8.4 Simultaneous recording of left and right ventricular pressures in chronic constrictive pericarditis. On longer R–R intervals there is a dip and plateau waveform in diastole. The end-diastolic pressures of both ventricles are high and virtually equal (arrowed). This helps to distinguish the condition from restrictive cardiomyopathy.

• Cardiac catheterization is necessary to differentiate the condition from restrictive cardiomyopathy. Atrial pressures are high and equal with prominent 'x' and 'y' descents in constriction. LVEDP = RVEDP (or virtually so) at any phase of respiration and both are high. Systolic function is usually normal in constriction, but may be impaired in severe cases (the constricted pericardium may involve the epicardium). There is a typical diastolic plateau waveform in both ventricles (rapid early filling then diastasis) (Figure 8.4).

Management

Although diuretic therapy may be of temporary benefit, pericardectomy is usually necessary. As much of the anterior wall of both ventricles as possible is freed. It is a procedure not without difficulties as the pericardium may be strongly adherent to the epicardial muscle. Freeing the AV groove is important if at all possible. The pericardium should be sent for histology and culture. A year's course of anti-tuberculous therapy may be necessary.

Balloon dilatation of the pericardium has been tried in a few cases with some success, avoiding the need for a limited thoracotomy, and this may be very useful as a palliative measure in patients with malignant disease.

9 Infective Endocarditis

This is no longer termed 'subacute bacterial endocarditis', as non-bacterial organisms are becoming an increasing cause of the condition. Infective endocarditis is a changing disease, but the advent of newer antibiotics has had little effect on mortality figures. The changes in the type of disease are due to several factors:
- the decline in rheumatic fever
- increasing incidence in older patients
- increased survival of patients operated upon for congenital heart disease
- prosthetic valve endocarditis
- different organisms: increasing number of staphylococcal and fungal infections
- antibiotic resistance
- drug addicts with tricuspid valve endocarditis.

Overall mortality is still said to run at about 15%, but is a great deal less for penicillin-sensitive *Streptococcus viridans* (approximately 5%), and a great deal more for prosthetic valve endocarditis (approximately 60%) where further surgery is usually required as part of the management. About 1500 cases of infective endocarditis occur in the UK per year.

9.1 Predisposing cardiac lesions

These are shown below. The haemodynamic situation that predisposes to infection is a high-pressure jet into a lower-pressure system through a narrow orifice resulting in endothelial wear and tear

Commonly in	Less commonly in	Virtually never in
Aortic valve disease (bicuspid or rheumatic)	HCM and subaortic stenosis	ASD Pulmonary valve stenosis
Mitral valve disease: Regurgitation > stenosis, Floppy valve	Previously normal valve	Divided PDA
	Jet lesion AV fistula	
Coarctation	Mural thrombus e.g. postinfarct	
Patent ductus arteriosous VSD		
Prosthetic valves Tricuspid valve in drug addicts		

(Rodbard's factors). Thus infective endocarditis is much more likely on a VSD than an ASD. Bacterial colonization occurs and platelet, fibrin and cellular accumulation follows, surrounding bacteria in a 'protective cocoon'.

There seems little doubt now that infective endocarditis can occur on a previously normal valve. In spite of this the logistics of antibiotic cover for dental procedures, etc. are such that it is at present advised only for those patients with known predisposing lesions listed in the table overleaf.

Other predisposing factors should also be remembered: patients at higher risk of infection from general medical conditions (e.g. diabetes, renal failure, haemodialysis and alcoholism), i.v. drug abusers are also at high risk. Overall about 5% of the total population is at risk.

9.2 Portals of entry

These are often unknown, but careful history taking may reveal one of the following in the previous few months:

• *Dental work* of any type: extraction, fillings or even scaling. Patients with poor dental hygiene are at risk and these are often the elderly, the immunosuppressed, patients with polycythaemia (congenital heart disease) or gingivitis associated with gum hypertrophy (e.g. phenytoin or nifedipine). Badly fitting dentures or dental braces may also be dangerous. Retained dental roots are a particularly common source of infection and the teeth are still the most common portal of entry.

• *Urinary tract infection*. Cystoscopy. Catheterization.

• *Respiratory infection*.

• *Enterococci* may gain access to the circulation via carcinoma of the colon, and present with infective endocarditis (e.g. *Streptococcus bovis*). Endoscopy is still contentious. It is unlikely following standard gastroduodenoscopy or even sigmoidoscopy.

• *Skin disease*. Purulent lesions. Burns.

• *Intravenous cannulation*. This is particularly a problem with CVP lines and may be a cause of infective endocarditis soon after valve replacement. It is especially likely in patients requiring CVP lines for more than 48 hours and in those with additional medical problems (e.g. jaundice, uraemia, additional steroid treatment). Strict aseptic procedures necessary for all CVP line insertions.

• *Gall bladder disease*.

• *Surgery*.

• *Abortion*. Operative > spontaneous.

• *Paturition*. Although a theoretically likely portal of entry, this is probably less of a risk factor than once thought.
• *Intravenous drug abuse*.
• *Fractures*.

The fact that the portal of entry is often unknown has led to virtually every invasive procedure being incriminated as a possible cause. As a result many probably 'innocent' procedures (e.g. gastroscopy) have been included. Sigmoidoscopy is possibly a cause of bacteraemia, and rectal biopsy should also be covered by antibiotics (see below). Basically all endoscopy procedures should be covered by antibiotics in patients with known predisposing lesions.

 ## Organisms responsible

Bacterial

• *Streptococcus viridans* group. Still the commonest cause although less so than in the past. Probably accounts for 40% cases now. They are a heterogeneous group including *S. milleri, S. oralis, S. mitis, S. mitior, S. mutans, S. salivarius* and other oral streptococci. *S. milleri* is present in mouth gut and vagina. It tends to form abscesses more frequently than other types.
• *Streptococcus bovis*. A normal inhabitant of the gut. Similar to the *viridans* group in its sensitivity to penicillin. May be associated with malignant or inflammatory bowel disease.
• *Enterococcus faecalis* and *Enterococcus faecium*. Approximately 10% cases. Usually in the elderly.
• *Staphylococcus aureus*. ⎫
• *Staphylococcus epidermidis*. ⎬ ⎫ approximately 25% cases
• Diptheroid bacilli. ⎬ especially postcardiac
• Microaerophilic streptococci. ⎭ surgery
• Much rarer bacteria can cause infective endocarditis, often with an insidious course and a long period of mild symptoms: e.g.
HACEK group of gram-negative bacilli (*Haemophilus–Actinobacillus–Cardiobacterium–Fikenella–Kingella*). Also called HB group of bacilli. Fastidious organisms requiring prolonged culture in 10% CO_2.
Anaerobic Gram-negative bacilli: *Fusobacterium, Bacteroides, Streptobacillus moniliformis, Propionibacterium acnes, Listeria monocytogenes, Brucella abortus, Legionella* and many others.
• *Coxiella burneti* (Q fever).
• *Chlamydia psittaci, Chlamydia trachomatis*.

Fungal

Candida, Aspergillus, Histoplasma.

Other organisms

? Viral infection (as yet unproven).

 Diagnosis and physical signs

An awareness of the possibility of infective endocarditis is vital, as the condition may occur in the absence of a fever or a murmur initially, especially if the patient is elderly or has received recent antibiotic therapy.

Infective endocarditis is also the great mimic, for the wide variety of physical signs may be mistaken for conditions as diverse as a collagen vascular disease, rheumatic fever, a non-specific viral infection, a primary neurological condition, mild haemolytic anaemia, left atrial myxoma or brucellosis.

Presentation

Typically the condition presents with:
* *Signs of infection.* Fever, night sweats, rigors. Weight loss and general malaise. Anaemia is expected. With chronic untreated infection there is additional clubbing and splenomegaly.
* *Signs and symptoms of immune complex deposition.* Microscopic haematuria is common and there may be frank glomerulonephritis. A generalized vasculitis can affect any vessel (e.g. brain, skin, kidneys, etc.). A toxic encephalopathy may occur. Retinal haemorrhages are common (flame- or boat-shaped). Roth spots (boat-shaped haemorrhages with a pale centre) on the retina occur in more fulminating or in untreated cases. Splinter haemorrhages on finger or toe nails. Arthralgia. Osler's nodes – painful pulp infarcts on fingers or toes, or on palms or soles. Janeway lesions – less common than Osler's nodes: painless flat erythema on palms or soles.
* *Signs of the cardiac lesion.* A new murmur is very significant, as is a change in the nature of an existing murmur. Auscultation daily is necessary in patients with infective endocarditis. Mild aortic or mitral regurgitation may not be audible.
* *Emboli.* These may be followed by abscess formation in the relevant organ. Common sites are: cerebral, retinal, coronary, splenic, mesenteric, renal or femoropopliteal arteries. In patients with right-sided endocarditis, pulmonary infarcts are often followed by lung

abscesses. A mycotic aneurysm may follow a cerebral embolus and present with subarachnoid haemorrhage. Possibly Osler's nodes have an embolic element also. Large emboli are common in fungal endocarditis. Embolic events may occur during or after antibiotic treatment, even in an apparently 'cured' case. Secondary abscess formation prevents bacteriological cure.

• *Complications of valve destruction or abscess formation.* This may result in increasingly severe valve regurgitation. Abscess formation can result in the dehiscence of the prosthetic valve sewing ring. A septal abscess (e.g. aortic valve endocarditis) produces a long PR interval leading to complete AV block. Aortic root abscesses may produce a sinus of Valsalva aneurysm, or involve the coronary ostia. Large fleshy vegetations may cause valve obstruction (e.g. aortic fungal endocarditis).

• *Left ventricular failure.* This is one of the commonest causes of death in infective endocarditis. Primary involvement of the myocardium occurs with reduction in contractility and non-specific ST–T-wave changes on the ECG. There may be an associated pericardial effusion or even pyopericardium. Left ventricular failure is exacerbated by additional valve dysfunction.

Investigations

• Three blood cultures from different venous sites at different times and at peak fever; 85–90% of cases will be cultured in this way

There is little point in performing arterial or marrow cultures if venous blood cultures are negative. Approximately 10% of cases are culture negative. Blood should also be cultured through a CVP line if there is one *in situ.* The CVP line is then removed and the tip cultured

• Routine full blood count and ESR. Normally the condition is associated with an anaemia, neutrophil leucocytosis and high ESR. None of these are absolute. A rising haemoglobin and falling ESR are useful signs of therapeutic success. Routine biochemistry, liver function tests, creatinine.

• CRP (C-reactive protein). An acute-phase protein released by the liver in response to cytokines from activated macrophages. Rises acutely with bacterial infection (much less with viral). A falling CRP is a good sign of infection coming under control.

• Microscopy of fresh urine for red cells. Microscopic haematuria is common early in the disease and should regress during treatment. Mid-stream urine analysis if indicated.

• Swabs of any skin lesion, drip site. Nasal swab.

- Dental X-rays. Orthopantomogram + special views as indicated.
- ECG and CXR at regular intervals (at least weekly).
- A lengthening PR interval on the ECG suggests an aortic root and septal abscess.
- Weekly echocardiography. Vegetations are not visualized until > 2 mm in size. Colour Doppler with transthoracic echocardiography is best for the identification of aortic regurgitation, a septal abscess or an acquired VSD. Transoesophageal echocardiography (TOE) is very useful for visualizing mitral valve vegetations, leaflet perforation and the possible development of an aortic root abscess which untreated becomes a root mycotic aneurysm. A subaortic LVOTO aneurysm will only be picked up by TOE. TOE with colour Doppler will identify an LVOTO to RA fistula. An example of vegetations on a native mitral and tricuspid valve is seen in Figure 9.1.
- Immune complex titres.

Culture negative endocarditis

About 10% of infective endocarditis may be culture negative.
Five reasons in order of probability are:

1 Previous antibiotic therapy. The longer the course of antibiotics prior to blood cultures the more likely the chance of cultures being negative. If the condition remains untreated, re-seeding of the blood may occur after several weeks from organisms still alive in the centre of the vegetations. Even a single dose of an antibiotic may result initially in negative cultures.

2 Wrong diagnosis. In culture negative cases it is important to think of alternative diagnoses and re-examine the patient. Many conditions mimic infective endocarditis: particularly collagen vascular disease, polymyalgia rheumatica, malignant disease, atrial myxoma, sarcoid, drug reaction, etc. There may be a non-cardiac infection in a patient who has a heart murmur, or there may be non-infective endocarditis (see **9.8**).

3 Fastidious organisms that require special culture media and conditions, e.g. organisms from the HACEK group (CO_2 incubation), nutritionally-dependent streptococci (*S. defectivus* and *S. adjacens* needing cysteine- or pyridoxine-enriched medium), *Brucella*, *Legionella*, *Neisseria*, L-forms or anaerobes.

4 Cell-dependent organisms, e.g. *Coxiella burneti* (Q-fever), *Chlamydia psittaci* or *C. trachomatis*. Check Q-fever and *Chlamydia* complement-fixing antibodies.

5 Fungi: consider especially in chronically sick patients who are

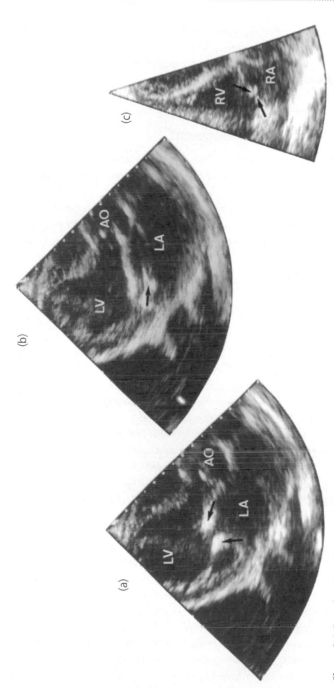

Figure 9.1 Transthoracic echocardiogram in infective endocarditis. (a) Diastolic frame of long axis view showing large vegetations on the mitral leaflets (arrowed). (b) Systolic frame of same patient showing prolapsing of the posterior mitral leaflet (arrowed). There was severe mitral regurgitation. (c) Apical four-chamber view of right heart showing small vegetations on tricuspid valve (arrowed).

immunosuppressed, who have been on prolonged intravenous feeding and those with prosthetic heart valves. Check *Aspergillus* precipitins and *Candida* antibodies. Most cases of endocarditis will have a raised titre to *Candida* antibodies (anamnestic response). A rising titre is more important.

9.5 Treatment management

There is nothing to be gained by waiting to see if cultures are positive. If the condition is suspected and investigations have been performed, treatment should start immediately.

If dental extractions are required these are ideally performed at the start of the course of antibiotics. This is not always practical and additional antibiotic cover is usually required in the middle of an established course. Culturing teeth is rarely useful as a large spectrum of oral flora results.

If a systemic embolus occurs it should be cultured and examined for hyphae.

Route

Intravenous therapy is essential initially. The choice rests between central and peripheral lines. Both have their advantages and must be inserted with strict aseptic techniques.

The central line (subclavian or internal jugular) should be changed weekly. The best central line is a tunnelled subclavian inserted via the infraclavicular route. The tunnel helps prevent spread of infection from the skin entry site. A tunnelled subclavian line does not require changing weekly if the entry site looks clean and it should last the whole antibiotic course with careful management.The catheter should be soft, pliable and not reach as far as the right atrium. The catheter in RA or SVC may cause infected mural thrombus. A stiff central line in the right atrium may perforate the wall. The central line skin entry site should be covered by a steri-drape (e.g. 'Opsite'). Covering with other dressings is not advised and povidone iodine on the entry site does not prevent infection.

Peripheral lines are less dangerous but more inconvenient and painful. The peripheral line should be changed every 72 hours if possible even if the vein has not thrombosed. This helps preserve the life of peripheral veins. The arm is immobilized, dilute antibiotic solution is used and a heparin flush (500 units in 5 ml 5% dextrose) given after each infusion helps preserve the vein.

The giving set should be changed daily with either system. For a patient on warfarin (e.g. mechanical prosthetic valves) a central line should not be inserted until the INR is < 2.0. Start with a peripheral line and i.v. heparin. Stop the warfarin temporarily. When the INR falls to < 2.0, insert central line and restart warfarin stopping the heparin when the INR > 2.5.

Length of course

There are no fixed rules. This depends on the patient's response to treatment, the sensitivity and nature of the organism, vegetation size on the echo, patient tolerance and drug access. There is a definite trend to shorter courses in sensitive 'friendly' organisms. The following are suggestions only.

- *Streptococcus viridans* group. If sensitive (MIC < 0.1 mg/l) 2 weeks i.v. therapy followed by 2 weeks oral amoxycillin. If insensitive, 4 weeks i.v. therapy.
- *Staphylococcus epidermidis*, 4–8 weeks i.v.
- *Staphylococcus aureus*, 4–8 weeks i.v.
- Q-fever, indefinite oral therapy.
- Fungal endocarditis, 3 months i.v. treatment followed by oral therapy.
- Prosthetic valve endocarditis. A minimum of 2 months' i.v. therapy should cure some cases. Most will need redo valve surgery, followed by a further month's i.v. treatment.

Choice of antibiotic regime

Once the diagnosis is considered likely treatment should be started before the blood culture results are known. Start with i.v. benzylpenicillin and gentamicin as detailed in section on penicillin-sensitive streptococci. If staphylococcal infection is likely (e.g. intravenous drug abusers or patients on haemodialysis) use vancomycin instead of penicillin. Always use at least two antibiotics for staphylococcal infection.

With a positive blood culture, guidance from a bacteriologist is essential, the choice depending on the organism antibiotic sensitivity. Antibiotic levels are necessary to check both the dose and the risk of toxicity (especially with the aminoglycosides and antifungal agents).

Plasma antibiotic levels are measured at trough (predose) and peak (15-min postintravenous dose). If the peak level is too high, the dose is reduced; if the trough level is too high, the interval between doses is increased.

Minimum inhibitory concentration (MIC) is estimated and provides a guide to dosage and drug choice. Therapy should aim to reach trough levels of at least 10 × MIC. In *Streptococcus viridans* infection if MIC is > 0.1 mg/l then the addition of an aminoglycoside to penicillin should be considered.

Do not stop treatment if the temperature fails to settle within a few days. This may take 2 weeks even with drug-sensitive organisms, but is more likely with large vegetations or abscess formation. If fever persists:

• check sensitivity of organism and drug levels
• echocardiography to check possible change in size of vegetations, aortic root or septal abscess
• other possible sources of fever
• consider adding another synergistic antibiotic
• surgery should be considered early for cases with persisting fever resistant to medical therapy.

A bactericidal antibiotic is used except in rare circumstances: tetracycline therapy in Q-fever endocarditis and high-dose erythromycin if there is penicillin and cephalosporin allergy. Probenecid is sometimes used to maintain high plasma amoxycillin levels when a patient is converted to oral therapy from i.v. penicillin.

The clinical response is a most useful guide to therapy. The regimes set out below are the doses suggested in a 70-kg adult with normal renal function. Doses must be reduced in smaller patients, elderly patients and those with renal failure.

All the antibiotic regimes listed below are by intravenous bolus injection unless otherwise specified, and are the shortest possible courses for the organisms discussed. Some patients may require longer courses depending on response to treatment. Gentamicin levels must be taken twice weekly with an 80 mg 12-hourly regime, and more often with an 8-hourly regime or if the serum creatinine is raised.

Antibiotics for patients not allergic to penicillin

Streptococcus viridans group and S. bovis (approximately 40% cases)

1 Fully sensitive to penicillin (MIC < 0.1 mg/l), with favourable conditions (see below):
Benzylpenicillin 1.2 g (2 MU) 4 hourly i.v. plus gentamicin 80 mg i.v. 12 hourly for 2 weeks. Followed by 2-weeks oral amoxycillin.
If this 2-week i.v. regime is to be considered there must be:

- no heart failure or conduction abnormalities
- no embolic phenomena
- native valve infection, not prosthetic
- small vegetations only
- response within 7 days of treatment with the temperature returning to normal.

2 Reduced sensitivity to penicillin (MIC > 0.1 mg/l) or less favourable conditions. Regime as in (1) above but continued for 4 weeks i.v. therapy.

Enterococci (approximately 10% cases)
Usually more resistant to penicillin than the *viridans* group (median MIC 2 mg/l).

1 Gentamicin sensitive (MIC < 100 mg/l).
Ampicillin or amoxycillin 2 g 4 hourly i.v. plus gentamicin 80 mg i v 12 hourly for 4 weeks.

2 Gentamicin highly resistant (MIC > 2000 mg/l).
Ampicillin or amoxycillin 2 g 4 hourly i.v. for at least 6 weeks.
Streptomycin may be added if the strain is sensitive to it.

Staphylococci
1 Penicillin sensitive (non-B-lactamase producers).
Benzylpenicillin 1.2 g (2 MU) i.v. for 4 weeks.
Plus fusidic acid 500 mg orally 8 hourly for 4 weeks.
Or plus gentamicin 80–120 mg 8 hourly for 1 week.

2 Methicillin sensitive (B-lactamase producers).
Flucloxacillin 2 g 4 hourly i.v. for 4 weeks.
Plus fusidic acid 500 mg orally 8 hourly for 4 weeks,
or plus gentamicin 80–120 mg 8 hourly for 1 week.

3 Methicillin resistant (B-lactamase producers and methicillin resistant).
Vancomycin initially 1 g by slow i.v. infusion over 100 min once or twice daily for 4 weeks. Blood levels determine dose. Aim for trough levels 5–10-mg/l and peak levels taken 1 hour post-dose up to 30 mg/l.
Plus fusidic acid 500-mg hourly orally for 4 weeks,
or plus gentamicin 80–120 mg 8 hourly for 1 week.

Antibiotics for patients allergic to penicillin

Streptococcus viridans group, S. bovis and enterococci
Either:
Teicoplanin 400 mg i.v. 12 hourly for three injections, followed by

400-mg i.v. daily for 4 weeks, plus gentamicin 80 mg i.v. twice daily for 2 weeks (*S. viridans* group and *S. bovis*) or 4 weeks (enterococci) or:

Vancomycin 1 g by i.v. infusion over 100 min once or twice daily for 4 weeks. Adjust dose to achieve trough levels of 5–10 mg/l and peak levels 1 hour postinfusion of about 30 mg/l, plus gentamicin regime as detailed with teicoplanin above.

Staphylococci

Vancomycin 1 g by i.v. infusion over 100 min once or twice daily for 4 weeks. Blood levels as detailed above for streptococci. Plus fusidic acid 500 mg 8 hourly orally for 4 weeks and/or gentamicin 80–120 mg 8 hourly for I week.

Gram-negative organisms

Ampicillin 2–4 g i.v. 6 hourly.

Gentamicin 80 mg i.v. 8 hourly initially.

Metronidazole 500 mg i.v. 8 hourly is added for uncontrolled anaerobic organisms (e.g. *Fusobacterium* or *Bacteroides endocarditis*).

Q fever (Coxiella burneti)

There are no rickettsiacidal drugs. Treatment should be regarded as indefinite if the drug regime is tolerated, as *Coxiella* may survive for years in the liver. Early surgery is advisable. Start drug treatment with doxycycline 100 mg bd orally plus either co-trimoxazole, rifampicin or a quinolone (e.g. ciprofloxacin). Monitoring successful therapy is difficult. Complement levels are unhelpful, the serum IgM levels may stay up with successful treatment, but the Phase 1 antibody titre should gradually fall.

Candida albicans or other yeast organisms

Large fleshy vegetations occur and tend to embolize, causing metastatic infection. Myocardial invasion occurs. Again early surgery is advised. Start treatment with 5-fluorocytosine (flucytosine) 3 g i.v. 6 hourly (50 mg/kg 6 hourly). Marrow depression and hepatic necrosis are the most dangerous side-effects. If flucytosine resistance develops add amphotericin B 250 µg/kg/day initially, increasing if renal function is satisfactory. Miconazole 600 mg i.v. 8 hourly is an alternative if renal function is poor. Oral fluconazole 50 mg daily is substituted after a successful course of i.v. treatment and surgery and continued for some months as late relapse may occur.

Aspergillus or other non-yeast fungi

This is rarely diagnosed in time and medical treatment alone is never successful. Early surgery is the only hope. Amphotericin B 250 µg/kg/day or miconazole 600 mg i.v. 8 hourly if poor renal function. Oral itraconazole 100 mg od for a month may be used following an i.v. course of amphotericin. It may in time prove more effective than amphotericin B. Where possible, fungal endocarditis should be treated with two drugs.

Recurrent fever during treatment

Fever recurrence after an initial successful period of medical therapy can pose a diagnostic problem. Four common reasons are:
- Development of the patient's sensitivity to an antibiotic. Most commonly with penicillin, but may occur with any antibiotic. Check for proteinuria and eosinophilia. Neutropenia is common. An interstitial nephritis may develop. The fever, nephritis and eosinophilia usually disappear rapidly if the antibiotic is stopped.
- Development of antibiotic resistance. Possible if the MIC is high and inadequate doses of the antibiotic are used initially. Change of antibiotic regime needed.
- Additional or uncontrolled infection. Remove central line if present and culture tip. Check chest, urine, etc. Consider occult pulmonary emboli (especially with tricuspid endocarditis), enlarging vegetations (on echo) or hidden abscess formation (e.g. around aortic root, septum or haematogenous spread to abdomen). Check abdominal ultrasound. (e.g. ? hepatic or renal abscess)
- Diagnosis still wrong. Consider other possibilities, e.g malignant disease or collagen vascular disease.

Antimicrobial side-effects and other problems

Penicillin

Allergy (fever, urticaria, arthralgia, rash); angioneurotic oedema; interstitial nephritis; sodium loading; encephalopathy; hypokalaemic alkalosis; neutropenia.

The last four are dose-dependent side-effects, usually quickly reversible on stopping the drug. They are rare, and are possible if > 24 g/day penicillin is used. With a history of penicillin allergy there is roughly a 10% chance of cross-sensitivity to cephalosporins.

Fusidic acid

Nausea and vomiting, jaundice and hepatotoxicity, microbial resistance.

Nausea and vomiting are very common, even with i.v. therapy, and may make it impossible to use the drug. Liver damage is reversible if the drug is stopped early. Microbial resistance develops quickly if the drug is used alone.

Aminoglycosides

Ototoxicity, nephrotoxicity.

About 10% of patients on these drugs develop VIIIth nerve damage. If long-term treatment is required, weekly audiometry is essential with calorics to detect early damage. Either the vestibular or auditory component may be damaged first or in isolation. High-frequency deafness may occur early without the patient noticing any side-effects. Beware the patient using the drip pole as a support, concealing ataxia. The suggested dose schedule is shown below. Doses are reduced in renal impairment.

Nephrotoxicity is exacerbated by concomitant use of frusemide, ethacrynic acid, cephaloridine and possibly some other cephalosporins. Frequent tests of renal function are necessary (serum creatinine three times per week). The urine is tested daily for protein, and urine microscopy performed to look for casts at regular intervals.

Guide to gentamicin dosage

There is a move to use lower doses of gentamicin. This helps avoid ototoxicity and expensive litigation. The drug is synergistic with penicillin and still very valuable at low serum levels.

• Adults with normal renal function: 80 mg i.v. 12 hourly initially. Adults < 60 kg in weight use 60 mg i.v. 12 hourly.

• Children with normal renal function: 3 mg/kg i.v. initially followed by 2 mg/kg i.v. 12 hourly.

• With renal impairment dose is reduced. Until drug levels are known dose is regulated corresponding to blood urea levels:

7–17 mmol/l: 80 mg 12 hourly

17–33 mmol/l: 80 mg daily

> 33 mmol/l: 80 mg alternate days or less

• Drug levels. Blood for these is taken from the opposite arm if a peripheral line is used. They are performed initially on the third day of treatment.

Trough level: taken just prior to gentamicin dose. The trough level is the most important measurement of all and must always be < 2 μg/ml.

Levels of 2–5 µg/ml mean drug accumulation and the dose interval should be increased.

Peak level: taken 15 min after i.v. dose. The level should be < 10 µg/ml. Preferably 6–10 µg/ml. The dose is reduced if the level exceeds this.

It is safest to restrict gentamicin therapy to just the first 2 weeks of treatment if possible.

Other drugs of great value in bacterial cases

1 *Amikacin:* in gentamicin-resistant cases. Dose 15 mg/kg/day in two doses 12 hourly.

2 *Tobramycin:* in mild renal impairment, as it is less nephrotoxic than gentamicin. Up to 5 mg/kg/day 8–12 hourly (similar to gentamicin).

3 *Vancomycin:* caution in any degree of uraemia. May be used as a single antibiotic. Maximum adult dose 2 g/day. Start with 500 mg i.v. 6 hourly. May be reduced to as little as 1 g/week in uraemia associated with endocarditis. Infusion may cause histamine release and the red man syndrome.

4 *Rifampicin:* not just an antituberculous drug, but toxicity in 20% of cases. Shock, renal failure, thrombocytopenia, hepatotoxicity, influenzal and respiratory symptoms. Oral therapy 450–600 mg daily before breakfast.

5 *Netilmicin:* this drug is less ototoxic than gentamicin or tobramycin and may supersede both. Dose for average size adult with normal renal function: 150 mg i.v. 12 hourly (total 4–6 mg/kg/day).

6 *Teicoplanin:* can be given as a once-daily dose either i.m. or preferably i.v. as 400 mg. It is much less ototoxic and nephrotoxic than aminoglycosides. It is particularly useful for *Staphylococcus epidermidis* and in combination with rifampicin for penicillin-resistant or hypersensitive cases. May also cause histamine release (similar to vancomycin).

Second-line drugs

1 *Lincomycin and clindamycin:* very effective in staphylococcal (and some anaerobic) infections. Pseudomembranous colitis limits their use. If it develops, vancomycin is effective given orally.

2 *Cephalosporin group:* may be useful in penicillin hypersensitivity. Nephrotoxicity a reputed problem with many and concomitant aminoglycoside use best avoided.

3 *Erythromycin:* bacteriostatic in low doses. May be useful in penicillin hypersensitivity.

Nephrotoxicity guide with antibiotic use in endocarditis

Antibiotic	Renal excretion	Site of damage	? Use in renal disease
Pencillin G	90% proximal tubular secretion	*Rare* Hypokalaemic alkalosis Hypersensitivity Interstitial nephritis	Yes, with dose reduction 1–2 g 6 hourly
Gentamicin	All glomerular filtration	Tubular necrosis 2–10% Binds to renal tissue	Yes, with great care taking drug levels Cephalosporins probably best avoided
Tobramycin	All glomerular filtration	Tubular necrosis in 1–2% Less than gentamicin	Safer than gentamicin in renal damage
Vancomycin	80% renal excretion	None	Yes, with dose reduction levels, from 1 g/day to 1 g/week
Amikacin	95% renal excretion	Probably similar to gentamicin	As with gentamicin levels
Cephalothin	70–80% renal excretion	Tubular necrosis	Aminoglycosides probably best avoided. Care in renal disease
Cephaloridine	85% renal excretion	Tubular necrosis	Avoid
Tetracyclines	Principally renal excretion	'Anti-anabolic effect' increases uraemia Old tetracyclines: Fanconi's syndrome	Avoid (except doxycycline)
Fusidic acid	Principally biliary excretion	None in kidney	Yes, no dose adjustment necessary
Amphotericin B	Slow renal excretion	Reduces renal blood flow (arteriolar constriction) Nephrocalcinosis, tubular damage: renal tubular acidosis, potassium wasting	Reduce dose (e.g. 0.25 mg/kg alternate days)

4 *Chloramphenicol:* best avoided in long courses unless desperate. Causes leucopenia, thrombocytopenia, irreversible aplastic anaemia, peripheral and optic neuritis, gut side-effects, erythema multiforme.

Monitoring therapy effects

1 Daily patient examination. The most important of all to detect new signs.

2 Daily weighing.

3 Six-hourly temperature chart.

4 Daily urine testing. Microscopy for RBCs and casts.

5 FBC, U and E and LFTs twice weekly as minimum. A steady or rising haemoglobin and falling CRP and ESR are good signs. The ESR is often the last variable to return to normal after a long antibiotic course in infective endocarditis. It may only return to normal a month or so after the course has finished. The CRP falls more quickly.

6 Antibiotic drug levels.

7 Weekly echocardiogram. Although vegetations are frequently not seen on the echo, a gradual change in valve configuration may be detected.

9.6 Other interventions and infective endocarditis

Anticoagulants and endocarditis

This is controversial with the risk of haemorrhage at the site of embolus impaction (e.g. mycotic embolus and subarachnoid or intracerebral haemorrhage). Anticoagulation does not prevent the development of vegetations.

It is best reserved for: patients with prosthetic (non-tissue) valves, pelvic vein thrombosis or gross deep-vein thrombosis, pulmonary embolism. Patients with mixed mitral valve disease and endocarditis already on anticoagulants should be continued on anticoagulants with a control INR of 2 : 1 approximately.

Cardiac catheterization

This is usually not necessary and was once thought to be absolutely contraindicated with the risk of dislodging friable vegetations. However, it may be useful in cases of aortic valve endocarditis with suspected abscess formation to obtain more information about the anatomy of the root by an aortogram with the catheter well above the valve. Also the significance of mitral regurgitation in the course of infective endocarditis may require cardiac catheterization with left ventricular angiography. Intravenous digital subtraction angiography of the aortic root can provide information about possible aortic root abscesses. Transoesophageal echocardiography is invaluable and obviates the need for aortography (page 487) in most cases.

Indications for surgical intervention
- Failure of antibiotics to control infection.
- Increasing valve regurgitation or destruction.
- Large fleshy vegetations, or increasing vegetation size on echocardiography.
- Valve obstruction due to vegetations.
- Lengthening of the PR interval: septal abscess formation.
- Paravalve abscess on echocardiography.
- Development of an aneurysm of the sinus of Valsalva.
- Endocarditis due to *Staphylococcus aureus*, Q-fever and most fungal cases.
- Systemic emboli.
- Most cases of prosthetic valve endocarditis.
- Relapse of infection after a full course of medical treatment.

If possible, a few days' antibiotics are given prior to surgery, but in very severe cases this may be only a few doses.

After valve replacement for infective endocarditis a full course of medical therapy should be given, of a length detailed earlier.

9.7 Prevention of infective endocarditis

Much of the evidence on which recommendations are made is based on animal work. The American Heart Association's recommendations of 1977 have been modified to allow a simpler regime, which is more likely to be followed. This prophylaxis is necessary for:
- any dental work
- any surgical procedure
- cystoscopy and urinary tract instrumentation
- prostatic biopsy (transrectal)
- insertion of permanent pacemakers.

Prophylaxis is not necessary prior to cardiac catheterization. There is no hard evidence that it is necessary prior to gastroscopy or sigmoidoscopy, but is advisable. Normally used prior to rectal or colonic biopsy and also prior to delivery.

It is safer to advise patients to have antibiotic prophylaxis prior to every dental appointment. If several visits to the dentist are required,

....

the same antibiotic regime should not be used within a month. Patients should be urged to visit the dentist regularly. The use of chlorhexidine gel (1%) applied to the gingival margin or chlorhexidine mouthwash (0.2%) 5 min prior to the dental work should reduce the severity of the

Antibiotic cover for patients with congenital heart disease or acquired valve disease receiving dental treatment or any operative procedure

1 Without anaesthetic or under local anaesthesia
Amoxycillin 3 g orally 1 hour before procedure.
For patients allergic to penicillin or who have had amoxycillin in the last month:
Either:
Clindamycin 600 mg as a single dose 1 hour before procedure.
or:
Erythromycin stearate 1.5 g orally before procedure plus 0.5 g 6 hours later. The 1.5 g dose may cause nausea and the single dose of clindamycin is better tolerated.

For children:
Age 5–10 years half adult dose for all three drugs above.
Age under 5 years: quarter of the adult dose.

2 Under general anaesthetic
Ampicillin 1 g i.v. with premedication (or amoxycillin 1 g in 2.5 ml 1% lignocaine i.m.) plus 0.5 g orally 6 hours later.
For patients allergic to penicillin or who have had amoxycillin or ampicillin in the last month:
Either:
Vancomycin 1 g slowly i.v. over 100 min plus gentamicin 120 mg i.v. just before induction.
or:
Teicoplanin 400 mg i.v. plus gentamicin 120 mg i.v. just before induction. This is the easiest regime.
or:
Clindamycin 300 mg in 50 ml N-saline over 10 min i.v. just before induction followed by clindamycin 150 mg orally or by i.v. injection over 10 min 6 hours later. This is not suitable for patients undergoing pelvic instrumentation, genitourinary or gastrointestinal procedures.

For children
Either:
Vancomycin 20 mg/kg plus gentamicin 2 mg/kg i.v.
or:
Clindamycin 150 mg i.v. (age 5–10 years) or 75 mg i.v. (age under 5 years) diluted as above.

3 Special risk patients
Patients with prosthetic heart valves or history of previous infective endocarditis.
Ampicillin 1 g plus gentamicin 120 mg i.v. with premedication plus amoxycillin 0.5 g orally at 6 hours.
For penicillin allergy use regime under **2** above.

bacteraemia. Intraligamental injections of local anaesthetics should be avoided as the high-pressure (0.2%) 5 min prior to the dental work

The regime shown in the table (page 391) is based on the recommendations of the endocarditis working party of the British Society for Antimicrobial Chemotherapy.

9.8 Non-infective endocarditis

Non-infective thrombotic endocarditis (marantic endocarditis)

Non-infective vegetations may occur on heart valves. This is sometimes called marantic endocarditis. They may, if large, be identified on echocardiography (> 5 mm in size) and may embolize. They occur in:
- mucinous adenocarcinomas of pancreas, lung and upper gastrointestinal tract
- other malignant disease, e.g. bladder, lung and lymphomas
- associated with a thrombotic tendency and peripheral microthrombi in small vessels in adult respiratory distress syndrome.

In cases of malignant disease there may be an associated migratory thrombophlebitis, disseminated intravascular coagulation and microangiopathic haemolytic anaemia. Often the condition is only discovered at autopsy.

Libman–Sacks endocarditis

First described in 1924 as an active verrucous endocarditis with verrucae or vegetations commonly affecting the aortic or mitral valves, chordae, papillary muscles and ventricular endocardium. Occasionally the tricuspid valve may be involved. It occurs as part of the spectrum of organ involvement of systemic lupus erythematosus (SLE) and, rarely, scleroderma. As with non-infective endocarditis, valve regurgitation is uncommon and the condition may only be diagnosed at autopsy (in ≤ 50% of cases of SLE). The vegetations are small and may be missed on echocardiography. They are much more likely in patients who have antiphospholipid antibodies in their serum. Valve cusps contain a large amount of mucopolysaccharide and it has been suggested that steroid therapy may be implicated.

Although valve involvement is common, severe valve regurgitation is not. Occasionally valve replacement is required.

10.1 Pulmonary hypertension (PHT)

Pulmonary hypertension exists when PA pressure exceeds 30/20 mmHg. Due either to an increase in flow through pulmonary vascular bed or to a reduction in calibre of pulmonary arterioles.

Common causes
• Left atrial hypertension: aortic and mitral valve disease, ischaemic heart disease, dilated cardiomyopathy, hypertrophic cardiomyopathy.
• Chronic pulmonary disease: chronic bronchitis and emphysema, pulmonary fibrosis.
• Chronic thromboembolism.
• High flow-reactive PHT, e.g. ASD, VSD, PDA.

Rare causes
• Primary pulmonary hypertension.
• Left atrial conditions: myxoma, cor triatriatum.
• Pulmonary veno-occlusive disease, pulmonary vein stenoses.
• Peripheral pulmonary artery branch stenoses.
• Chronic hypoxia: Pickwickian syndrome, high altitude, pharyngeal obstruction, neuromuscular disorders, e.g. polio, myasthenia.
• Restrictive cardiomyopathy and constrictive pericarditis.

There is a considerable fall in pulmonary vascular resistance in the first 24 hours of life when the ductus closes and the PVR continues to fall for the first few months.

Chronic PHT is associated with intimal thickening ('onion skinning') of pulmonary arterioles and medial hypertrophy in larger arteries. Vessels may be totally occluded by the endothelial proliferation and secondary thrombosis occurs.

Variability of PHT
Various factors may alter pulmonary artery pressure and these are relevant to treatment. The most important is the role of oxygen in regulating pulmonary vascular tone.

Increasing PHT	Decreasing PHT
Hypoxia, high altitude	Oxygen
Acidosis	Acetylcholine
Hypercapnia	Hydralazine
High haematocrit	Alpha-blocking agents
Prostaglandin $F_{2\alpha}$ and A_2	Prostaglandin E and I_2
? Histamine	Pirbuterol
Alpha-agonists	Calcium antagonists
	Nitrates, nitric oxide

Elevated haematocrit is important in patients with cyanotic congenital heart disease and the Eisenmenger syndrome.

10.2 Pulmonary embolism

Symptoms

• Dyspnoea. Acute-onset dyspnoea is typical. In retrospect mild dyspnoea may precede the acute attack by a day or two. In a few cases dyspnoea presents as acute bronchospasm.
• Pain. Sudden-onset pleuritic chest pain probably occurs with smaller emboli. Involvement of the diaphragmatic pleura causes shoulder-tip pain. Pain may be primarily abdominal.
• Cough. Persistent dry cough is common.
• Haemoptysis. Streaky or frank. Haemoptysis may persist with resolution of the infarcted segment.
• Sweating, fear and apprehension.
• Syncope occurs with massive pulmonary embolism. Pre-syncope and transient episodes of hypotension may occur with smaller ones. Overall mortality is approximately 8–10%.

Signs

A restless, centrally cyanosed, sweaty, distressed and dyspnoeic patient.
JVP raised with prominent 'a' wave if in SR.
Tachycardia, low-volume pulse, transient rhythm disturbance.
RV: $S_{3/4}$ gallop.
Accentuated delayed P_2.
Fever.
Chest signs: rales, later a pleural rub.
Leg signs: only about one-third of patients have evidence of deep-vein
    thrombosis (DVT) with phlebitis, oedema, etc.
Cardiac arrest and sudden death.
   Many of these signs are non-specific and a high index of suspicion should be maintained for patients at risk, e.g.
• history of previous DVTs
• patients on prolonged bed rest
• post-myocardial infarction (page 205)
• patients on diuretics – haemoconcentration
• patients with CCF – low flows
• post-operative patients: especially pelvic, prostatic, hip and leg surgery
• polycythaemic patients

- pelvic inflammatory or malignant disease
- prolonged travel: lengthy flight or train journey.

Smaller pulmonary emboli may be missed clinically, presenting as a flick in the temperature chart, mild dyspnoea and transient AF, SVT or just ventricular ectopic beats.

ECG changes (not specific for pulmonary embolism)

Typical acute right ventricular strain shows as: S_1 Q_3 T_3 pattern in standard leads, incomplete or complete RBBB, T wave inversion in anterior chest leads (see Figure 12.8).

Other possibilities to note: right axis shift. Rhythm changes: ectopic – atrial or ventricular, AF or SVT. ST–T changes with ST depression over inferior leads. All these may be transient.

Chest X-ray changes

There may be very little to see on the CXR of patients with small pulmonary emboli.

Features to look for include in the acute stage: elevated hemidiaphragm, pulmonary oligaemia in one or more segments, large pulmonary artery conus or enlargement of a single hilar artery with rapid pruning or tapering.

Later on (from 24 hours to 1 week) if pulmonary infarction occurs the CXR may show: pulmonary infiltrates, plate atelectasis, small pleural effusions or pleural thickening.

Super-added infection in an infarcted segment may cause cavitation.

Echocardiography

In acute pulmonary embolism will show a dilated RV. Doppler estimation of the PA pressure will be possible if good images are obtained and tricuspid regurgitation is present (see page 478).

Making the diagnosis

This may be difficult. Small emboli may be easily missed. Diagnosis is based on the following factors.

- Patient at risk.
- History and physical signs.
- ECG and CXR.
- *Blood gases:* the Po_2 should be < 80 mmHg (< 10.6 kPa) due to ventilation/perfusion (V/Q) mismatch. Large pulmonary emboli result in severe hypoxia, hypocapnia and metabolic acidosis – a 'mixed' picture.
- *Ventilation/perfusion scan:* this is a useful test for recurrent small emboli that may be missed by pulmonary angiography. The ventilation

scan must be normal. The diagnosis is difficult in the presence of chronic obstructive airways disease, severe emphysema or bronchopneumonia. Segmental perfusion defects in the presence of normal ventilation scan are strongly suggestive of pulmonary emboli.

Tomography of the perfusion study in various planes is useful. The CXR should be available to the interpreter of the scan. Follow up scans may show rapid resolution of the perfusion defects due to lysis of the thrombus.

• *Pulmonary angiography:* this is generally performed in the sicker patient in whom the diagnosis is still uncertain or who will probably require streptokinase therapy as the catheter can be left in the PA for 48–72 hours following angiography if necessary.

Angiograms should show vessel 'cut-offs' or obvious filling defects in the artery. There should be segmental filling defects in addition. Chronic thrombo-embolic pulmonary hypertensive patients will have large proximal arteries with tortuous distal vessels with peripheral pruning.

• *Spiral CT Scanning with contrast:* a valuable alternative to pulmonary angiography.

Investigations of less value
• *Cardiac enzymes.* Pulmonary infarction causes elevation of LDH and sometimes SGOT and bilirubin.
• *Leg venograms,* [125]I fibrinogen scanning, Doppler ultrasonography. Tests to document peripheral leg vein thrombus merely prove an association. They cannot make a diagnosis of pulmonary emboli.

Differential diagnosis
The commonest condition to be confused with acute pulmonary embolism is inferior myocardial infarction. Both cause chest pain, elevated neck veins and similar ECG changes. Transmural inferior infarction causes ST-segment elevation, and pulmonary embolism more commonly causes ST-segment depression in inferior leads. Patients with inferior infarcts are generally not dyspnoeic.

Other causes of pulmonary hypertension should be considered.

10.3 Management of pulmonary embolism

The acute attack is managed with anticoagulation, and thrombolytic therapy in more severe cases. Pulmonary embolectomy is rarely necessary. Attention is then focused on preventive measures.

General measures

Oxygen and analgesia are usually required. The severe apprehension associated with large pulmonary emboli will require opiate analgesia.

Volume loading. In more severe cases plasma or colloid substitutes should be given even with a raised venous pressure. This may help increase right ventricular stroke volume in severely compromised patients. Start with 500 ml plasma and repeat if necessary.

Anticoagulation

This is all that is required with mild-to-moderate embolization as natural lysis occurs in the lung spontaneously. Heparin is not directly thrombolytic.

Heparin 10 000 units i.v. stat followed by heparin 5000 units i.v. 2–4 hourly. A continuous infusion of heparin probably reduces bleeding complications (dose = 1000 units/hour). After 1 week if no further emboli have occurred then oral anticoagulants are started and the heparin stopped 2 days later. Heparin dose is monitored by APTT estimations. Oral anticoagulants are continued for 3 months only in the first instance unless there are recurrent emboli.

Recurrent emboli are rare in patients treated with anticoagulation alone.

Thrombolytic therapy

This is reserved for more seriously ill patients who appear unlikely to survive 24–48 hours or who have two or more lobar arteries occluded on angiography.

Thrombolytic therapy has been shown to resolve emboli faster than heparin, to lower the pulmonary artery pressure more than heparin, and appearances on repeat pulmonary angiography and lung scanning show greater improvement with thrombolytic therapy than with heparin.

The improvement is greatest with massive pulmonary emboli. No trial has shown a greater reduction is mortality of thrombolytic therapy over heparin.

Urokinase or tPA are more expensive than streptokinase, but may be necessary if streptokinase reactions occur (fever, rashes and allergic reactions are more common with streptokinase).

Prior to streptokinase therapy, blood is taken for the following tests: full blood count, haematocrit; platelet count, INR, APTT, fibrinogen titre and FDPs. Tests are repeated during therapy (every 4 hours if possible).

For more details of thrombolytic agents and their action see **5.9**, page 194.

Streptokinase dose (Kabikinase, Streptase)

Hydrocortisone 100 mg i.v. stat. streptokinase 250 000 units in 100 ml N-saline infused into PA or peripheral vein over 30 min. Then: streptokinase 100 000 units hourly up to 72 hours maximum. Heparin is then gradually restarted over the next 12 hours.

The streptokinase dose is controlled by the fibrinogen titre. A titre falling below 1 : 4 in saline may require a decrease in streptokinase dose (e.g. by 50 000 units/hour). The thrombin time should be prolonged by two- to fourfold normal value.

The main control, however, is the clinical state. Prolonged thrombin times do not predict bleeding complications.

Complications of streptokinase

• Allergic reactions are common. Rise in temperature is expected; rashes and pruritus are common. Nausea, vomiting, flushing and headaches may occur. Acute hypotension may occur with the first dose. Hydrocortisone and volume replacement are necessary.
• Bleeding complications. Local bleeding at catheter entry sites is expected, and a fall in haemoglobin is common on treatment. Heparin increases the bleeding risk. Pressure on a local bleeding site is all that is generally necessary. A pledget soaked in EACA (ε-aminocaproic acid) may help.

Streptokinase is stopped with major bleeding complications and fibrinogen replacement started (fresh frozen plasma, cryoprecipitate or fresh blood).

The effects on stopping are usually reversed after 1–2 hours when emergency surgery could be contemplated if absolutely necessary. In a desperate situation with continued bleeding, fibrinolytic inhibitors (EACA) or kallikrein inactivator (Trasylol) can be tried.

Contraindications to streptokinase

See **5.9**.

Urokinase (Abbokinase, Ukidan)

If this is available and streptokinase has produced unacceptable side-effects or there has been a known recent streptococcal illness, urokinase can be substituted (it is not antigenic). Urokinase

4400 i.u./kg/hour infusion over 12 hours. Approximately 15 ml solution/hour, up to 200 ml.

Fibrin-specific thrombolytic agents (see 5.9)

rt-PA and APSAC are two fibrin-specific thrombolytic agents with fewer bleeding complications than streptokinase. They are used primarily for coronary thrombolysis, but they should also be considered for patients with large pulmonary emboli who have had streptokinase in the past with the persistence of neutralizing antibodies.

Pulmonary embolectomy

This is rarely necessary. It carries a high mortality (23–57%) in various series especially if the operation is performed very early. (Two-thirds of patients who die from pulmonary embolism do so in the first 2 hours anyway.) Surgical mortality is lower if no cardiac arrest has occurred.

It should be considered in patients with cardiogenic shock who: have had 1 hour maximum medical therapy; in whom streptokinase is contraindicated; or who are unlikely to survive the next hour.

Cardiac massage should be prolonged in an arrest due to massive pulmonary embolism as it may help to fragment the thrombus. Pulmonary embolectomy can only remove large proximal thrombus, while streptokinase may in addition deal with smaller peripheral thrombi.

Prevention of pulmonary emboli

Low-dose subcutaneous heparin has been shown in several trials to prevent pulmonary emboli following surgery (e.g. 5000 units s.c. 2 hours pre-operatively, then 5000 units s.c. 8 hourly for 7 days). A combination of dextran 70 given at the end of surgery plus the use of pneumatic leggings has also been shown to reduce postoperative pulmonary emboli. Early mobilization is vital.

Most cases of recurrences of pulmonary emboli will be prevented by oral anticoagulants.

Various operations on the IVC below the renal veins have attempted to prevent PE (plication, ligation, filters, umbrellas, etc.). This is only of temporary benefit as large collateral channels rapidly develop. It may be life saving in rare instances.

10.4 Anticoagulants in pregnancy

This is covered in detail under section on prosthetic valves, **3.8**, page 112.

10.5 Primary pulmonary hypertension

Described in 1950 by Paul Wood, this is a rare disease: annual incidence approximately 1 per 200 000 to 1 000 000 population. It is commoner in young women. Endothelial dysfunction has been identified in primary pulmonary hypertension, either as a cause or effect. Lung biopsies have shown reduced expression of nitric oxide synthase (and hence endothelium-derived relaxinant factor, EDRF), reduced levels of prostacyclin (PGI_2) and increased endothelin-1, all contributing to hypertrophy and thrombus in the microvasculature. Larger central vessels may also contain thrombus.

Clinical factors implicated include: chronic small pulmonary emboli; collagen vascular disease (association with Raynaud's phenomenon); allergic vasculitis (polyarteritis nodosa; drugs (aminorex fumarate, an anorexic agent); bush tea – *Crotalaria fulva*, alkaloid ingestion by West Indians; hormonal influences (female sex predominance, association with the Pill, presentation during or after pregnancy, etc.); association with cirrhosis.

Symptoms are similar to patients with pulmonary emboli; increasing dyspnoea and syncope.

Signs to note are: mild central cyanosis, prominant 'a' wave in JVP especially after mild effort. RV heave (left parasternal); RV S_4 and S_3 in later stages; palpable pulmonary artery pulsation in second left interspace; pulmonary ejection click (best with patient holding breath in expiration); loud and often palpable P_2. Listen for a diastolic murmur of pulmonary regurgitation (Graham Steel) and a systolic murmur of tricuspid regurgitation.

ECG shows severe RV strain (T-wave inversion in V1–V3), right-axis deviation and incomplete or complete RBBB. Usually in sinus rhythm.

CXR shows a normal size heart with enlarged pulmonary artery conus and central pulmonary arteries, but pruned peripheral arteries. Lung peripheries look dark and oligaemic.

Echocardiography confirms pulmonary hypertension (see page 478 for calculation), RV hypertrophy and pulmonary and tricuspid regurgitation. Exclude occult left heart problems as a possible cause of PHT: mitral or aortic valve disease, atrial myxoma, cor triatriatum, etc.

Cardiac catheterization is necessary only to check the effect of drug treatment on pulmonary and systemic vascular resistance (page 513), or as a possible work up to transplantation.

Management

Mean survival is 5 years from diagnosis: a depressing condition to manage, with no definite aetiology, and much of the therapy palliative.

• *Anticoagulation.* Routine. Shown to improve survival in Mayo Clinic series of 1984.

• *Calcium antagonists.* High doses of long-acting drugs are needed but only about a quarter of patients will respond with a fall in PVR. Gradual increase in dose advisable unless monitored with Swan–Ganz catheter *in situ.* Typical doses needed are: nifedipine 180–240 mg daily or diltiazem 720 mg daily. Systemic hypotension may be a problem. Responders have improved prognosis.

• *Domiciliary oxygen* may help patients who can still be managed at home.

• *Prostacyclin* (PGI_2, epoprostenol) infusion via a tunnelled central line. Shown to improve symptoms, haemodynamics and survival. Generally reserved for the more severe or deteriorating case when it may be used as a bridge to transplantation. Infusion dosing is performed with right heart catheterization. Start at 2 ng/kg/min increasing by 2 ng/kg/min every 15 min. Increments are stopped when arterial pressure falls by 40%, or HR increases by 40%, or patient develops intolerant symptoms: nausea, vomiting, headache, etc. Reduce maximum dose by 2 ng/kg/min to achieve maximum tolerable dose.

• *Atrial septostomy.* Creating a right to left shunt. This may help by decompressing the right heart and improve LV filling and cardiac output.

• *Transplantation.* Offers the only real hope of long-term survival. Heart and lung, double lung or single lung transplants are possible and severe RV dysfunction may recover once the afterload is reduced with a new lung. One-year survival following lung transplantation is about 70% and recurrence in the transplanted lung has not been seen. Surgical mortality is higher than for other conditions and obliterative bronchiolitis more common.

Spontaneous improvement does occur but is very rare. Future pharmacological directions include the use of endothelin-receptor antagonists or nitric oxide precursors.

Systemic hypertension

Definition

Blood pressure rises with age, with cold environment or anxiety, with effort, and varies with the time of day (lowest at 4.00 a.m. rising rapidly by 9.00 a.m.). With mild hypertension the blood pressure is taken twice or more before calling a patient 'hypertensive'. With more severe hypertension this is not necessary. Systolic and diastolic pressure are of equal importance.

Blood pressure

Age (years)	Normal	Borderline	Definite
17–40	< 149/90	150/95	> 160/100
41–50	< 150/90	160/95	> 160/100
≥ 60	< 160/90	165/95	> 170/100

Pitfalls in measurement

A long cuff is needed to encircle the arm. Too small a cuff or too fat an arm results in spuriously high readings. The patient should be calm having had 5-min rest and abstained from drinking coffee and smoking. The blood pressure should be measured to the nearest 2 mmHg in the seated position. It is preferable to use Korotkow Phase 5 (disappearance of the sounds) for the diastolic reading rather than Phase 4 (muffling of the sounds).

Significance of hypertension

Hypertension is associated with an increased risk of CVA, cardiac failure, myocardial infarction, occlusive peripheral arterial disease and renal failure. Each increment of 10 mmHg systolic pressure reduces life expectancy. Successful blood pressure control reduces mortality from CVA and renal failure (but not definitely myocardial infarct deaths). Each reduction in systolic pressure of 6 mmHg reduces the CVA risk by 40%.

Mild hypertension should be treated even if there is no organ damage.

Typical symptoms

Headache: frontal or occipital are typically worse in the morning. May have migraine. Dyspnoea on effort progressing to orthopnoea or PND. Angina (increased muscle mass + coronary disease) and/or claudication. Nocturia even if off diuretics. Possibly haematuria and/or dysuria in history. History of transient ischaemic attacks. Mild visual disturbance. Epistaxes.

Signs to note

Blood pressure in both arms. Synchrony of radial and femoral pulses. Check all peripheral pulses. Arterial bruits: carotid, aortic, renal. LV hypertrophy. ? S_3 present. Fundal examination: AV nipping, haemorrhages, exudates, papilloedema. Check for proteinuria.

Causes

- Essential: 95% of cases.
- Renal disease, glomerulonephritis, pyelonephritis, polycystic disease, hydronephrosis.
- Renal artery stenosis (atheromatous plaques or fibromuscular hyperplasia).
- Coarctation of the aorta.
- Phaeochromocytoma.
- Primary hyperaldosteronism (Conn's syndrome).
- Cushing's syndrome.
- Iatrogenic drug therapy: glucocorticoids, carbenoxolone, MAOIs, sympathomimetics, oestrogens.
- Acromegaly.
- Hypercalcaemia.
- CNS disturbances: raised intracranial pressure, familial dysautonomia.
- Postoperative: especially cardiopulmonary bypass.
- Pre-eclampsia.
- Pseudohyperaldosteronism (Little's syndrome)

Investigations

Almost all patients will have essential hypertension (? family history) and the necessary investigations are: FBC, U and E, creatinine (preferably U and E off diuretics). Urine testing: protein, blood, sugar (if positive, urine culture) CXR, ECG.

A routine IVU is not necessary. It should be considered in patients with a history of renal disease and in those who are most likely to have renovascular hypertension:

....

- onset of hypertension under the age of 30 years
- accelerated hypertension or deteriorating renal function
- hypertension after renal trauma, or an episode of renal pain
- presence of a renal bruit.

The estimation of 24-hour urine VMA is expensive and the test should be done in all cases of hypertension + glycosuria, patients with a history of paroxysmal hypertension, sweating, palpitations, episodes of hypotension, or the young patient. Three 24-hour urine VMAs are required with the patient on a vanilla-free diet and preferably off all drugs (normal range up to 35 μmol/24 hours). Urine saves must be done before the IVP. A test with a single 24 h urine collection is now diagnostic (see page 407).

Renovascular hypertension (renal artery stenosis)

Features suggesting this on an IVU are a disparity of renal size by > 2 cm, delayed appearance of dye on the affected side with increased density of dye later on that side. With a positive IVU the following investigations may be considered necessary to demonstrate that the abnormal kidney is the cause of the hypertension.

- Captopril-enhanced renal scintigraphy is a reliable and safe investigation. A Technetium labelled DTPA renogram is performed before and after a 12.5 mg dose of captopril. Renal function drops sharply on the affected side.
- Digital subtraction arteriography (DSA) of the renal vessels. This is preferable to direct intubation of the renal arteries themselves and a flush descending aortogram with DSA is usually all that is needed. The investigation of choice.
- Plasma renin activity (peripheral blood) lying and after 1 hour standing.
- Renal vein renin ratio. Simultaneous sampling with the patient off beta-blockade. A ratio of > 1.5 : 1 (abnormal to normal) is significant. Differential ureteric sampling is now rarely needed in the majority of patients.

Phaeochromocytoma

The majority of these tumours occur in the adrenal medulla arising from neurochromaffin cells. Extramedullary tumours (paragangliomas or ganglioneuromas) can occur anywhere along the sympathetic chain, posterior mediastinum, or heart. About 5% are associated with the multiple endocrine neoplasia syndrome (MEN) type II, or with the Von Hippel–Lindau syndrome (retinal and cerebellar haemangiomas) or in neurofibromatosis (Von Recklinghausen's disease). These neuroendocrine tumours can secrete a variety of polypeptides, e.g. calcitonin, parathormone, calcitonin gene-related peptide (CGRP), vasoactive intestinal peptide (VIP, causing watery diarrhoea and hypokalaemia) or neuropeptide Y.

Symptoms are often paroxysmal with episodes of palpitation, angina, headaches, dizzyness, sweating and visual disturbance. There may be intense peripheral vasoconstriction producing a pale, mottled cold skin. Postural hypotension may occur with volume depletion. Acute pulmonary oedema may occur due to a catecholamine-induced myocarditis plus hypertensive LVF.

ECG is usually abnormal, with variable T-wave inversion in chest leads and signs of left ventricular hypertrophy.

Urine testing: may have catecholamine driven glycosuria.

Diagnosis

Urinary catecholamines. The estimation of urinary adrenaline, noradrenaline and dopamine has superseded the old estimation of urinary vanillylmandelic acid (VMA) which is less sensitive. Until recently diagnosis rested on three 24-hour urine collections as hormone release is pulsatile. However, it is possible to screen for a phaeochromocytoma by comparing the catecholamine concentration in a single 24-hour urine sample with the urine creatinine, avoiding the problem of multiple or incomplete urine collections. Urine collection in acid bottles.

Normal ranges	Adrenaline	Noradrenaline	Dopamine
24-hour urine total	8–150 nmol	50–570 nmol	0–3240 nmol
Catecholamine/ urine creatinine	≤ 15 nmol/mmol urine creatinine	≤ 50 nmol/mmol urine creatinine	≤ 338 nmol/mmol urine creatinine
Plasma	0.1–1.2 pmol/ml	0.5–3.5 pmol/ml	
Platelet	0.03–0.7 pmol/mg platelet protein	0.33–3.2 pmol/mg platelet protein	

Adrenal venous blood contains adrenaline : noradrenaline in a 4 : 1 ratio. High adrenaline levels suggest an adrenal tumour. Very high noradrenaline levels compared with adrenaline suggest an extramedullary tumour.

- Abdominal ultrasound. If adrenal tumour is not visualized consider:
- CT scan and/or MRI scan of adrenals, 5% of the tumours are multiple (may be bilateral) and approximately 5% are malignant.
- IVU with tomography of the adrenals. Urine collections should precede the IVU.

• Pentolinium suppression test. Plasma catecholamines should be suppressed by 2.5 mg pentolinium. Failure of suppression is a positive test, but false-positive results can occur in renal failure.
• Clonidine suppression test. Following 0.3 mg clonidine orally, plasma catecholamines should fall to < 500 pmol/ml in 3 hours.
• MIBG scan. Iodine-123 meta-iodobenzylguanidine is a guanethidine analogue, and is taken up by presynaptic adrenergic neurones. Dense uptake occurs in phaeochromocytoma tissue. It is a very valuable imaging method for extramedullary tumours.
• With modern imaging techniques, further investigations are rarely necessary. More dangerous investigations such as arteriography or adrenal venous and IVC sampling are only performed after adequate alpha- and beta-blockade with intra-arterial pressure monitoring.

Therapy prior to invasive investigation or surgery

A minimum of oral phenoxybenzamine 10 mg tds and propranolol 80 mg tds is needed for 2 weeks, starting the phenoxybenzamine first. Diuretics should be avoided as there is already volume depletion. Long-acting calcium antagonists may be used. Gradual control of blood pressure is important. Sudden falls could provoke retinal or cerebral infarction. Persistent hypertension in spite of adequate alpha- and beta-blockade may be due to other peptides (e.g. endothelin, neuropetide Y) secreted by the tumour. Further control of hypertension is managed during investigation or surgery by i.v. phentolamine, hydralazine or trimetaphan (see page 228).

Immediately after tumour removal, intense vasodilatation may occur requiring close attention to volume replacement. Central venous and intra-arterial pressure monitoring are essential.

Malignant phaeochromocytoma will require long-term alpha- and beta-blockade, additional chemotherapy, and attempts to block further catecholamine secretion with α-methyltyrosine or ^{131}I-MIBG.

Treatment

General measures

Weight reduction, reducing alcohol intake and increasing exercise have all independently been shown to reduce blood pressure in hypertensive patients. Discourage adding salt to food (but patients may use it in cooking). Women on the Pill should be advised to switch to a different form of contraception if treatment is not quickly successful. Patients with severe hypertension (> 230/130) should be admitted for bed rest and carefully monitored treatment.

Drug treatment

Patients should be advised that almost all anti-hypertensive therapy has some side-effects. Treatment will be necessary for life in most cases. Stopping therapy usually results in the blood pressure climbing again. Drug treatment should be tailored to the individual patient and there is no single ideal regime.

Diuretics

Thiazides increase salt and water excretion but can cause hyperuricaemia, hypercalcaemia, hypokalaemia, hypertrigyceridaemia and lower high-density lipoprotein (HDL) cholesterol. They may cause impotence. Frusemide is not a good drug for hypertension unless used with captopril, or unless there is a degree of renal failure. Spironolactone is most useful for primary hyperaldosteronism. Vasodilators and beta-blocking agents are discussed in Chapter 5.

There is a gradual shift away from diuretics and beta-blockade as initial treatment to drugs with fewer long-term side-effects: calcium antagonists, ACE inhibitors or apha-1-blockers. The table summarizes the effects of these five groups of drugs on metabolic and other variables.

Parameter	Diuretic	Beta-blocker	Calcium antagonist	ACE inhibitor	Alpha-1-blocker
LDL cholesterol	–	–/0	0	0	+
HDL cholesterol	0	–	0	0	+/0
Triglycerides	–	–	0	0	+
Glucose Intolerance	–	–	0	+	+
Activity	0		0	0	0
LV hypertrophy	0	+	+	+	+
Blood pressure	+	+	+	+	+

0 No effect, – deleterious effect. + beneficial effect.

Angiotensin-receptor antagonists (see also page 234)

These drugs are tolerated well by patients who find the cough induced by ACE inhibitors intolerable. As they are specific for the AT_1-receptor bradykinin levels are not increased, and there is no first-dose effect (gradual onset of action). They reduce but do not completely inhibit aldosterone release, so hyperkalaemia is less likely than with ACE inhibitors. They have a mild uricosuric action.

It can be seen that while all classes of drugs reduce blood pressure, diuretics and beta-blockers have the worst metabolic profile. Most

patients can be managed on an ACE inhibitor, or an angiotensin-receptor antagonist, or a long-acting calcium antagonist as a single agent, e.g.:
- Calcium antagonist: amlodipine 5-10 mg od, or nifedipine LA 30–60 mg od, or verapamil SR 120–240 mg od.
- ACE inhibitor: enalapril 2.5–5.0 mg od or bd (maxixmum dose 20 mg bd), or lisinopril 2.5–5.0 mg od (maximum dose 40 mg od) or ramipril 1.25 mg od (maximum dose 10 mg od). Diuretic needed with bigger doses (see page 231)
- Angiotensin II receptor antagonist, e.g. losartan 50–100 mg od or valsartan 80–160 mg od.
- Alpha-1 blocking agent: doxazosin 1 mg od (maximum dose 16 mg od). This has a longer half-life than prazosin and tachyphylaxis is not a problem.
- Beta-blocking agent: indicated for the hyperactive or anxious patient, or the patient with a previous history of myocardial infarction. Atenolol 50–100 mg od.
- Imidazoline (I_1)-receptor agonist. Moxonidine 200–400 µgm daily. Centrally acting. Reduces sympathetic outflow lowering peripheral resistance. Like clonidine but does not activate alpha-2 receptors. Avoid in severe renal or cardiac failure.

With more resistant hypertension different classes of drugs are used in combination. Always consider patient compliance with failing treatment.

ACE inhibitors and angiotensin receptor antagonists are contraindicated in renal artery stenosis. Interglomerular filtration pressure is maintained in renal artery stenosis by increased tone in the efferent arteriole (mediated by angiotensin II). ACE inhibitors and angiotensin receptor antagonists may prevent this autoregulatory mechanism and glomerular filtration may fall sharply, precipitating renal failure.

With severe malignant hypertension, complete bed rest and parenteral therapy are needed with intra-arterial pressure monitoring:
- nitroprusside i.v. dose regime on page 227 or
- labetalol 200 mg in 200 ml N saline infused at 1–2 mg (1–2 ml)/min.

Failure to control blood pressure

There are many reasons for this. In order of probability:
- Inadequate treatment regime. Some patients will require several different drugs together using doses low enough to avoid side-effects as much as possible.

- Compliance. Failure to take the drugs because of side-effects. This is common particularly in men who may become impotent on therapy.
- The elderly arteriosclerotic patient. Old rigid arteries do not dilate well. Care must be taken not to be too enthusiastic about blood-pressure control in this age group. Acute reduction in pressure will reduce cerebral perfusion and may cause syncope or a CVA.
- Excessive salt intake. Patients must be told to avoid all added salt, and to avoid salty foods.
- Renovascular hypertension.
- Rarely 'surgical' lesions, e.g. phaeochromocytoma.

Surgery

Is necessary for coarctation, phaeochromocytoma, uncontrolled primary hyperaldosteronism and some cases of renal artery stenosis if angioplasty is not an option.

Renal angioplasty is more successful in fibromuscular hyperplasia than in arteriosclerotic vessels. There is a risk of renal artery dissection or acute occlusion. Prior to stenting the cure rate for dilatation of fibromuscular hyperplasia was about 50%, but only about 20% for successful dilatation in arteriosclerotic vessels. Proximal and ostial renal artery stenoses until recently have been managed surgically. Stenting all these lesions is now increasingly popular and successful, but as with coronary stenting in-stent restenosis may occur.

Surgery involves either renal endarterectomy, autotransplantation, aorto-renal saphenous vein bypass or nephrectomy. The splenic artery can be used to replace the renal artery as it is usually free of atheroma. Removal of a small kidney does not necessarily result in improvement in blood pressure.

Dissecting aneurysm of the thoracic aorta

This commonly occurs in men aged 40–70 years and is frequently fatal if untreated. Fifty per cent die within 48 hours, 70% in 1 week and 90% in 3 months. It is three times as common in men, more so in Afro-Caribbean than Caucasians, and rare in oriental races. It is usually a spontaneous event and a history of trauma is unusual. Predisposing factors include:

- hypertension (distal > proximal)
- bicuspid or unicommissural aortic valve
- coarctation of the aorta
- pregnancy

- Turner's or Noonan's syndrome
- Marfan's syndrome (see page 425)
- other connective tissue disorders, e.g. Ehlers–Danlos syndrome, SLE, relapsing polychondritis, giant cell aortitis
- surgical aortotomy sites.

Pathophysiology

A combination of high intraluminal pressure and medial damage seems to be the prime factor (e.g. cystic medial necrosis in Marfan's syndrome). Syphilis causes saccular aortic aneurysms not dissections, and atheroma is usually associated with saccular aneurysms. Cause of medial damage is unknown (a genetic mucopolysaccharide deficiency in Marfan's syndrome, possibly ischaemic necrosis due to occlusion of vasa vasorum in other cases).

Presentation

- *Pain*. The commonest form of presentation. A sudden-onset literally tearing sensation felt in the chest. Usually retrosternal radiating through to the back, neck and left chest. The pain may be similar to ischaemic cardiac pain. It is very severe. Leaking dissections will produce pleuritic pain in addition. Dissection round a coronary ostium may produce an additional myocardial infarct.
- *Symptoms from arterial involvement:*

CNS: monoplegia, paraplegia (spinal artery occlusion), hemiplegia, stupor to loss of consciousness, visual disturbances, speech disturbance.

Gastrointestinal: abdominal pain (mesenteric artery dissection), haemorrhage (bowel infarction or aorto-intestinal fistula), dysphagia (oesophageal compression).

Renal: renal pain, haematuria (renal artery dissection) or anuria.

Limb: pain and pallor in any limb.

- *Pleuritic pain:* aneurysm leaking may also cause haemoptysis.
- *Giddiness or syncope:* either cerebral effect or secondary to effective volume loss, e.g. retroperitoneal haematoma.
- *Dyspnoea* (LVF, massive haemothorax, pleural effusions, pulmonary haemorrhage).

Aortic dissection may thus mimic clinically a wide variety of conditions from a CVA, acute appendicitis, acute pancreatitis, perforated peptic ulcer, saddle embolism as well as myocardial infarction or pulmonary embolism. A patient may present with one ischaemic and one paralysed limb simultaneously.

Physical signs and examination

The patient may be in great pain, shocked, cyanosed and sweating profusely. The blood pressure may be high, normal or low.

The most important things to check are:

Blood pressure in both arms; all peripheral pulses, their presence and equality (a change in the nature of the pulses may be a valuable clue); there may be arterial bruits, arterial tenderness or palpable aneurysms.

Presence of aortic regurgitation.

Sign of tamponade (page 364), pericardial rub itself is unusual. SVC obstruction rarely confuses the issue, as it is commoner with saccular aneurysms.

Signs of LVF, pleural effusions; staining of chest or abdomen (haemorrhage from leaking aneurysm is an ominous sign).

Abdominal signs, rigidity, palpable mass – ? pulsatile, abdominal tenderness is common.

CNS signs, fundal examination, hypertensive changes; Horner's syndrome; urinary retention; limb movement and sensation; general state of consciousness; ? Marfan habitus.

Chest X-ray

Widening of the upper mediastinum is strongly suggestive of a dissection, but not diagnostic. An unfolded aorta with a tortuous descending aorta may resemble a dissection.

Fluid in the left costophrenic angle associated with a wide mediastinum is a particularly ominous sign.

Classification

The original De Bakey classification is shown in Figure 10.1.

Type I The ascending and descending aorta are involved usually into the abdomen. The 'walking stick' distribution.

Type II Involvement of ascending aorta only. The least common. May occur in Marfan's syndrome.

Type III Involvement of descending aorta only distal to the left subclavian downwards. The most favourable type prognostically.

This classification was proposed in 1965 and is less used now. More recently Shumway has proposed a more simple classification into two types only:

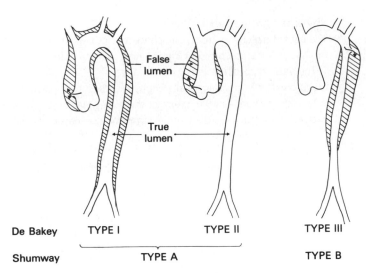

Figure 10.1 Thoracic aorta dissection – classification.

Type A (Proximal) Ascending aorta involved } Shumway
Type B (Distal) Ascending aorta not involved } classification

The Shumway classification has largely taken over from the De Bakey.

Management

Stage 1
Pain relief, i.v. diamorphine as required. ECG monitoring, chest X-ray. Establish two CVP lines and radial artery pressure if possible. Cross-match 10 units blood, as volume replacement may be necessary if aneurysm leakage has occurred. Plasma should be given initially, followed by whole blood. Dextran 70 may have to be used. Echocardiography is employed to visualize the aortic root and to check for pericardial fluid. Transoesophageal echocardiography is diagnostic.

Stage 2

Correction of hypertension if present. Wheat in 1965 realized the importance of lowering both mean systolic pressure and the dP/dt. This he accomplished by trimetaphan i.v. 1–2 mg/ml, guanethidine 50 mg bd and reserpine 1–2 mg i.m. A variety of other drugs have been used since, e.g. methyl-dopa, beta-blocking agents and diuretics.

The simplest regime is i.v. nitroprusside (page 227). It is easier to control, having a very short half-life. Frequent checks on acid–base balance are necessary to check for a metabolic acidosis.

Peak systolic pressure should be < 120 mmHg and mean aortic pressure < 90 mmHg.

Stage 3
Diagnostic method depends on technology available.

Transoesophageal echocardiography. This is proving very useful in the diagnosis of dissection and is particularly good at visualizing the dissection flap in the descending aorta.

Emergency aortography. Once the diagnosis is suspected, this may be necessary. It should be performed under heavy sedation or general anaesthesia. A pigtail catheter from the femoral route is preferable and usually this catheter stays in true lumen. Separate aortic root and aortic arch injections with follow through to descending aorta are necessary. The patient should be on i.v. nitroprusside or similar drugs prior to the injections: the force of the injection of large volumes of contrast media into a dissected root has occasionally proved fatal. Renal film should be taken at the end of the procedure.

Magnetic resonance imaging. When generally available, this will probably prove to be the safest, quickest and most reliable method of diagnosis. The danger of an aortic injection is avoided and no X-irradiation needed.

CT scan. This investigation is proving increasingly useful in aortic dissection but is not always available on an emergency basis. A double lumen can be visualized and the dissection flap. It may not, however, be quite as good as aortography for visualizing the origin/point of entry of the dissection, but is very helpful in making the diagnosis and determining the extent of the dissection. It is obviously safer than aortography.

Stage 4

Type A. Surgery is the treatment of choice for Type A dissections and medical treatment alone carries a bad prognosis. Cardiopulmonary bypass with coronary perfusion. The ascending aorta is transected, the two cuffs of true and false walls are sutured together at both sides of the transection and then end-to-end anastomosis performed, sometimes with a Dacron interposition graft. The aortic valve often becomes competent again once it is resuspended, making aortic valve replacement unnecessary. Occasionally a root replacement is necessary using a tube valve conduit with re-implantation of the coronaries and the original aortic wall buttressed around the graft.

If the great vessels are involved, surgery becomes difficult with a greater risk of post-operative stroke. Cardiopulmonary bypass is set up and the patient profoundly cooled to 18°C. Circulatory arrest is performed and the great vessels joined to an arch graft on a single pedicle flap.

Type B. Medical management initially, unless complications develop such as an infarcting organ or limb, leaking aneurysm or extension with unremitting pain. If the dissection re-enters above the diaphragm it is possible to replace the descending thoracic aorta with a Dacron graft (using a temporary proximal-to-distal aorta bypass). Difficulties with this operation are the distal anastomosis and the possibility of paraplegia due to damage to the anterior spinal artery branches.

Involvement of the abdominal aorta in a Type B dissection is much more of a problem, and medical treatment is advocated initially. However, local surgery at the aortic bifurcation may be necessary to save ischaemic legs.

10.8 Cardiac myxoma

This may occur in any cardiac chamber but most commonly in the left atrium. It is typically a gelatinous friable tumour attached to the atrial septum by a short pedicle. It is three times more common in the left atrium than the right. Untreated, it is usually fatal, although disease progression may be very slow over a period of years. The tumour often prolapses through the mitral or tricuspid valve and can cause sudden obstruction to blood flow. Fragments of the tumour easily break off and cause systemic emboli. Multiple tumours occur very rarely. There is also a very rare familial form associated with lentiginosis (multiple freckles) or HCM.

Symptoms
The atrial myxoma commonly presents in one of four ways in order of frequency:
• *Dyspnoea*. This may be of gradual onset or sudden severe pulmonary oedema.

- *Systemic emboli.* Any organ may be involved, e.g. brain (fits, hemiplegia, etc.), myocardial infarction, acute ischaemia of a limb, etc.
- *Constitutional upset.* Weight loss, fever, myalgia (low albumen and raised globulin with a high ESR are often associated).
- *Sudden death.* The atrial myxoma is found at post-mortem occluding the mitral valve orifice.

Physical signs

The left atrial myxoma most closely mimics mitral stenosis but there are one or two pointers suggesting a myxoma:

- the patient is in sinus rhythm. Atrial dysrhythmias are rare
- signs of mitral stenosis may be transient and only occur if the tumour approaches the mitral valve orifice. Sometimes postural changes will influence the murmur
- there is no opening snap
- there may be an early diastolic plop as the tumour prolapses through the valve.

Right atrial myxomas are more difficult to pick up clinically. There may be signs suggesting right ventricular dysfunction (raised JVP, oedema, etc.) or pulmonary infarction from emboli. A tricuspid diastolic flow murmur is often difficult to hear.

Investigations

Chest X-ray shows a small heart with enlargement of the left atrial appendage and possible pulmonary oedema. There is no mitral valve calcification. In long-standing cases, calcification may occur in the tumour itself.

Echocardiography is diagnostic. Two-dimensional echocardiography (Figure 12.19b) will be diagnostic in almost all cases of prolapsing myxoma. Transoesophageal echocardiography will give more accurate information of the size and site of the myxoma.

Cardiac catheterization is now virtually never required. In cases of left-sided myxomas where there is diagnostic doubt after echocardiography, pulmonary angiography with follow through to the left heart may help. Direct left heart catheterization should be avoided as this may dislodge friable material from the myxoma. With right-sided myxomas, if there is doubt following echocardiography, digital subtraction angiography from a peripheral venous injection is helpful.

Histology

This may be obtained from analysis of peripheral embolic material.

Although the tumour embolizes frequently, it does not grow in its peripheral site.

Differential diagnosis
The following conditions should be considered in a patient with a mitral murmur, mild pyrexia, weight loss, abnormal plasma proteins and high ESR:
- rheumatic mitral stenosis
- infective endocarditis
- systemic lupus erythematosus
- reticulosis
- cor triatriatum
- left atrial thrombus.

Treatment
Following echocardiographic diagnosis, surgical removal of the myxoma should be performed as soon as possible using cardiopulmonary bypass. Occasionally atrial septectomy and an interatrial patch are required. Recurrence of the myxoma is extremely rare but patients should be followed up for the first 5 years.

11 The Heart in Systemic Disease

11.1 Acromegaly

Increased growth hormone (GH) from a pituitary tumour results in increased synthesis of insulin-like growth factors (IGF I and II) from the liver. Diabetes occurs in about 50% of cases. Cardiovascular changes are:

• systemic hypertension in 30%. Total exchangeable sodium increased. Some have increased aldosterone levels. All have increased sensitivity to angiotensin II. The hypertension is usually mild and controllable medically

• left ventricular hypertrophy present in more than half the cases

• hypertrophic cardiomyopathy. This is independent of hypertension or coronary disease. It may be massive, with interstitial fibrosis and changes very similar to hypertrophic obstructive cardiomyopathy. Patients will need managing exactly on the same lines (see **4.2**). Subaortic myotomy/myomectomy may be needed for severe cases

• diabetes mellitus may result in small vessel disease

• coronary disease is more frequent due to hypertension, diabetes and raised plasma free fatty acid levels.

11.2 AIDS (acquired immune deficiency syndrome)

Clinical evidence of cardiac involvement only occurs in about 10% of cases, although at autopsy 25% of cases may have cardiac disease. Typical problems are:

• dilated cardiomyopathy picture. Myocarditis may occasionally be due to a wide variety of opportunistic infections (e.g. toxoplasmosis, histoplasmosis, cytomegalovirus) but is usually due to the human immunodeficiency virus (HIV) itself. Symptoms from congestive cardiac failure may be incorrectly attributed to pre-existing lung disease

• pericardial effusion. May lead to tamponade and require aspiration

• ventricular arrhythmias

• non-bacterial thrombotic endocarditis (marantic endocarditis)

• infective endocarditis, e.g. *Aspergillus*

• metastatic involvement from Kaposi's sarcoma

• right ventricular failure (recurrent chest infections causing pulmonary hypertension).

Treatment is only palliative. Pericardial aspiration, standard treatment for cardiac failure or drug therapy for specific opportunistic infection.

Amyloidosis

Amyloid fibrils are derived from a monoclonal immunoglobulin light chain (kappa or lambda) or its N-terminal fragment. Circulates in the blood as Bence-Jones protein and deposited in the tissues as beta-pleated sheet fibrils. May be deposited in any tissue.

Histologically identifiable by staining orange/pink with Congo red, exhibiting green/yellow birefringence in polarized light and a characteristic fibrillary structure under electron microscopy.

Immune origin amyloid (formerly primary amyloid): AL-type protein

Restrictive cardiomyopathy (see **4.3**, page 135)
Amyloid deposits in the myocardium give the muscle a 'rubbery rigidity'. Infiltration between myocardial cells results in a small stiff heart with high LVEDP and RVEDP while systolic function remains normal until late in the disease. Small pericardial effusions may occur, but the typical picture is of congestive cardiac failure with a normal sized heart on the CXR. Coronary artery occlusion may occur with amyloid deposits in the arterial wall. Tachyarrhythmias are common, atrial fibrillation producing a rapid deterioration with a stiff ventricular muscle. Sinus arrest and AV block may require pacing. Mild AV valve regurgitation occurs but valve replacement is rarely indicated. Pulmonary infiltration is common.

Clinical findings show a raised JVP with prominent 'x' and 'y' descents and a possible Kussmaul's sign (inspiratory filling of the neck veins). The apex is usually impalpable but an S_4 and/or early S_3 may be heard. The picture is very similar to constrictive pericarditis which is the chief differential diagnosis (see page 366).

Other non-cardiac features include the following: macroglossia, peripheral neuropathy, postural hypotension, large joint arthritis, renal involvement, waxy skin deposits, spontaneous purpura and ecchymoses.

ECG shows low voltage with Q waves in anterior or inferior leads simulating old infarction. There may be sinus arrest, AF or degrees of AV block. Echocardiography shows a concentrically thickened myocardium with a speckled appearance, 'granular sparkle', on two dimensional imaging. There may be an insignificant pericardial effusion. Initially early diastolic filling is impaired with EA reversal (see page 484), but later in the course of the disease this 'pseudonormalizes' as diastolic filling becomes more restrictive. Cardiac catheterization shows a typical diastolic dip and plateau wave form in both ventricles. However RVEDP and LVEDP differ usually by > 7 mmHg in all phases of respiration in contrast with constrictive pericarditis where they are the same. Diagnosis is confirmed by endomyocardial biopsy. A serum amyloid protein (SAP) scan will give an idea of the amyloid load in other viscera.

There is no specific treatment for a depressingly relentless condition but low-dose chemotherapy (e.g. with melphalan and prednisone) may produce some regression in cardiac amyloid if continued for > 1 year. This combination is superior to colchicine. Patients with cardiac amyloid may be very sensitive to digoxin. Amiodarone is used for paroxysmal tachyarrhythmias, pacing for sinus arrest and AV block plus diuretics for systemic or pulmonary oedema.

Cardiac transplantation is not contraindicated in cardiac amyloid but should only be considered if the patient is likely to survive > 5 years with regard to visceral infiltration. Attempts should then be made to reduce the fibril precursors with chemotherapy.

As with multiple myeloma autologous peripheral blood stem cell transplantation has been successful in a few cases.

Senile cardiac amyloid: ASC_1 amyloid protein

Amyloid deposits (again probably of immune origin) are very common in the atria of the elderly and may be the cause of atrial arrhythmias in this age group. Senile cardiac amyloid is more common in black patients than white, and in a few may be associated with a familial defect in a gene coding for transthyretin.

Smaller deposits may be found in the ventricles and aorta of patients at autopsy but these are rarely of pathological significance.

Reactive amyloid (formerly secondary amyloid): AA-type amyloid protein

Amyloid deposition secondary to chronic inflammatory disease: tuberculosis, leprosy, chronic rheumatoid arthritis, Crohn's disease, bronchiectasis, paraplegia (urinary infections), etc. Infiltration in liver, spleen and kidney occurs but the heart is much less commonly involved.

Systemic oedema is more likely to be due to nephrotic syndrome than heart failure.

Ankylosing spondylitis

Progressive inflammatory disease of the vertebral column, sacro-iliac, hip, shoulder and manubriosternal joints, with chronic back pain and eventual fusion and calcification of the intervertebral discs and anterior spinal ligament. Ninety per cent in men. High incidence of the human leucocyte antigen HLA-B27 histocompatibility antigen. Cardiac involvement in 10% of cases. Secondary amyloidosis in about 6%:

* conduction disturbance leading to AV block
* aortic regurgitation less common, due to aortic root dilatation (medial necrosis).

Permanent pacing and aortic valve replacement may sometimes be needed in the same patient.

Arteritis and valve granulomata do not occur, unlike rheumatoid cardiac disease.

Endomyocardial fibrosis (EMF)/Loeffler's eosinophilic endocarditis

These are now thought to be the same condition, causing a restrictive cardiomyopathy. EMF is a tropical disease common in equatorial African rainforests. Its aetiology is unknown, but a recurrent febrile illness suggests an infective origin, with new cases more apparent in the rainy season. Only a mild eosinphilia is present and common anyway in these regions, with worm infestation.

The cardiac effects of Loeffler's eosinophilic syndrome and eosinophilic leukaemia are similar. Eosinophils in the myocardium degranulate and cause fibrosis, particularly of the endocardium. The ventricular cavity becomes smaller, with encroaching fibrosis and eventually there is complete obliteration of the apex of either or both ventricles. Secondary thrombosis occurs over this endocardial fibrosis, with systemic emboli. There is marked AV valve regurgitation with involvement of the papillary muscles. There may be a pericardial effusion and conduction problems with advanced disease.

The clinical picture depends on which ventricle is involved. The symptoms may be predominantly right-sided with ascites and peripheral oedema, left-sided with pulmonary oedema and systemic emboli, or both.

Cardiac catheterization and endomyocardial biopsy will confirm the diagnosis. Degranulated eosinophils may be found between the myocardial cells. Pressure measurements in the right heart in advanced disease show a 'tube-like' heart with identical pressures in PA, RV and RA. Angiography shows typical apical obliteration by fibrous tissue.

Management
Patients with severe eosinophilia should receive steroids and/or hydroxyurea. Heart failure is managed on conventional lines. Severe AV valve regurgitation warrants valve replacement and some cases have been improved by endocardial resection.

Haemochromatosis

Should be considered in any young man with a dilated cardiomyopathy. Occasionally presents as a restrictive type of cardiomyopathy. Increased iron absorption with iron overload results in iron deposition in the myocyte sarcoplasm with subsequent cell death and fibrosis. HLA-A3 and HLA-B14, histocompatibility antigens, are common. Additional features are liver disease, diabetes, skin pigmentation, hypopituitarism with hypogonadism, arthritis similar to rheumatoid and pseudogout. A similar illness may occur following repeated blood transfusions (e.g. for sickle cell anaemia, aplastic anaemia or thalassaemia major) with cardiac haemosiderosis.

Clinical picture of CCF, usually with a large heart. Atrial fibrillation is common, ventricular arrhythmias and heart block less so. Iron does not deposit in the conducting system.

Diagnosis is usually made by liver biopsy or sternal marrow. Endomyocardial biopsy will show up iron stores on Prussian blue staining. Raised serum iron, low iron binding capacity and high serum ferritin levels (often > 1 g/ml with normal range 18–300 ng/ml or µg/l).

Treatment for haemochromatosis heart disease is venesection to remove iron over 1–2 years. Documented improvement in LV function has occurred both with venesection and desferrioxamine mesylate infusions to chelate the iron.

Marfan's syndrome

An autosomal dominant condition with a prevalence of 1 in 10 000, probably due to mutations in the gene coding for fibrillin synthesis on chromosome 15. Over 70 different mutations have been found in this gene. This wide diversity of mutations accounts for the different phenotypes in Marfan syndrome, but as yet it is not possible to predict the phenotype from the specific mutation. The mutations result in reduced fibrillin synthesis or early fibrillin degradation. Either sex, 87% die from cardiovascular abnormalities.

Diagnosis is still based on finding two or more of the classical clinical signs in the musculoskeletal system, the CVS and the eyes. Possible findings are listed below.

- Tall thin patient: dolichostenomelia. Arm span greater than height.
- Arachnodactyly: long tapered fingers.
- High-arched palate.
- Musculoskeletal problems, e.g. scoliosis, pectus excavatum, protrusio acetabulae, causing early hip joint osteoarthritis.
- Hypermobility of joints and skin laxity. History of joint dislocation.
- Possible history of pneumothorax. Apical bullae occur.
- Eye problems: ectopia lentis – lens dislocates upwards. Iridodonesis. Usually manageable with corrective spectacles. Lens may need extraction. Increased incidence of myopia, retinal detachment, strabismus.
- Floppy mitral valve. Mild-to-severe mitral regurgitation. Chordal rupture. (See page 79.)
- Dilatation of aortic root with consequent aortic regurgitation.
- Aortic dissection. See **10.7**, page 411.

One of the most used signs has been the metacarpal index: the lengths of the second to fifth metacarpals are added and divided by the sum of their minimum widths. In Marfan's syndrome this index is > 8.5.

In childhood, the commoner problems are the development of a progressive scoliosis, which may need surgical correction possibly with a Harrington rod, and the correction of visual difficulties.

Later problems include progressive mitral regurgitation and/or dilatation of the aortic root.

The aorta in Marfan's syndrome

The whole aorta may demonstrate cystic medial necrosis. The weakened media allows the aorta to stretch even in the normotensive patient. The typical site for the Marfan aortic aneurysm is just above the aortic valve, with the aorta returning to more normal dimensions at the origin of the innominate artery, forming a sort of 'onion' shape. However, any part of the aorta may become aneurysmal in time. Stretching of the aortic annulus (annulo-aortic ectasia) causes aortic regurgitation. Aortic dissection may occur.

Regular echocardiography is essential at least annually, to check aortic root dimensions. Transoesophageal echocardiography is useful if available. A composite aortic root and valve replacement (Bentall's operation) is indicated once the aortic root dimension is > 5.5 cm on echocardiography, whether or not the patient has symptoms. All patients with Marfan's syndrome should be on beta-blockade reducing aortic dP/dt and hopefully the rate of progression of the aortic aneurysm.

Forme fruste Marfan

This term has been used to describe patients with one feature of the syndrome: e.g. annulo-aortic ectasia. The genetic defect of this alone has not been identified but it may progress in the same way as a true Marfan aorta.

11.8 Myxoedema

Commonest in the elderly due to Hashimoto's thyroiditis. Women > men. May be due to surgery, radio-iodine or drugs (amiodarone, lithium). Typical findings are the exact opposite of thyrotoxicosis. A low metabolic rate, raised SVR, hypodynamic circulation with low cardiac output. Patients may have:

• weight gain, cold intolerance, dry skin and hair, lethargy, menorrhagia, constipation, memory loss leading to frank dementia, myotonic jerks

• typical facial appearance: puffy eyes, eyebrow thinning, dull expression

• sinus bradycardia. Low pulse pressure

• pericardial, pleural, peritoneal and synovial effusions with high protein content. Pericardial effusions accumulate slowly and tamponade is rare

• coronary disease. Low-density lipoprotein (LDL) cholesterol is raised. Ischaemia may often be silent

• ECG low voltage: long QT interval, conduction defects, bradycardia. Permanent pacing may be needed.

Again easily missed diagnosis in the elderly. Check free T$_4$ (low) and TSH (must be elevated for the diagnosis).

Management

Dose of L-thyroxine, 50 µg daily up to 200 µg daily if indicated. Thyroid replacement requires great care in patients with coronary disease. Start at thyroxine 25 μg daily and increase very slowly (monthly or less). Patients with severe coronary disease should have coronary bypass grafting before replacement therapy.

Postcoronary bypass management can be difficult. Epicardial pacing wires are useful. Patients are sensitive to hypnotics and analgesics. They do not respond to fluid challenge by increasing cardiac output. Pulmonary oedema may develop at relatively low LA pressures as capillary permeability is increased. Fluid input must be tightly controlled as there is a tendency to dilutional hyponatraemia.

11.9 Rheumatoid arthritis

Symmetrical synovial thickening and inflammation leading to an erosive arthritis. Women > men. Loss of articular cartilage leads to joint subluxation and destruction coupled with weakening of ligaments and tendons. Generalized illness with fever, normochromic normocytic anaemia, possibly with splenomegaly (Felty's syndrome), Sjögren's syndrome and later secondary amyloidosis.

The heart is one of many organs involved in the extra-articular complications of rheumatoid arthritis. Cardiac involvement is not common and may be asymptomatic.

• *Pericarditis:* the commonest form of cardiac involvement. Usually benign fibrinous pericarditis, often an asymptomatic pericardial rub associated with pleural involvement. Pericardial effusions may need aspiration. Occasionally leads to constriction.

• *Myocardial involvement:* rheumatoid nodules within the myocardium can rarely cause LV dysfunction. Conduction system involvement leading to complete AV block.

• *Valve lesions.* Small nodules on valves (aortic > mitral) can cause aortic regurgitation.

• *Coronary arteritis* is rare.

Other organ involvement

• *Lung:* pleural effusion, multiple pulmonary nodules, progressive interstitial fibrosis leading to honeycomb lung and pulmonary hypertension. Rheumatoid plus pneumoconiosis (Caplan's syndrome).

• *Vasculitis:* Raynaud's phenomenon. Digital arteritis with focal pulp infarcts. Chronic leg ulcers. Gastrointestinal haemorrhage. Mesenteric or renal arteritis. Mononeuritis multiplex.

• *Nervous system:* peripheral neuropathy. Nerve compression, e.g. carpal tunnel syndrome.

- *Eye:* iridocyclitis (juvenile arthritis). Scleritis leading to scleromalacia perforans.

Management

Conventional treatment for cardiac complications if symptomatic. Most patients will already be on specific anti-inflammatory agents. It is not known whether steroid therapy in acute fibrinous pericarditis helps prevent later constriction.

11.10 Sarcoidosis

A multisystem granulomatous disease with a prevalence of about 20 per 100 000 in the UK. Equal sex distribution. Commoner in the Irish and West Indians. About 5% of cases of generalized sarcoid have overt cardiac involvement, but cardiac involvement occurs in about 25% of cases of widespread sarcoid at postmortem.

Any part of the heart may be involved. Common sites are LV or RV free wall, interventricular septum, papillary muscles, AV node and His–Purkinje system. Uncommonly, atrial muscle, pericardium, valve tissue or great vessels may be infiltrated. In order of frequency patients present with:

- complete AV block (20–30% of cases). Stokes–Adams attacks. Often in young age group.
- ventricular tachycardia or extra-systoles
- supraventricular arrhythmias
- chest pain simulating ischaemia
- sudden death in about 15%
- acute myocarditis-like picture
- congestive cardiac failure with extensive infiltration.

Complete heart block may be transient. It is often rapidly reversible on steroid therapy but is an absolute indication for permanent pacing whatever the results of steroids. Myocardial infiltration may produce Q waves on an ECG simulating old infarction. Mural thrombus can occur over infiltration sites. AV valve regurgitation occurs in 8% of patients but papillary muscle infiltration is a commoner cause than granulomata on the valve. Old healed ventricular scars may cause small aneurysms. Diffuse myocardial involvement can cause a restrictive cardiomyopathy.

There is no single imaging technique that reliably picks up cardiac sarcoid, and granulomatous deposits may be microscopic and missed on endomyocardial biopsy. Treatment may involve permanent pacing, steroid therapy for acute attacks (not curative) and anti-arrhythmic therapy. Known ventricular aneurysms are not a contra-indication for steroids. Digoxin is safe.

11.11 Scleroderma

Progressive systemic sclerosis. Women > men. Fibrous thickening and degeneration of skin with changes also in heart, lung, gastrointestinal tract and kidneys. Focal necrosis and subsequent fibrosis result from recurrent spasm of the small arterioles and intimal proliferation.

• Thickening and tightening of the skin, particularly in the fingers and face (mask-like). Loss of skin creases. Necrosis, scarring and tapering of the fingertips (sclerodactyly) with acrocyanosis. Restriction of finger movement and claw hand. Skeletal muscle atrophy.

• Raynaud's phenomenon.

• Lung involvement. Pulmonary fibrosis and pulmonary hypertension. Stiff lungs. Reduced transfer factor (KCO).

• Renal involvement with progressive renal failure and systemic hypertension. Gastrointestinal tract involvement with atrophy and fibrosis: dysphagia hypomotility of small bowel, bacterial overgrowth, malabsorption.

• CREST syndrome calcinosis, Raynaud's, oesophageal involvement, sclerodactyly and telangiectasia.

• Pericarditis in 20%. May develop large effusions, or later pericardial constriction.

• Myocardial involvement: focal fibrosis is the end result of myofibrillar degeneration and contraction band necrosis. Large epicardial coronaries are usually normal. Microvascular intimal proliferation contributes to spasm-induced ischaema. The end result may be dilated or restrictive cardiomyopathy-type picture.

• Primary valve disease is very rare (unlike other collagen vascular diseases).

• Conduction defects. Pacing with a DDD unit may be necessary (dilated or stiff LV).

Management

The condition is relentless with symptomatic control all that can be offered. Large doses of calcium antagonists such as nifedipine help the Raynaud's symptoms as well as controlling hypertension and possibly delaying progression of pulmonary hypertension. Conventional treatment for cardiac failure plus pacing may be needed.

11.12 Systemic lupus erythematosus

Multi-organ chronic inflammatory disease typically with fever, polyarthralgia and arthritis, erythematous rash including facial 'butterfly' rash, pleurisy, pericarditis, anaemia, thrombocytopenia, splenomegaly, renal failure and CNS involvement. Much commoner in young women. Drug-induced lupus (e.g. from procainamide) rarely causes CNS or renal disease. Cardiac involvement is common.

• Pericarditis: the most frequent form of cardiac involvement. As with rheumatoid, often silent. May be recurrent or need pericardial aspiration. Tamponade or later constriction can occur.

• Valve disease: Libman–Sacks endocarditis (see page 391). TOE studies have shown valve involvement in 60% of patients with SLE usually on the aortic and mitral valves. Therapy for SLE does not prevent valve vegetations, and they cannot be used as a marker for successful therapy. Valve involvement is usually silent. Patients with definite vegetations in SLE should be advised to have antibiotic cover for dental procedures, etc. as the Libman–Sacks endocarditis may become secondarily infected.

• Myocarditis is rare. LV failure is more likely to be due to hypertension or anaemia.

• Coronary arteritis is rare. Fibrinoid necrosis in small intramural vessels, with secondary thrombotic occlusion. Possible increase in classical atheromatous coronary disease in younger patients due to associated hypertension.

Other organ involvement

• Skin: symmetrical rash on face, hands, fingertips. Malar butterfly rash not all that common. Periungual telangiectasia. Discoid lupus lesions. Reversible alopecia. Hyperpigmentation or vitiligo. Purpura. Urticaria.

• Joints: similar distribution but less destructive than rheumatoid.

• Lung: pleurisy with or without effusion. Basal atelectasis.

• Raynaud's phenomenon.

• Lupus nephritis: hypertension and progressive renal failure are common.

• CNS: CVAs are common and may be due to vasculitis, emboli or intracerebral haemorrhage. If the CT scan shows an infarct and if there is no evidence of vasculitis elsewhere anticoagulation should be considered. Other CNS involvement includes depression, fits, cranial nerve palsy and peripheral neuropathy. Retinal lesions include white cytoid bodies.

• Sjögren's syndrome.

Management

Steroids for acute exacerbation of the illness with possible additional azathioprine or cyclophosphamide. Non-steroidal anti-inflammatory agents where possible for recurrent pericarditis. Valve replacement rarely necessary for Libman–Sacks non-infective endocarditis. Renal failure commonest cause of death.

11.13 Thyrotoxicosis

Thyroxine increases cardiac beta-receptors (effects similar to catecholamine excess) but acts separately also.

Results in an increased total blood volume, metabolic rate, heart rate, stroke volume, cardiac output, coronary and skeletal muscle blood flow, contractility, LVEDV, rate of diastolic relaxation and atrial excitability. Results in a decreased SVR, diastolic filling time and contractility reserve (no increase in LVEF on exercise). Patients may have:

- weight loss, heat intolerance, eye signs with proptosis, ophthalmoplegia, chemosis, etc. amenorrhoea
- tachycardia. High sleeping pulse rate. Wide pulse pressure
- loud heart sounds. S_3. Exertional dyspnoea
- ejection systolic flow murmur: high stroke volume
- hyperdynamic apex
- pleuropericardial rub with hyperkinetic heart
- AF in 9–22% (normal population 0.4%)
- systemic embolic risk
- angina even with normal coronaries. Rarely, myocardial infarction
- high-output failure. Large heart may resemble dilated cardiomyopathy. Similar to chronic anaemia.

In the elderly thyrotoxicosis is easily overlooked. There may be no eye signs or obvious goitre. Total T_4 and T_3 levels may be normal even in the thyrotoxic patient in cardiac failure as peripheral conversion of T_4 to T_3 is reduced, and TBG levels are low reducing total T_4. Therefore measure free T_4 (high) and TSH (low) in any patient with AF of unknown cause.

Management

- Rate control: digoxin alone is rarely enough. Additional beta-blockade or verapamil needed. Avoid beta-blockers with ISA. Large doses may be needed (increased clearance). If large heart on CXR, avoid beta-blockade and calcium antagonists, just use digoxin, diuretics and antithyroid drugs. For the rare thyroid storm propranolol is given i.v. 0.1 mg/kg slowly over 10 min.

- Start carbimazole 10–15 mg tds or propylthiouracil 100 mg tds.
- Avoid cardioversion until the patient is definitely euthyroid.
- Anticoagulate until back in SR.

Left ventricular function should improve with successful treatment and the heart becomes smaller on the CXR but it may never return completely to normal.

12 Cardiac Investigations

12.1 Electrocardiography

The electrical axis

The normal mean QRS axis in the frontal plane is –30° to +90°. The normal T-wave axis in the frontal plane should be within 45° of the mean frontal QRS axis, i.e. the QRS–T angle should be < 45°. The hexaxial reference system is shown below.

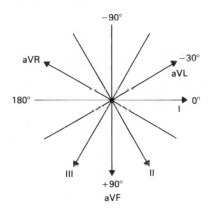

The following gives a quick calculation of the mean frontal QRS axis: find the isoelectric lead; the QRS axis is at right angles to this. Find the lead at right angles to the isoelectric lead from the hexaxial reference system. If the QRS is positive this lead is the electrical axis, if it is negative the axis is 180° away.

Left axis deviation = –30° to –90°.

Right axis deviation = +90° to +180°.

The quadrant –90° to 180° = extreme right or extreme left axis deviation.

Right-axis deviation	Left-axis deviation
Infancy	Left anterior hemiblock
RV hypertrophy	LV hypertrophy
Acute RV strain: pulmonary embolism	LBBB
Cor pulmonale	Primum ASD
Secundum ASD	Tricuspid atresia
RBBB	Cardiomyopathies
Fallot, severe PS	
TAPVD	

Intervals

Normal PR interval: 0.2 s.

Normal QRS duration: 0.1 s.

Normal Q wave is < 0.04-s wide and < 25% of the total QRS complex.

The QT interval must be corrected for heart rate (QTc):

$$\text{Normal QTc} = \frac{QT}{\sqrt{R\text{–}R \text{ interval}}} = 0.38\text{–}0.42 \text{ s}$$

Heart rate calculation from R–R interval. At standard paper speed of 25 mm/seach big square = 0.2 s. Count the number of 'big squares' between each R wave.

R–R interval (s)	Number of large squares	Heart rate (beats/min)
0.2	1	300
0.4	2	150
0.6	3	100
0.8	4	75
1.0	5	60
1.2	6	50
1.4	7	43
1.6	8	37

For intracardiac electrophysiological measurements see **7.8**, page 308.

Hypertrophy

Atrial hypertrophy and the P wave

The normal P-wave axis is +30° to +80° in the frontal plane. It is normally < 2.5 mm in height. Right atrial depolarization occurs first and causes the initial P-wave deflection. Left atrial depolarization causes the terminal deflection.

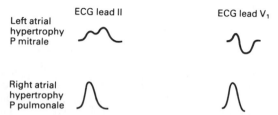

ECG lead II   ECG lead V$_1$

Left atrial hypertrophy P mitrale

Right atrial hypertrophy P pulmonale

Ventricular hypertrophy

There is no single marker of ventricular hypertrophy on the ECG. Several factors are taken into consideration (electrical axis, voltage, delay in the intrinsicoid deflection and ST–T wave changes) and then the ECG is correlated with the patient's condition. Relying on a single marker of ventricular hypertrophy, e.g. ventricular voltage, may not be reliable. A thin chest wall in young men results in a large voltage. A thick chest wall may mask it.

Right ventricular hypertrophy	Left ventricular hypertrophy
Right axis deviation > 90°	Left-axis deviation > −30°
RV1 + SV6 > 11 mm	SV1 or V2 + RV5 or V5 or V6 > 40 mm
RV1 or SV6 > 7 mm	SV1 or V1 or RV5 or V6 > 25 mm
R/S V1 > 1	RI + SIII > 25 mm
R/S V6 < 1	R in I or aVL > 14 mm
T-wave inversion V1–V3 or V4, ST depression	T-wave inversion in I, aVL ST depression V4–V6
Delay in intrinsicoid deflection in V1 > 0.05 s	Delay in intrinsicoid deflection in V6 > 0.04 s
P pulmonale	P mitrale

Factors influencing chest lead voltage
- LV cavity size.
- LV muscle mass.
- Presence of pericardial fluid.
- Lung volume in front of heart.
- Chest wall thickness.

Examples of acute RV strain are shown in Figure 12.8, and LV hypertrophy in Figure 12.1.

Right ventricular hypertrophy in children
The neonate has right ventricular predominance on the ECG with dominant R waves in V1 and aVR and deep S waves in V6. The pattern gradually swings leftwards through childhood and has reached adult configuration by the age of 15 years. By the end of the first week T waves are negative in V1 and V2 and positive in V5 and V6. By 1 month, the positive R wave in aVR has disappeared. The dominance of the RV in the first 3 months makes the diagnosis of pathological RV hypertrophy difficult and serial ECGs may be needed.

Presence of a Q wave in V1
Delay in intrinsicoid deflection in V1 > 0.04 s in the absence of RBBB
R/S or R/Q in aVR > 1
QRS axis > 120°
P pulmonale with P wave > 3 mm in II
R/S in V1 7 (at 3 months); R/S in V6 0.5 (at 3 months)

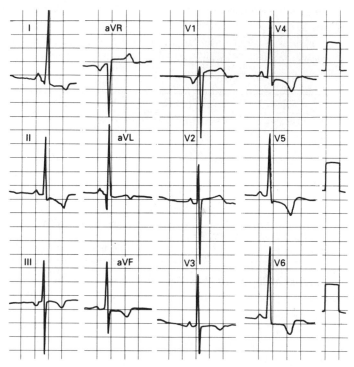

Figure 12.1 ECG in severe left ventricular hypertrophy taken from patient with HCM.

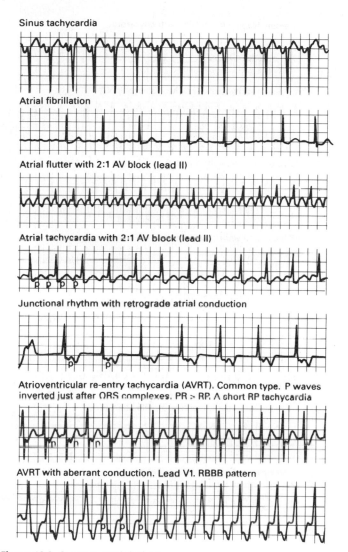

Figure 12.2 Common atrial rhythms.

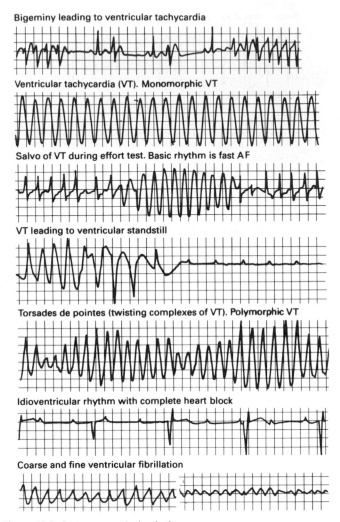

Figure 12.3 Common ventricular rhythms.

Sinus arrest

Sinus arrest with idioventricular escape rhythm

First degree heart block (AV block)

Second degree AV block. Wenckebach type. Mobitz type I AV block

Second degree AV block. Mobitz type II AV block

Second degree AV block. 2:1 AV block

Third degree AV block. Complete AV block

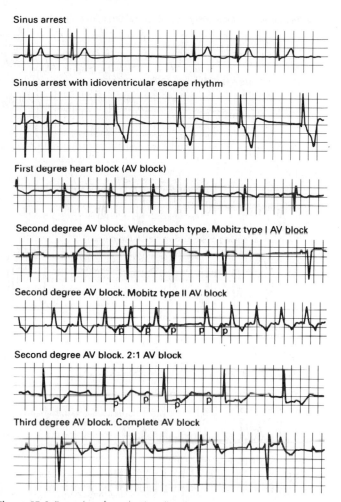

Figure 12.4 Examples of conduction disturbances.

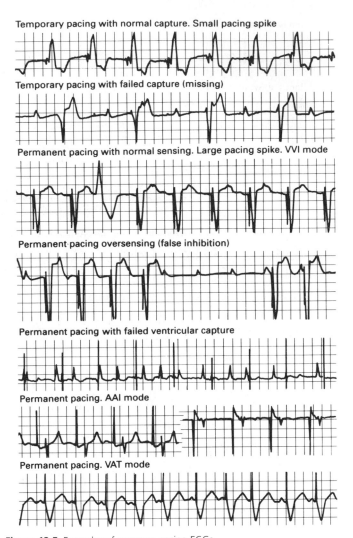

Figure 12.5 Examples of common pacing ECGs.

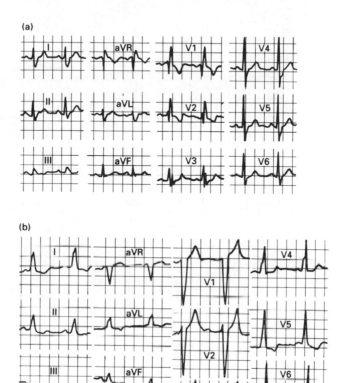

Figure 12.6 (a) Right bundle branch block, (b) left bundle branch block.

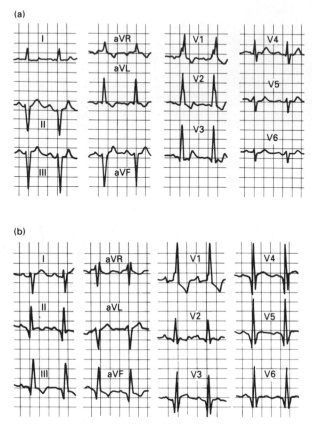

Figure 12.7 Bifascicular blocks: (a) right bundle branch block and left anterior hemiblock, (b) right bundle branch block and left posterior hemiblock.

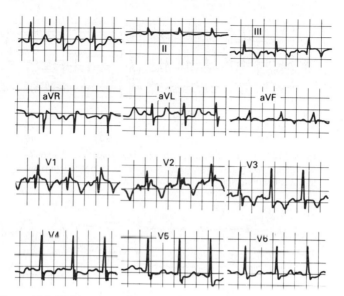

Figure 12.8 ECG in acute pulmonary embolism. This shows typical S_1, Q_3, T_3 pattern, incomplete RBBB and RV strain.

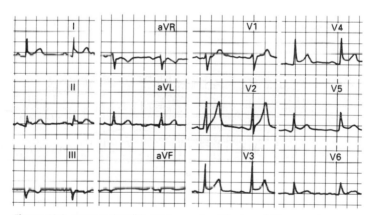

Figure 12.9 Acute pericarditis. Widespread saddle shaped ST segment elevation.

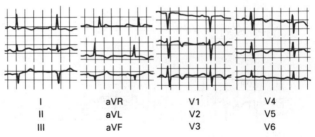

I	aVR	V1	V4
II	aVL	V2	V5
III	aVF	V3	V6

Figure 12.10 Acute anterior subendocardial ischaemia. Anterior T-wave changes only due to severe LAD stenosis. Enzyme elevation needed with this type of ECG to document infarction.

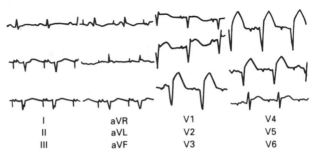

I	aVR	V1	V4
II	aVL	V2	V5
III	aVF	V3	V6

Figure 12.11 Acute transmural anterior myocardial infarction. Typical anterior Q wave with ST-segment elevation. Atrial pacing.

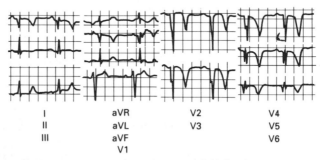

I	aVR	V2	V4
II	aVL	V3	V5
III	aVF		V6
	V1		

Figure 12.12 Recent transmural anterior myocardial infarction.

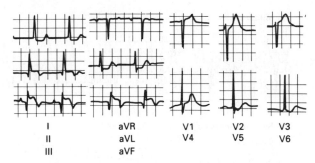

I	aVR	V1	V2	V3
II	aVL	V4	V5	V6
III	aVF			

Figure 12.13 Acute transmural inferior myocardial infarction. This shows typical Q waves and raised ST segments in inferior leads. There is variable sinus and nodal rhythm. Reciprocal or mirror image ST depression in I and aVL.

Acute	Recent	Old
2–5 days	2–6 months	6 months
ST segment	T wave inverted	Just Q
elevation		waves

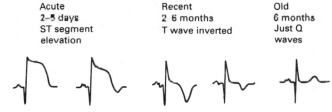

Figure 12.14 Evolution of ST segments following myocardial infarction. Persistent ST segment elevation after 3 months suggests an LV aneurysm.

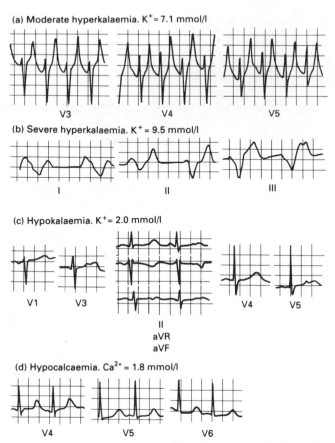

Figure 12.15 Electrolytes and the ECG. (a) Moderate hyperkalaemia produces tall peaked T waves. (b) Severe hyperkalaemia produces gross widening of the QRS also with a resulting 'sine wave' appearance. P waves disappear. (c) Hypokalaemia produces prominent U waves with small T waves resulting in an apparently long QT interval. The T wave is often lost in the U wave. (d) Hypocalcaemia produces a long QT interval with small T waves, while hypercalcaemia produces a short QT interval with normal T waves.

Combined ventricular hypertrophy

The effects of both RV and LV hypertrophy on the ECG may cancel each other out and the QRS complexes appear normal. Suspect it if:
LV hypertrophy + right axis.
RV hypertrophy + left axis.
LV hypertrophy + dominant R in V1 and aVR and deep S in V5.
RV hypertrophy + large Q and R waves in V5 and V6.

12.2 Exercise testing

The reliability, limitations and uses of exercise testing have been carefully established in recent years. Although the sensitivity and specificity of treadmill exercise testing have been widely studied it has also been realized that the results of an exercise test must be interpreted with reference to Bayes' theorem. The prevalence of coronary artery disease in the population under study is very important. The predictive accuracy of a positive test increases with increasing prevalence of the disease in the population. For a definition of terms see table on page 452.

Assume exercise test with 80% sensitivity and 75% specificity

Patient	Pre-test likelihood of coronary disease	Predictive accuracy of positive test
Asymptomatic man	5%	14–36%
Man with angina pectoris	90%	97%

Use in asymptomatic patients

It can be seen that exercise testing is of little value in screening asymptomatic subjects. The ST-segment response to exercise in this group has a poor predictive accuracy. In this group with a low pre-test likelihood of coronary disease, a positive test is often a false-positive test.

Use in symptomatic patients

In the high-risk group (e.g. men with angina) a positive test confirms a clinical diagnosis. A negative test may well be a false-negative test and has a low correlation with the absence of coronary disease.

Thus exercise testing in patients with cardiac symptoms has major limitations from the diagnosis point of view (coronary disease vs. normal coronaries). Nevertheless it has great value in the assessment of cardiac function and the evaluation of symptoms.

Definition of terms

Term	Explanation	How calculated
Sensitivity	Percentage of all patients with coronary artery disease who have an abnormal exercise test	$\dfrac{TP}{TP + FN} \times 100$
Specificity	Percentage of negative exercise tests in normal patients without coronary artery disease	$\dfrac{TN}{TN + FP} \times 100$
Predictive accuracy	Percentage of positive exercise tests that are true positives	$\dfrac{TP}{TP + FP} \times 100$
False-positive response	Percentage of total positive exercise tests that are false-positives (occurring in normal patients)	$\dfrac{FP}{TP + FP} \times 100$ (or 100% − predictive accuracy)
False-negative response	Percentage of total negative exercise tests that are false-negatives (occurring in patients with coronary artery disease)	$\dfrac{FN}{TN + FN} \times 100$ (or 100% − sensitivity)
Risk ratio	Predictive accuracy related to false-negative response (predictive error)	$\dfrac{TP}{TP + FP} \Big/ \dfrac{FN}{TN + FN}$

TN, total negatives; TP, total positives; FN, total false-negatives; FP, total false-positives.

Uses of exercise testing
- Confirmation of a diagnosis of coronary disease in a group with a high pre-test likelihood of the disease.
- Evaluation of cardiac function and exercise capacity.
- Prognosis following myocardial infarction.
- Serial testing in evaluation of medical or surgical treatment.
- Detection of exercise-induced arrhythmias.
- Useful in rehabilitation and patient motivation.

Patient safety
The patient should have avoided cigarettes or a recent meal prior to the test. A physician should be present at all exercise tests or in the immediate vicinity. The procedure is extremely safe provided strict criteria for stopping the exercise test are followed. Reported mortality rates are < 1 in 10 000 tests.

A defibrillator must be instantly available. A complete trolley of cardiac resuscitation equipment should be on-hand, including intubating equipment and full range of cardiac drugs. Although cardiac resuscitation is very rarely necessary during or after exercise testing, occasional patients may develop refractory ventricular tachycardia requiring cardioversion.

Contraindications to exercise testing
Exercise testing should be avoided in the following cases.
- Severe aortic stenosis.
- Acute myocarditis or pericarditis.
- Any pyrexial or 'flu'-like illness.
- Severe left main stem stenosis or its equivalent.
- Left ventricular failure or congestive cardiac failure.
- Adults with complete heart block.
- Unstable or crescendo angina.
- Frequent fast atrial or ventricular arrhythmias.
- Renal failure.
- Orthopaedic or neurological impairment.
- Dissecting aneurysm.
- Uncontrolled hypertension.
- Thyrotoxicosis.
- The test is obviously avoided in any frail, elderly or sick patient.
- Acute myocardial infarction. In patients who are fully mobile and capable of climbing one flight of stairs, exercise testing may be

Table of standard treadmill protocols showing speed and elevation

Stage	Bruce (mph)	(%)	Sheffield (mph)	(%)	Naughton (mph)	(%)	Ellestad (mph)	(%)	Balke 3.0 (mph)	(%)	IMC 3.4 (mph)	(%)	Rehabilitation (mph)	(%)
1	1.7	10.0	1.7	0.0	1.0	0.0	1.7	10.0	3.0	6.0	3.4	0.0	2.0	0.0
2	2.5	12.0	1.7	5.0	2.0	0.0	3.0	10.0	3.0	8.0	3.4	4.0	2.5	0.0
3	3.4	14.0	1.7	10.0	2.0	0.0	4.0	10.0	3.0	10.0	3.4	8.0	2.5	3.0
4	4.2	16.0	2.5	12.0	2.0	3.5	5.0	10.0	3.0	12.0	3.4	12.0	2.5	6.0
5	5.0	18.0	3.4	14.0	2.0	7.0	5.0	15.0	3.0	14.0	3.4	16.0	2.5	9.0
6	5.5	20.0	4.2	16.0	2.0	10.5	6.0	15.0	3.0	16.0	3.4	20.0	2.5	12.0
7	6.0	22.0	5.0	18.0	2.0	14.0			3.0	18.0				

Stage 3 of the Sheffield protocol onwards is the same as Stage 1 onwards of the Bruce protocol.

performed under careful supervision at about 7–10 days post-infarction, i.e. the day before hospital discharge.

Which exercise test?

It is now known that graduated treadmill exercise testing is superior to bicycle ergometry or step testing. Greater limits of exercise are achieved and maximal oxygen uptake is higher with treadmill testing than with other methods. Some patients are unable to pedal a bicycle efficiently, and many stop with 'tired legs' before reaching desired target heart rates.

There are numerous treadmill protocols with variations in increasing speed and gradient. Many centres start the test with a preliminary 'warm-up' period of 3 min (1.0 mph at 5% elevation).

There is no particular advantage of one protocol over another. Many centres use the Bruce protocol as its higher stages (6 and 7) are much more demanding than some other protocols. (More gradual protocols are available for less fit patients, e.g. those used in cardiac rehabilitation.) Most tests are now performed continuously. The blood pressure is recorded at every stage.

ECG leads and lead systems

Many exercise tests are spoiled through inadequate skin preparation. The shaved skin should be cleaned with alcohol or acetone-soaked gauze. The cleaned skin is gently abraded with dry gauze, sandpaper, sterile needle or dental burr. Silver/silver chloride pre-gelled electrodes are then applied (e.g. Cambmac medicotest or Sentry medical products). The electrodes and leads are secured by micropore tape. Electrically screened leads should be used.

The sensitivity for recording significant ST depression increases as more leads are used. Cardiac centres have now moved from a standard V5 lead to 10- or 12-lead ECG recording. The percentage of all positive cases of ST-segment depression post-exercise recorded using these leads is shown in the following table:

ECG lead	Percentage
V5 alone	89%
V5 V6	91%
V4 V5 V6	93%
V3 V4 V5 V6	95%
II V3 V4 V5 V6	96%
II AVF V3 V4 V5 V6	100%

Oxygen consumption

The relation between heart rate and oxygen consumption is linear for most patients during exercise. The slope of the relation is less for the fitter and more athletic patients (i.e. greater oxygen consumption for less increment in heart rate). Maximum oxygen consumption is a good measure of maximum cardiac performance and is usually measured in ml O_2/kg/min or metabolic equivalents (METS). Resting O_2 consumption is approximately 3.5 ml O_2/kg/min which = 1 METS.

In a male athlete V_{O_2} max. is approximately 70–80 ml O_2/kg/min, and 60 ml O_2/kg/min for a female athlete.

Table of oxygen consumption at stages of exercise in various protocols in ml O_2/kg/min

Stage	Bruce	Sheffield	Balke 3.0
1	17.5	8	18.0
2	24.5	12	21.0
3	34	17.5	24.0
4	46	24.5	28.0
5	56	34	32.0

Thus at Stage 5 of the Bruce protocol (= Stage 7 of Sheffield protocol) oxygen requirement is 56 ml O_2/kg/min or 16 METS.

End points and when to terminate the exercise test

1 The test should be stopped when target heart rate has been achieved. This may be maximum heart rate for age or sub-maximal (commonly 85% of maximum predicted heart rate).

Age-adjusted target heart rates

Age (years)	Submaximal heart rate (85% max)	Maximal heart rate
30	165	194
35	160	188
40	155	182
45	150	176
50	145	171
55	140	165
60	135	159
65	130	153

A useful mental guide for heart rate (maximum) is for men, 220 − age; for women, 210 − age.

2 The test should be stopped prior to maximum or sub-maximal heart rate if any of the following symptoms or signs occur:

- progressive angina pectoris
- undue dyspnoea
- vasoconstriction with a clammy sweaty skin
- fatigue
- musculoskeletal pain
- feeling of faintness
- atrial fibrillation or atrial tachycardia
- premature ventricular contractions with increasing frequency
- ventricular tachycardia
- progressive ST-segment depression ⎤ with or without
- progressive ST-segment elevation ⎦ chest pain
- failure of HR or BP to rise with effort, this is very important and applies even in patients on beta-blocking agents
- excessive rise in peak systolic pressure (> 230 mmHg)
- electrical alternans
- development of LBBB
- development of AV block.

Sometimes the greatest ECG abnormalities occur during the recovery period when the patient is lying down. Young unfit patients may develop a profound vagal bradycardia postexercise requiring atropine. A period of 10–15 min is usually long enough for recovery. All haemodynamic criteria (heart rate and blood pressure) and ECG should have returned to the pre-exercise state before the patient is moved.

Exercise testing and drugs

Digoxin frequently causes a false-positive exercise test and ST-segment changes at rest are common. If possible the drug should be stopped at least 1 week prior to exercise. Digoxin is not thought to cause false-negative responses.

Beta-blocking agents do not need to be withdrawn prior to exercise, and sudden withdrawal may be dangerous. The maximum heart rate response and maximum workload achieved will be reduced from normal. However, there is evidence that beta-blockade may help in converting false positive results to negative, and allow true positive results to remain positive.

A single dose of a beta-blocking agent may be taken 1.5–2 hours prior to the test if the patient is not on beta-blockade already and thought to have a false positive test. Beta-blockade will increase the specificity and predictive accuracy of the exercise test but reduce its sensitivity.

Exercise testing following myocardial infarction

In the absence of the contraindications listed, exercise testing may be safely performed following myocardial infarction and before hospital discharge (at about 7–10 days postinfarction), although exercise testing is usually delayed until about 1 month postinfarction. A limited treadmill test is useful in predicting recurrent angina or sudden death in the first year postinfarction. It helps to identify patients who need coronary angiography. Poor prognostic factors are shown on page 193.

What represents a positive test?

1 ST-segment depression (see Figure 12.16)

There must be ≥ 1.0 mm ST-segment depression 80 ms after the J point, using the PQ segment as the baseline in six consecutive cycles. If the J point is not clearly visible, the nadir of the S wave may be used instead. It does not matter if the ST segment is downsloping, horizontal or upsloping at the 80-ms point. Sometimes all three may occur in the same patient in different leads, and the ST segment changes should preferably to be in more than one lead anyway. Some centres prefer to use 1.5-mm ST depression 80 ms after the J point if the ST segment is upsloping. If 1.5- or 2.0-mm ST depression is taken as the necessary hallmark of a positive test, the sensitivity of the test will fall, but the predictive accuracy will increase. T-wave inversion alone is valueless.

The PQ junction is taken as the baseline as this junction is normally depressed on exercise below the classical isoelectric line. The Ta wave (P-wave repolarization) on exercise may extend through the QRS and

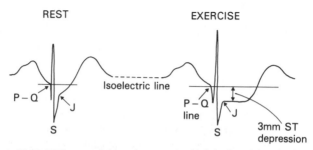

Figure 12.16 ECG at rest (left) and on exercise (right). The PQ iunction line is below the isoelectric line and is taken as the baseline for ST-segment analysis. The complex on the right shows 3-mm ST-segment depression 80 ms after the J point. If the J point is not clearly seen, the nadir of the S wave may be used.

influence the ST segment even in normal patients. Hence the need for the 80-ms delay after the J point for test interpretation.

Although the degree of ST segment depression is the diagnostic hallmark of a positive exercise test it is also important to note:

• how many and in which leads it occurs
• the heart rate at which it first appears
• its persistence in the recovery period.

Some equipment now integrates the area of ST-segment depression (in microvolt-seconds). It is also possible to run exercise tests using signal averaging of the QRS complex. This produces clear recordings with no electrical or myographic interference. However, the equipment is expensive, and meticulous attention to satisfactory electrode placement is all that is really necessary. Typically positive exercise tests are shown in Figure 12.17.

2 *ST-segment elevation* (Figure 12.18)
May occur during exercise in leads with Q waves and has the same significance as ST depression in other leads. It is due to systolic outward wall movement over the infarct area.

3 *Chest pain*
Taken in association with ST depression, chest pain increases the sensitivity of the exercise test to approximately 85% in a cohort of symptomatic patients. The nature of the pain is important. Unilateral chest pain is unlikely to be angina. Patients who experience 'walk through' or 'second wind' angina do not normally do so on an exercise test as the workload is progressive and not steady.

Other criteria below are not as useful as the ST segment in predicting coronary disease. However, they are important correlates of a positive test and increase the sensitivity of the test still further when combined with ST segment analysis.

4 *Increase in R-wave voltage* (Figure 12.17 bottom panel)
In the normal patient, R-wave voltage decreases during exercise. Immediately postexercise R-wave voltage is at its smallest and then gradually returns to normal during the recovery period. The reduction in R-wave voltage is thought to be due to the reduction of left ventricular end-diastolic volume with increasing exercise in the normal patient. The relation of QRS voltage to LV blood volume is the Brody effect. LV volume also decreases on standing up from the supine position.

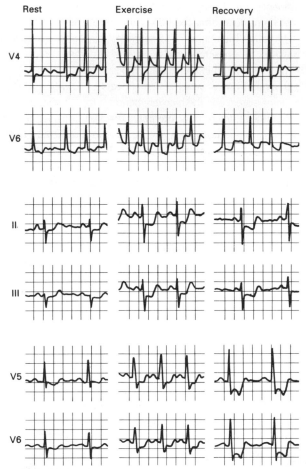

Figure 12.17 Changes in ST segments. This shows three examples of positive ST-segment depression. The top panel shows upsloping and downsloping ST-segment depression in different leads. The second panel shows a positive test persisting after beta-blockade. The bottom panel shows ST-segment depression getting progressive worse into the recovery stage. R-wave voltage increases. See page 459.

In patients with coronary disease R-wave voltage usually remains unchanged or increases, especially in those with poor LV function. R-wave changes may be useful in patients with LBBB where ST changes lack sensitivity or specificity.

Unfortunately the R wave is not only related to LVEDV but to other

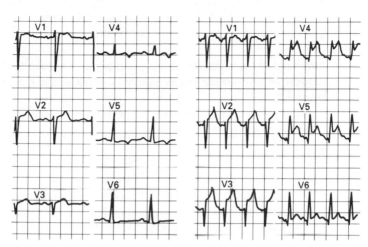

Figure 12.18 ST elevation during exercise test.

factors also (e.g. respiration). R-wave voltage is best averaged for several cycles and leads rather than taking a mean of a single lead (e.g. V5).

5 Inverted U waves

Leads in which U waves are well seen may show U-wave inversion in patients with coronary disease. The changes may be transient and at peak exercise only. They are characterized by a concave depression in the T–P segment. The U wave is usually overlooked in exercise testing.

6 Abnormal systolic blood pressure response

Failure of the systolic blood pressure to rise during exercise is an important indicator of an abnormal LV and is an indication to stop the test. A decrease in systolic blood pressure during exercise is even more specific of severe coronary artery disease – assuming there are no valve lesions and the patient is not on vasodilators.

7 Development of ventricular arrhythmias (Figure 12.3)

The development of ventricular arrhythmias is not specific for coronary artery disease. Ventricular ectopics (> 10/min), multifocal ectopics, ventricular tachycardia, etc., associated with ST-segment depression and chest pain are more specific.

8 Auscultating changes

Auscultation should be performed immediately in the recovery period.

New mitral regurgitation or a fourth heart sound ($S_{4)}$) is highly significant.

Summary of variables developing during an exercise test suggestive of multiple vessel coronary disease and a poorer prognosis

• ST depression: at low heart rate (< 130/min off beta-blockade), > 2 mm in several leads, downsloping, persisting > 5 min into recovery period.
• Blood pressure response: failure to rise or falling > 10 mmHg.
• Ventricular arrhythmias developing at low exercise load.
• Poor exercise tolerance: inability to complete Bruce protocol Stage II or equivalent and a positive test with inappropriate tachycardia.

Patients with these results are generally referred for coronary angiography.

False-positive results

An enormous number of conditions may be associated with false-positive exercise tests. They are particularly common in patients with a low pre-test likelihood of coronary artery disease (e.g. asymptomatic young women). Known associations of false positive results in patients with normal coronaries are:
• hyperventilation
• prolapsing mitral valve
• hypertrophic cardiomyopathy
• dilated cardiomyopathy
• hypertension with LV hypertrophy
• LBBB
• aortic stenosis
• young women with chest pain
• WPW syndrome
• drugs, e.g. digoxin, antidepressants
• anaemia
• coronary artery spasm
• hypokalaemia
• hypersensitivity to catecholamines
• observer variability.

Hyperventilation as a cause of a false-positive test can be excluded by asking the standing patient to hyperventilate for 30 s prior to the exercise test. Patients with sympathetic overactivity, emotional liability and resting tachycardia are very likely to have a false positive test. This functional condition has been called the hyperkinetic heart syndrome. Beta-blockade may abolish resting T-wave abnormalities on the ECG in these patients and will increase the specificity of the test by preventing the false-positive result.

12.3 Echocardiography

Echocardiography is now a standard non-invasive cardiac investigation following the early pioneering work of Edler and Hertz in 1953.

Pulsed ultrasound of high frequency is generated by a piezo-electric crystal, which acts as both transmitter and receiver. Transmitted pulses of sound are produced by the transducer and reflected sound is converted back to an electrical signal and recorded.

The higher the frequency of the ultrasound used the greater the resolution of the image (with the shorter wavelength), but tissue attenuation (absorption of ultrasound) is greater.

Properties of ultrasound commonly used in cardiology

Frequency
2.25 MHz in adults
5 MHz in children (where tissue attenuation is less)

Focal length
7.5 cm
10 cm for more obese patients, or patients with emphysema

Repetition rate
1000/s, each transmitting and receiving period lasts for 1 ms only, of this period only 1 µs is taken up in transmission and the rest in 'listening'

Velocity of sound in human tissue
1540 m/s, distances can be recorded in centimetres rather than time

Velocity of sound in silastic (ball valve)
980 m/s

Types of scan (Figure 12.19)

A-mode (amplitude modulation)
The returned ultrasound signals are displayed on the oscilloscope as a series of vertical lines. The amplitude/height of each line represents the

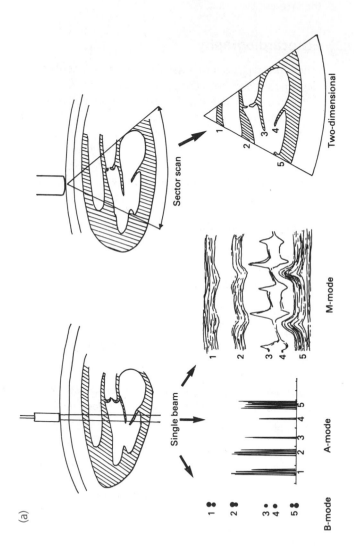

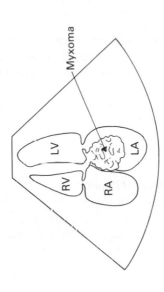

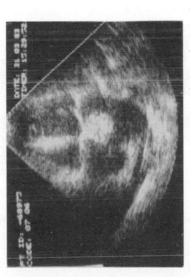

Figure 12.19 (a) Diagrammatic representation of types of echocardiogram. The numbers refer to the same structure in each type of scan: 1, anterior right ventricular wall; 2, interventricular septum; 3, anterior mitral leaflet; 4, posterior mitral leaflet; 5, posterior left ventricular wall. (b) An example of a two-dimensional scan in the four-chamber view, showing a left atrial myxoma.

strength of the returning signals. The base is represented as distance (cm) from the transducer.

B-mode (brightness modulation)
The peaks of the A-mode scan are represented as a series of linear dots whose brightness represents the echo intensity.

M-mode (motion mode)
The B-mode scan is displayed on light-sensitive paper moving at constant speed to produce the conventional permanent record – a single dimension/time image.

Two-dimensional ('realtime')
A two-dimensional image of a segment of the heart is produced on the screen: a cine image or moving tomographic cut that can be stored on videotape. Frozen images can be hard copied. The two-dimensional image is produced either by rotating the scanning head rapidly through 80–90° (single crystal) or by a phased array (multicrystal) scanning head. In the phased array system the ultrasound crystals are excited in sequence or phase to produce a fan-shaped wave front.

The original multicrystal head in linear format (as used in abdominal ultrasound) is unsuitable for cardiac imaging as the ribs interfere with the ultrasound beams.

Two-dimensional echocardiography cannot be covered in this book. Several conditions are much better visualized by a two-dimensional study than by M-mode. These include most congenital heart disease, LV aneurysm, intraventricular thrombus, LA myxoma, septal defects and small shunts, which can be detected by the 5% dextrose microbubble injection technique. An example of an LA myxoma seen on a two-dimensional scan is shown in Figure 12.19b.

Several views are needed in a single two-dimensional study. The four commonest are long-axis and short-axis views, the four-chamber view and the subcostal view. Suprasternal views are useful in children for visualizing the great vessels.

Normal echocardiographic values in an adult
Ventricular and atrial dimensions (ID, internal dimension):

LVIDd (end diastole): 3.5–5.6 cm
LVIDs (end systole): 1.9–4.0 cm } see Figure 12.20
Posterior LV wall thickness: 0.7–1.1 cm (at end diastole)
RVID (end diastole): 0.7–2.6 cm

....

Posterior LV wall excursion (amplitude): 0.8–1.2 cm

Interventricular septal thickness: 0.7–1.2 cm

LAID (end systole): 1.9–4.0 cm

Ratio of septum to posterior wall thickness = 1.3:1

Aorta and aortic valve:

Aortic root internal diameter: 2.0–3.7 cm

Aortic valve opening: 1.6–2.6 cm

Mitral valve:

E–F slope (closure rate): 70–150 cm/s

E point to septal distance: 0–5 mm

D–F distance: 20–30 mm

Ventricular function:

Ejection fraction: 0.62–0.85

Velocity of circumferential fibre shortening of LV (V_{cf}) = 1.1–1.8 circ/s

Formulae used in echocardiographic calculations of left ventricular function

LVEDV = $(LVIDd)^3$ = $(Dd)^3$ ml (for normal ventricles)

LVESV = $(LVIDs)^3$ = $(Ds)^3$ ml

Stroke volume = $Dd^3 - Ds^3$ ml

$$\text{Ejection fraction} = \frac{Dd^3 - Ds^3}{Dd^3} \, 100\%$$

$$V_{cf} = \frac{Dd - Ds}{Ds \times LVET} \text{ circ/s}$$

LVET is measured from carotid pulse (see systolic time intervals).

Example from Figure 12.20:

Dd = 5.0 cm Dd^3 = 125

Ds = 2.9 cm Ds^3 = 24.4

Dd is taken as the maximum diastolic diameter at the point of augmentation due to the A wave – at the timing of the R wave of the ECG (see Figure 12.20).

$$\text{Ejection fraction} = \frac{125 - 24.4}{125} \times 100 = 80\%$$

It is important in calculations of LV function from echocardiograms to obtain good endocardial echoes from both septum and posterior left

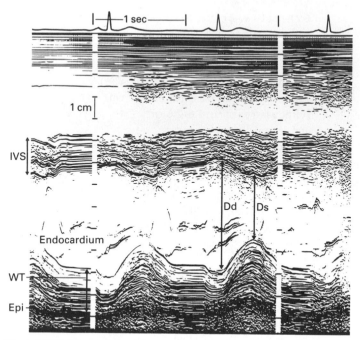

Figure 12.20 Echocardiograph in an adult to show measurement of ventricular dimensions.

ventricular wall. The epicardium is a denser band of echoes visible at the back of the posterior left ventricular wall (PLVW). The ratio of interventricular septal thickness (IVS) to posterior wall thickness (endocardium to epicardium at end diastole) may be calculated and should be less than 1.3 : 1.

Common patterns of mitral valve movement on M-mode echocardiogram (Figure 12.21)

1 The normal mitral valve in sinus rhythm. At point D the anterior and posterior mitral leaflets separate. The anterior leaflet has the greater excursion which can be measured (D–E distance). The E point is the point of maximal opening and the anterior leaflet virtually touches the septum in the normal ventricle. In LV failure there is separation of the septum to E point and the greater the E point to septal distance the worse the LV function.

The mitral valve immediately starts to close again to the F point. The E–F slope is a measure of the rate of mitral valve closure. Normal E–F

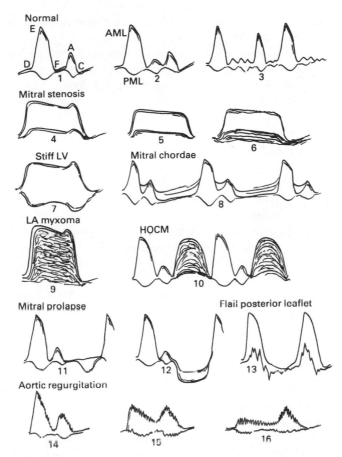

Figure 12.21 Common patterns of mitral valve movement on M-mode echocardiogram.

slope is 70–150 cm/s. It is reduced in mitral stenosis. The mitral valve re-opens at end diastole with the A wave. The leaflets meet at point C at the onset of systole. The movement of the posterior leaflet mirrors the anterior leaflet, but its excursion is less. It is more difficult to record on the M-mode echo.

2 The normal mitral valve with a slower heart rate in sinus rhythm. The movements are as in **1**, but an extra excursion is seen in mid-diastole after the F point. This is normal and just represents mid-diastolic flow into LV.

3 The normal mitral valve in AF. Here the A wave disappears and the excursion of the E point varies depending on the R–R interval. Little fibrillation waves may be seen between the main mitral excursions.
4 Mitral stenosis in sinus rhythm. The mitral anterior leaflet excursion is reduced. The slope of mitral valve closure (E–F slope) is greatly reduced and in severe cases may be horizontal, giving a castellated appearance to the mitral valve. In mobile mitral stenosis still in SR a small A wave may be seen. The posterior leaflet moves anteriorly and may also exhibit an A wave.
5 Mitral stenosis in AF in a more severe case. The A wave disappears (compare with **4**), and excursion is reduced.
6 Calcific mitral stenosis. Multiple hard horizontal bars on the posterior leaflet suggest calcification.
7 Stiff LV excursion of the anterior leaflet and the diastolic closure rate may be reduced. However, the posterior leaflet moves posteriorly. In sinus rhythm there may be a slight delay in coaptation of the leaflets to the C point (patients with high LVEDP).
8 Mitral chordae. These may be seen as the transducer is angled towards the apex. Horizontal parallel lines appear above the coapted anterior and posterior leaflets.
9 LA myxoma. A very characteristic appearance. Multiple echoes filling in the space behind and below the anterior leaflet. There may be an initial clear space before the echoes appear, i.e. the valve opens first, and then the tumour pops down into the mitral orifice. Differential diagnosis includes mitral valve vegetatons, mitral valve aneurysm and LA thrombus.
10 HCM. The mitral valve may be normal in diastole. In systole the entire mitral apparatus moves anteriorly producing the characteristic bulge illustrated. This abuts the septum producing LVOTO. It is called the SAM (systolic anterior movement).
11 Mitral prolapse. A common echo finding in an asymptomatic patient (see mitral regurgitation). This diagram shows late systolic prolapse of the posterior leaflet. The point of separation of the anterior and posterior leaflets in mid systole will coincide with the mid-systolic click if present. The late systolic murmur follows.
12 Pansystolic prolapse. This is a more severe variety and is associated usually with symptomatic mitral regurgitation.
13 Flail posterior leaflet. Ruptured chordae can result in chaotic movement of the posterior leaflet. The important diagnostic point is anterior movement and fluttering of the posterior leaflet in diastole.
14–16 Grades of aortic regurgitation: mild, moderate and severe. Mild

aortic regurgitation causes diastolic fluttering of the anterior leaflet only, with normal mitral valve excursion. As regurgitation becomes more severe, mitral valve excursion is reduced (premature mitral valve closure) and both anterior and posterior leaflets flutter. In very severe cases the mitral valve hardly opens until the A wave.

Common patterns of aortic valve movement on M-mode echocardiogram (Figure 12.22)

1 Normal. The aortic cusps in diastole form a central closure line (CL). With left ventricular ejection the cusps separate to the edge of the aortic wall: the right coronary cusp anteriorly (RCC) and the posterior non-coronary cusp (PCC) posteriorly. The aortic valve in systole assumes a parallelogram shape. The left ventricular ejection time can be measured from the point of cusp opening to cusp closure if good echoes are obtained.

2 Normal. In this diagram the left coronary cusp is included and is

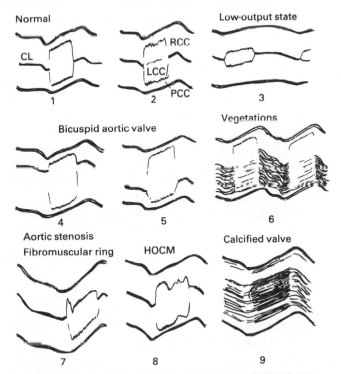

Figure 12.22 Common patterns of aortic valve movement on M-mode echocardiogram.

rarely seen. Systolic fluttering of the aortic cusps is not necessarily abnormal and may occur with high- or low-output states or causes of turbulence (e.g. subvalve stenosis).

3 Low-output state. Separation of the aortic cusps is limited, but the cusps are normal. Anterior and posterior movement of the aorta is diminished – the aorta is barely swinging compared with **1** and **2**.

4 and **5** Bicuspid aortic valve. Although the cusps separate normally the closure line is eccentric and may be either anterior (**4**) or posterior (**5**). Approximately 15% of bicuspid valves have a central closure line, and this sign cannot be relied on diagnostically. In addition a tricuspid aortic valve with a subaortic VSD and prolapsing right coronary cusp may produce an eccentric closure line. Once a bicuspid valve is heavily calcified it cannot be distinguished from a tricuspid calcified valve by echocardiography.

6 Vegetations. These will only be visualized echocardiographically if they are > 2 mm. Small granular vegetations will be missed. Large aortic valve vegetations will be seen in both systole and diastole as dense horizontal lines. They may be confused with aortic valve calcification. Usually aortic valve vegetations are not continuous in systole and diastole, and are often seen only in diastole. Aortic valve calcification usually produces denser more continuous linear echoes. Unfortunately, there is no absolute guide to their distinction.

7 Fibromuscular ring (discrete subaortic stenosis). There is immediate systolic closure of the aortic valve, best seen on the right coronary cusp. Often valve opening never returns to normal during the rest of systole. Compare this with hypertrophic obstructive cardiomyopathy (**8**) where premature aortic valve closure also occurs, but later in mid systole. The two conditions may occur together. The fibromuscular ring is best visualized on two-dimensional imaging.

8 HCM. Premature aortic valve closure occurs in mid systole when septum and mitral apparatus meet to produce LVOTO. Mid-systolic aortic valve closure *per se* is not diagnostic of HCM. It may occur in other conditions (e.g. mitral leaflet prolapse, aortic regurgitation, DCM, VSD, DORV).

9 Calcific aortic stenosis. Dense linear echoes usually continuous through systole and diastole are produced by one or more cusps. In more severe cases the entire aorta may be filled with these echoes and no discrete cusp movement is visible.

The pulmonary valve
The most difficult valve to visualize with the echo. Usually the posterior

leaflet only is seen, and during pulmonary valve opening the echo often disappears to reappear as the valve closes.

Diagrammatic examples of pulmonary valve movement are shown in Figure 12.23.

1 Normal. Atrial systole is transmitted to the pulmonary valve and causes a small posterior movement or A wave. Systolic opening occurs next (B–C). The valve drifts slightly anteriorly to point D later in systole and then closes rapidly (D–E). In diastole the valve drifts slowly posteriorly (E–F slope) in the presence of a low PA pressure before the next A wave.

2 Pulmonary hypertension. The A wave disappears and so does the normal posterior drift of the E–F slope. The E–F line is horizontal or may even be reserved. There is frequently coarse systolic fluttering of the pulmonary valve and mid-systolic closure.

3 Pulmonary stenosis. The A wave becomes increasingly prominent as the pulmonary stenosis becomes more severe. Unfortunately the size of the A wave is not a completely reliable guide to the severity of the pulmonary stenosis.

Infundibular pulmonary stenosis produces diastolic and systolic fluttering of the pulmonary valve from turbulence. The A wave disappears as the subpulmonary obstruction prevents its transmission to the valve.

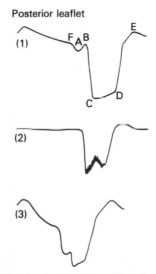

Figure 12.23 Pulmonary valve appearances on M-mode echocardiogram. (1) Normal, (2) pulmonary hypertension, (3) pulmonary stenosis.

....

The tricuspid valve

Best visualized with two-dimensional imaging in the short axis. Doppler studies may show tricuspid regurgitation. For calculation of PA pressure using the tricuspid regurgitant jet, see page 478. On M-mode imaging mitral and tricuspid valve movements are very similar with tricuspid closure occurring up to 40 ms after mitral closure. With wide right bundle branch block, closure may be delayed up to 65 ms. In Ebstein's anomaly, in which tricuspid and mitral echoes are often seen well at the same time, tricuspid closure is delayed still further.

Many features of mitral valve disease echocardiographically also apply to the tricuspid valve (e.g. visualization of vegetations, posterior tricuspid leaflet prolapse).

In primum ASD with AV canal defect there may be a free floating leaflet across the ventricular septal defect component. Either the mitral or tricuspid component of the valve may be seen to cross into the septum.

Septal movement

The septum normally acts as part of the left ventricle with posterior movement in systole (see example under LV function). Some conditions result in paradoxical septal motion in which the septal's posterior movement is delayed; it moves anteriorly in systole acting as part of the RV. The main causes are the following:

• RV volume overload: atrial septal defect, tricuspid regurgitation, pulmonary regurgitation, partial or total anomalous pulmonary veins, Ebstein's anomaly
• delayed or abnormal activation: LBBB, WPW syndrome, ventricular ectopics
• septal abnormalities: ischaemic heart disease, dilated cardiomyopathy
• pericardial disease: pericardial effusion, constrictive pericarditis, congenital absence of pericardium
• open heart surgery: even in the absence of a conduction defect.

Checking connections in congenital heart disease

Two-dimensional and Doppler echocardiography have in many cases obviated the need for invasive investigation. Among the many factors that need to be assessed at echocardiography are:

• Aortic–mitral continuity. The posterior wall of the aorta should be continuous with the anterior mitral leaflet. Absence of aortic–mitral continuity is seen in double-outlet right ventricle, some patients with Fallot's tetralogy and truncus arteriosus.

- Aortic–septal continuity. The anterior aortic wall is normally continuous with the. interventricular septum. Overriding of the aorta can be seen in Fallot's tetralogy in the two-dimensional long axis.
- Which AV valve is continuous with which great vessel? In transposition of the great vessels (TGA) the posterior AV valve (mitral) is continuous with the posterior pulmonary artery. The anterior tricuspid valve is continuous with the aorta. Distinction of the great vessels depends on size (larger aorta in adults), venous injections of contrast (5% dextrose) in children and the recognition of a possible end-diastolic A wave on the pulmonary valve. Unfortunately, both AV valves may look identical and the distinction of the great vessels is important.

Pericardial effusion

The echocardiogram is very useful for detection of pericardial effusion. Pericardial fluid accumulates anterior to both ventricles and anterior and lateral to the right atrium. The pericardial reflection behind the left atrium limits the extension of effusion behind the left atrium and the pericardium tends to be adherent posteriorly. Pericardial fluid tends to be limited on the left side at the AV groove.

Thus an echo taken at ventricular level may show fluid in front of the RV wall and behind the posterior LV wall (Figure 12.24). Smaller

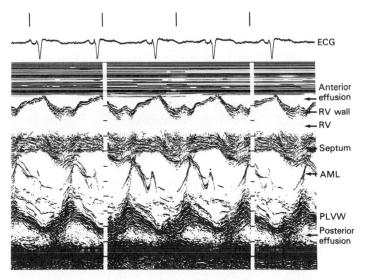

Figure 12.24 Pericardial effusion seen both anterior to the RV wall and posterior to the LV wall.

effusions may only be visualized posteriorly. Usually an echo at the level of the aortic valve shows fluid anteriorly, but none behind the left atrium for the reasons given above.

The effect of the swinging heart inside the bag of fluid may produce paradoxical septal motion, pseudomitral prolapse and electrical alternans on the ECG (see page 365).

Two-dimensional echocardiography shows the effusion clearly and the size of the effusion is the best predictor of tamponade. Diastolic collapse of the RV and/or the RA may occur and the presence of diastolic collapse is an indication for pericardial aspiration. Fibrinous strands and exudates may be seen in chronic inflammatory effusions. A loculated pleural effusion may be mistaken for pericardial fluid.

Doppler ultrasound

Doppler echocardiographic equipment compares the frequency of transmitted ultrasound with the received ultrasound frequency reflected off moving blood cells. Cells moving directly towards the transducer will result in a higher frequency ultrasound, and cells moving away from the transducer, a lower frequency.

This Doppler shift frequency is used to estimate the velocity of blood

i.e. $f_D = \dfrac{2f(V \cos \theta)}{c}$

where f_D = Doppler shift frequency
V = velocity of blood
θ = angle between transmitted and reflected sound
f = transmitted frequency
c = velocity of sound

Doppler ultrasound has revolutionized cardiac diagnosis particularly in paediatric cardiology and has obviated the need for cardiac catheterization in many cases. It has proved very useful for estimating the severity of many cardiac lesions, e.g.:

• aortic, mitral and pulmonary valve gradients and areas
• PA pressure (e.g. in children with VSDs)
• VSD closure (rising peak velocity of jet)
• PDA
• coarctation
• subaortic stenosis, infundibular stenosis
• pulmonary artery branch stenosis
• severity of valve regurgitation.

Modes of Doppler ultrasound used in cardiology

1 Pulsed wave (PW). Useful for identifying the exact site of stenosis, leak, etc. Not useful, however, for quantitative measurements. Pulsed Doppler cannot detect high-frequency Doppler shifts as the pulse repetition frequency is limited. This results in 'aliasing' in which the signal may wrap around and appear on the other side of the baseline. This may introduce confusion as to the true direction of flow.

2 Continuous wave (CW). Needed to quantitate valve stenoses, etc. Aliasing does not occur. Blood flowing away from the transducer is represented as a spectral display below the baseline, and blood flowing towards it as a display above the baseline.

3 Colour Doppler. This colour codes for the direction of ultrasound shift: e.g. red indicating blood moving towards the transducer, blue indicating blood moving away from the transducer.

This enables the echo technician to localise much more quickly the site and direction of abnormal blood flow (e.g. prosthetic valve regurgitation). It is not so useful in quantitating the severity of lesions.

The normal Doppler examination

Normal blood velocity. In adults (and children) in metres per second:
- tricuspid valve 0.3–0.7 m/s
- pulmonary valve 0.5–1.0 m/s
- mitral valve 0.6–1.3 m/s
- aortic valve 0.9–1.7 m/s.

Children with innocent murmurs have higher velocities in the ascending aorta. Low velocity in the ascending aorta is due to a low cardiac output or a wide aorta (e.g. Marfan's syndrome). Higher velocities occur in higher flow situations (e.g. postexercise, anxiety) or in the right heart with left-to-right shunts.

Normal valve regurgitation. Doppler examination has established that a very mild degree of regurgitation occurs through normal pulmonary and tricuspid valves. This regurgitation has a low peak velocity (e.g. < 1 m/s through the pulmonary valve). Tricuspid and pulmonary regurgitation are more common in cases with pulmonary hypertension, older children or RBBB.

Laminar vs. turbulent flow. With laminar flow all the velocities of the blood cells are similar and a thin waveform with minimal spectral broadening is produced. With turbulent flow, multiple different velocities are recorded and the Doppler signal is filled in with marked spectral broadening. See Figures 12.28 and 12.29.

Estimation of PA pressure. First a good recording of tricuspid regurgitation is obtained using CW Doppler. Peak velocity of the tricuspid regurgitation is measured (say 2 m/s). Then peak RV pressure = $4V^2$ of peak tricuspid regurgitation velocity (= 16). Add an extra 5 for estimated RA pressure, then peak RV pressure = 21 mmHg = peak PA pressure assuming no pulmonary stenosis.

Valve gradients
With good apical views using continuous wave, Doppler aortic and mitral valve gradients can be estimated. A suprasternal view of the aortic valve is needed in children (not possible in adults). Even using continuous wave Doppler, it is possible to underestimate the aortic valve gradient if the cardiac output is low, the maximum jet is not recorded or the angle between the ultrasound beam and the blood jet > 20°.

• Aortic valve: peak gradient, Figure 12.25.

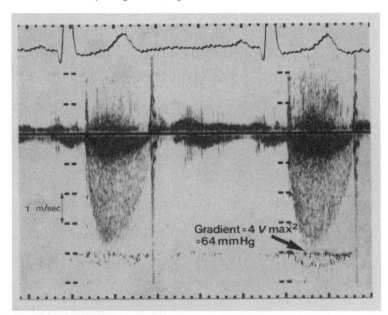

Figure 12.25 Continuous wave Doppler signal in a patient with moderate aortic valve stenosis (apical view). Peak velocity = 4 m/s (V_{max}). Peak systolic gradient = $4 V_{max}^2$ = 64 mmHg.

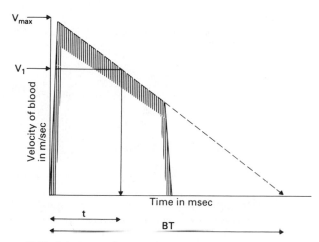

Figure 12.26 Calculation of mitral valve gradient and valve area from a diagrammatic apical continuous wave Doppler signal. See text.

Peak systolic gradient = 4 V_{max}^2 where V_{max} is the measured peak velocity in m/s.
- Mitral valve: peak gradient = 4 V_{max}^2. Use CW from the apex.

Mitral valve area:

Measurement of pressure half time is needed to calculate mitral valve area (Figure 12.26).

V_1 = 0.7 x V_{max}, and occurs at the time (t) when the pressure gradient has fallen to half its maximum value, t = pressure half time.

Mitral valve area = 220/t

$\qquad$ = 759/BT, where DT is the base time of the slope extrapolated to zero.

$\qquad$ (t = 0.29 × BT)

These formulae cannot be used for the tricuspid valve.

Doppler mitral valve studies and diastolic function
(Figures 12.28 & 12.29)

Flow patterns through a normal mitral valve depend on left ventricular stiffness, atrial systolic function and rhythm, the phases of respiration and heart rate (Figure 12.27). Using the apical four-chamber view with the sample volume in the mitral valve orifice (as in Figure 12.28) numerous variables are derived. Approximate normal ranges are shown in the table on page 484.

Figure 12.30 shows the measurement of these indices in a diagrammatic trace.

Sinus rhythm.
Mild mitral stenosis. Peak velocity 1.07 m/s. Pressure half time 114 ms.
Valve area 1.92 cm². Prominent A waves

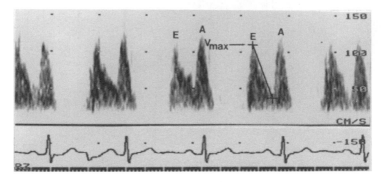

Severe mitral stenosis. Peak velocity 2.0 m/s. Pressure half time 211 ms.
Valve area 1.04 cm²

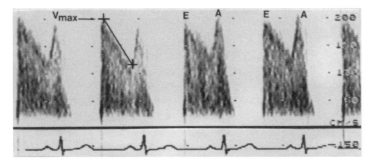

Atrial fibrillation.
Severe mitral stenosis. Peak velocity 2.0m/s. Pressure half time 180 ms.
Valve area 1.22 cm². Note loss of A wave

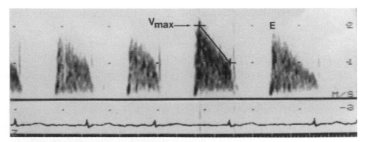

Figure 12.27 Continuous-wave Doppler echo in mitral stenosis.

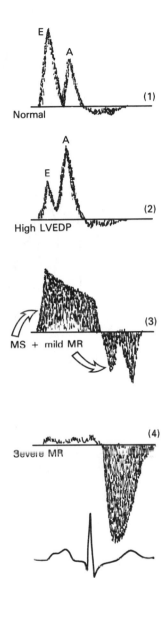

(1)

Normal

(2)

High LVEDP

(3)

MS + mild MR

(4)

Severe MR

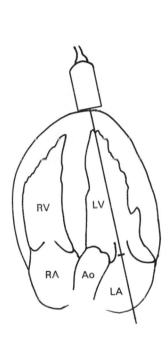

Figure 12.28 Apical continuous-wave Doppler echocardiography with sample volume in mitral valve orifice. (1) Normal laminar flow with minimal spectral broadening, A = contribution of atrial systole. (2) Normal laminar mitral flow but with high LVEDP. Early flow velocity E is reduced, but late velocity is increased with the A wave. (3) Mixed mitral valve disease. Turbulent flow in both directions produces multiple velocities and spectral broadening. The signal above the baseline is towards the transducer (stenotic jet), and the signal below is the regurgitation jet away from the transducer. (4) Severe mitral regurgitation. Complete envelope of turbulent flow. Early peak velocity of severe regurgitation.

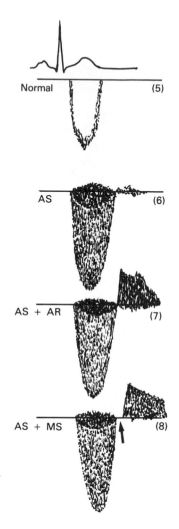

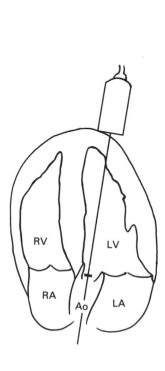

Figure 12.29 Apical continuous-wave Dopper echocardiography with sample volume in aortic valve orifice. (5) Normal velocity profile with laminar flow. (6) Aortic stenosis. Increased peak velocity with turbulent flow through the aortic valve. (7) Mixed aortic valve disease. Turbulent flow in both directions, the stenotic component being away from the transducer with its signal below the baseline, and the regurgitant component above. Forward and reversed flow are continuous. (8) Aortic and mitral stenosis with no aortic regurgitation. The two jet signals are not continuous with a small gap between (arrowed). This helps to distinguish the signals of mitral stenosis from aortic regurgitation.

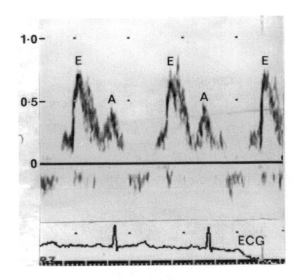

Calculation of diastolic indices from diagrammatic transmitral flow pattern

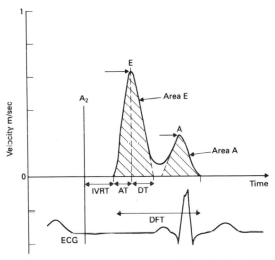

Figure 12.30 Pulsed-wave Doppler echo of normal mitral valve and calculation of diastolic indices from diagrammatic transmitral flow pattern. A_2, aortic valve closure; IVRT, isovolumic relaxation time; AT, acceleration time; DT, deceleration time; DFT, total diastolic filling time. Arrows at E and A indicate PE and PA, respectively.

....

Recently it has been found that none of these indices are as sensitive to early increases in diastolic stiffness (due to LV hypertrophy) as measurements made from acoustic quantification.

Acoustic quantification (AQ)

The endocardial border of the left ventricle can be continuously outlined on a four-chamber view. This automatic border detection produces an LV area or volume/time curve (similar to the volume/time curve of LV angiography). Abnormalities can be demonstrated on area/volume curve filling rates by acoustic quantification even when the mitral flow Doppler pattern is still normal. It appears to be a very sensitive technique for early diastolic dysfunction.

Variables derived from transmitral diastolic Doppler flow recording. See Figure 12.30.

Variable	How derived	Normal range
PE	Peak early filling velocity (cm/s)	78 ± 15
PA	Peak late filling velocity (cm/s)	48 ± 12
E/A ratio		1.6 ± 0.2
E area or integral	Rapid early (passive) filling velocity–time integral (area under the E portion of the Doppler profile) (cm^2)	0.1 ± 0.03
A area or integral	Late (active) filling velocity–time integral (area under the A portion of the Doppler profile) (cm^2)	0.06 ± 0.01
Total filling integral	E area + A area (cm^2)	0.16 ± 0.04
E area/A area		1.7 ± 0.4
E area/total area	Rapid early filling contribution to total filling, or early filling fraction	0.62 ± 0.05
A area/total area	Late fllling contribution to total filling, atrial filling fraction	0.37 ± 0.07
IVRT	Isovolumic relaxation time (ms). Time between A_2 and onset of Doppler filling	48–65
Acceleration time	AT. Time from onset of diastolic flow to E point (ms)	70–90
Deceleration time	DT. Time from E point to point where the E–F slope hits the baseline (ms)	105–180
DFT	Total diastolic filling time (ms)	300–520

Transoesophageal echocardiography (TOE)

This technique has proved of enormous diagnostic value in many aspects of both paediatric and adult cardiology. It has become an essential part in the management of prosthetic valve endocarditis, the search for the source of systemic emboli, the diagnosis of aortic dissection or in the assessment of mitral valve repair intra-operatively (Figure 12.31).

Standard transthoracic echocardiography (TTE) has been limited by poor tissue penetration of high frequency transducers (5 MHz) although good definition (resolution) is better with these. Adequate transthoracic images can be very difficult to obtain even with the lower frequency 2.25–2.5 MHz transducer in obese patients, or those with emphysema or chest deformities. Structures at the back of the heart may be missed altogether.

Cardiac structures best imaged by transoesophageal echocardiography

Structure	Possible abnormality
Right atrium	Thrombus, myxoma, pacing wire, central line
Left atrium	Thrombus, myxoma, spontaneous contrast
Left atrial appendage	Thrombus
Pulmonary veins	Anatomy, flow direction
Atrial septum	PFO, ASD, atrial septum aneurysm, shunts
Mitral valve	Anatomy, vegetations, strands, regurgitant jets, chordal rupture
Mitral valve prosthesis	Possible dehiscence, thrombosis, vegetations regurgitant jets, xenograft tears
Aortic valve prosthesis	Posterior ring abscess, valve dysfunction as in mitral
Ascending and descending aorta	Aortic dimensions, dissection, atheroma, patent duct
Coarctation	Site severity, gradient, possible post dilatation aneurysms

Intra-atrial thrombus

TOE is essential prior to mitral valvuloplasty (page 76) and prior to DC cardioversion for atrial fibrillation if there is any doubt about the possibility of thrombus in the atrial appendage or in those patients who have not received prior anticoagulation (page 319). Patients with spontaneous echo contrast (Figure 12.31) should also be anticoagulated first. TOE is less valuable in the search for a possible embolic source from the clinically normal heart although it is a frequently demanded investigation for this problem.

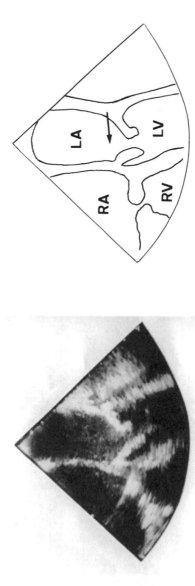

Figure 12.31 Transoesophageal echocardiography in a woman with mitral and tricuspid stenosis showing spontaneous echo contrast in the left atrium (arrowed). RA = right atrium; RV = right ventricle; LA = left atrium; LV = left ventricle.

Prosthetic valve endocarditis

TOE is able to detect small vegetations missed on TTE as it has a higher resolution image. All mechanical valves have a tiny puff of regurgitation through the centre of the valve as the ball or disc or discs close. Any regurgitant jet on the side of the valve is pathological and can easily be seen with TOE. Valve dehiscence, thrombosis or paravalve abscess are well seen. Acoustic echoes from the mechanical valve struts prevent good visualization of the posterior aortic root in patients with an aortic valve replacement, and the back of the mitral valve and left atrium in patients with a mitral prosthesis.

A negative TOE does not exclude infective endocarditis. Patients with infective endocarditis must have a TTE at least weekly and a TOE if their condition deteriorates. The two techniques are complemetary not mutually exclusive.

Aortic dissection

TOE is the investigation of choice in possible aortic dissection (**10.7** page 415) as it avoids the risks of aortography. The site and extent of the dissection is seen as both ascending and descending thoracic aorta are imaged. Sometimes the tear or entry site can be seen with Doppler which will show flow in the false lumen. It is important that the procedure is performed with careful blood pressure monitoring and with adequate sedation. Acute rises in systolic pressure must be avoided.

Mitral valve repair

TOE can prove very helpful intraoperatively in assessing the degree of

---

Disadvantages of transoesophageal echocardiography

Cost: Omniplane probe about £24 000. Annual renewal needed in a busy unit
Doctor nurse and technician required
Patient must be fasted and consented
Longer procedure
Sedation or general anaesthetic occasionally required in adults as in children
Cidex sterilization system needed for the probe
Unsuitable patients:
    chronic obstructive airways disease
    severe pulmonary hypertension (hypoxic risk)
    LVF: only if ventilated
    oesophageal pathology (stricture, varices, etc.)
    cervical spine pathology (e.g. rheumatoid arthritis)

---

mitral regurgitation before and after mitral repair for severe mitral regurgitation (floppy valve, ruptured chordae).

TOE in ITU
TOE in ventilated patients is safe and useful in patients in ITU, e.g. in patients with low cardiac outputs, suspicious murmurs, or sepsis from an unknown source.

12.4 Cardiac catheterization

The advent of two-dimensional and Doppler echocardiography has reduced the need for cardiac catheterization in both congenital and adult heart disease. Newer forms of angiography, such as digital subtraction angiography and radionuclide angiography together with magnetic resonance imaging, may reduce the need still further. However, it still plays a vital role in cardiac diagnosis. There has been a rapid increase in the use of intervention techniques that avoid the need for cardiac surgical treatment, e.g.:

Congenital heart disease
• Rashkind balloon septostomy in TGA. Balloon dilatation of coarctation, Mustard baffle, pulmonary venous obstruction, Blalock anastomosis, valve stenosis, etc.

Percutaneous transluminal coronary angioplasty (PTCA)
• Native coronary vessels, vein grafts, internal mammary grafts.
• Streptokinase infusion into main pulmonary artery in massive acute pulmonary embolism or into the coronary artery in acute myocardial infarction or during PTCA.

Valvuloplasty
• Balloon dilatation of all four valves is now a recognised procedure.
   Cardiac catheterization is usually merely a diagnostic procedure with well-defined mortality and morbidity risks. Since coronary arteriography was introduced by Mason Sones in 1962, great advances in techniques and equipment have occurred.

Mortality and morbidity
Mortality in most centres is now approximately 0.1% in patients having

coronary arteriography. The deaths occur in patients with the most severe coronary disease.

There is a definite morbidity relating to arterial entry site complications. The American Collaborative Study on Coronary Artery Surgery (CASS) published in 1979 suggested that the femoral entry site was safer. The brachial approach was only safe if the operator performed 80% or more of his procedures from the arm.

Most cardiologists are able to catheterize from either route with no morbidity.

What to tell the patient

The patient is told why the test is necessary and an explanation of what is involved and why local anaesthetic is preferred. The reasons that general anaesthesia is usually unnecessary are as follows: it interferes with haemodynamics and oxygen saturations; patients cannot indicate if they develop angina or other symptoms; patients are usually required to perform respiratory manoeuvres, coughing, etc.; patients are sometimes required to perform exercise during the test.

The procedure should be painless, although the patient should be warned of the hot flush associated with angiography, and the very small risks should be explained.

Which route?

This is a matter of operator preference. Usually, however, the right brachial route is often used for:
• patients on anticoagulants (unless a sealing device is used in the femoral artery)
• coarctation of the aorta (or axillary cut-down in babies)
• patients with intermittent claudication or those who have had aorto–iliac surgery
• occasionally aortic valve stenosis as a dominant lesion
• hypertensive patients with high peak systolic pressures, as femoral haemostasis may be difficult.

The femoral route is usually preferred for patients with:
• atrial septal defects and
• most congenital heart disease
• young women with atypical chest pain who may have small brachial arteries and a tendency to arterial spasm
• patients with Raynaud's phenomenon
• several (two or more) previous brachial catheterizations
• presence of a right subclavian bruit.

Premedication

Some form of premedication is important, as anxious patients may become vagal on arrival in the catheter laboratory or after withdrawal of the catheters. Anxiety may provoke angina before the procedure even starts in patients with ischaemic heart disease. The following is a suggested regime:

Adults

Diazepam 10–20 mg orally 1–2 hours precatheter. A further dose (Diazemuls) may be given i.v. prior to the catheter if the patient is still anxious. Fentanyl 25–50 mg i.v. is a useful additional analgesic given just before the catheter.

Children (up to 20 kg) 30 mins precatheter
Peth. Co. 0.06–0.08 mls/kg i.m. Max dose 1.5 mls i.m.
Peth. Co is Pethidine 25 mg, Promethazine 6.25 mg, Chlorpromazine 6.25 mg per 1 ml.
Children (20–40 kg)
Morphine 0.2 mg/kg ⎫
Hyoscine (Scopolamine 10 µgm/kg ⎬ i.m. 30 min precatheter
                                    ⎭

   Adults do not usually require general anaesthesia if these doses are used, but paediatric cases usually have a general anaesthetic. Patients should be starved for > 4 hours precatheter. Their cardiac medication should not be discontinued, except for diuretics which are best avoided on the morning of catheterization.

   Polycythaemic patients with cyanotic congenital heart disease are at risk (if the haemoglobin level is > 18 g/100 ml) of both arterial and venous thrombosis. A few days prior to cardiac catheter the patients should be admitted for venesection, with concurrent plasma exchange if the haemoglobin exceeds this level (see **2.10,** page 60).

Renal failure

Patients with renal failure (creatinine > 200 µmol/l) should receive an infusion of N saline prior to cardiac catheterization or they will develop contrast nephropathy and rapidly deteriorating renal failure following the catheter. This is particularly necessary prior to PTCA as they may receive a large dose of contrast. Unless the patient has been in pulmonary oedema pretreat with 1 litre N saline over 12 hours pre catheter and repeat on return to the ward following the procedure. Daily renal function tests needed until the creatinine starts to fall.

Coping with catheter complications occurring on the ward

1 Haemorrhage

Leg. This is controlled by firm pressure. A Johns Hopkins bandage is not effective and just obscures the puncture site. Firm pressure above the puncture site will help control the development of a haematoma. If the bleeding is not controlled after 30 min:

• Check the clotting screen. If the patient is on warfarin, fresh frozen plasma may help. Vitamin K is not recommended as it makes subsequent anticoagulation very difficult. If the patient has just had heparin then check the APTT, as protamine reversal may help (dose = protamine 10 mg/1000 units heparin administered).

• Is the patient hypertensive? High peak systolic pressure will exacerbate bleeding.

• Call for help. Very rarely, femoral artery repair may be necessary for a false aneurysm. A hard tender pulsatile lump over the puncture site developing after cardiac catheterization suggests a false aneurysm. The diagnosis can be confirmed by ultrasound imaging.

Firm pressure with an ultrasound probe on the neck of the aneurysm for about 20–30 min can result in the false aneurysm thrombosing, avoiding the need for surgical repair in most cases. The majority of femoral false aneurysms can be dealt with in this way if the neck of the false aneurysm is small. It is painful, the patient will need sedation and analgesia. Occasionally a false aneurysm thromboses spontaneously. The risk is greater with the larger sheaths used for PTCA (especially atherectomy or rotablation). However the use of devices to occlude the femoral artery puncture site (e.g. Vasoseal, Angioseal) is of great value in these cases. Their use reduces haemorrhagic complications and allows for early mobilization, but expense precludes their routine use.

Arm. The same principles apply. However, in this case the artery has been repaired by direct suture. Bleeding is often venous oozing only. Firm brachial pressure should not occlude the radial pulse. Protamine is not usually given following brachial artery catheterization. Any haematoma development will require exploring and resuturing of the brachial artery.

2 Infection

Postcatheter pyrexia is usually due to a dye reaction and settles within 24 hours. Persisting pyrexia should be investigated and treated on usual lines with blood cultures, urine cultures, etc. prior to antibiotics.

12 Cardiac investigations

12.4 Cardiac catheterization

....

A tender pink area around the brachial cut-down should be treated with complete rest (arm resting on a pillow), and oral amoxycillin 500 mg tds and flucloxacillin 500 mg qds for 5 days.

3 Dye reaction

This is commonly mild, causing: skin reaction, erythema, urticaria or even bullous eruption, nausea and vomiting, headache, hypotension, pyrexia, rigors. Very rarely, it causes more severe reactions: fits, transient cortical disturbance, e.g. cortical blindness, anaphylactic shock.

• Urticaria and skin reaction are usually helped by intravenous antihistamines (e.g. chlorpheniramine 10 mg i.v.) and more severe cases by additional intravenous hydrocortisone 100 mg.

• Nausea, vomiting, i.v. metoclopramide 10 mg.

• Hypotension, i.v. fluids may be necessary, especially in patients who have been excessively diuresed or who have had a lot of dye (e.g. > 3 ml/kg).

• Pyrexia and rigors are usually transient. Rest and sedation are all that is necessary.

• Anaphylactic shock. Occurs in the catheter laboratory rather than the ward, and should be treated by urgent volume replacement with intravenous plasma substitute or N-saline, hydrocortisone 200 mg i.v., adrenaline 1 in 1000, 1 ml slowly s.c.

• Cortical disturbances are rare and again usually transient. They are not necessarily embolic, and may in part be due to vascular spasm or an osmotic effect of the dye. Fits are controlled as in grand mal epilepsy with i.v. diazepam.

4 Cyanotic attacks

These typically occur in the small child with Fallot's tetralogy and severe infundibular stenosis. The combination of metabolic acidosis, hypoxia and hypovolaemia predispose to infundibular shutdown or spasm. Catecholamine release secondary to pain and/or fear will also exacerbate this. Treatment depends on reversing these factors:

• propranolol 0.025–0.1 mg/kg i.v., or

• morphine sulphate 0.1–0.2 mg/kg i.v. in severe cases

• check the arterial acid–base balance. If the base deficit is or exceeds −5 give i.v. $NaHCO_3$ 8.4% as:

$$\frac{body\ wt\ (kg)}{6} \times base\ deficit,\ then\ repeat\ the\ blood\ gases$$

- exclude hypoglycaemia on above sample
- oxygen via a face mask
- placing the child in a knee–chest position acts in the same way as 'squatting' by cutting off acidotic venous return from the legs, as an initial manoeuvre it may help while drugs are being prepared.

5 The lost radial pulse

This should be dealt with in the catheter laboratory at the time. If the patient is hypotensive, volume replacement with i.v. heparinization may help. Nitrates are of little benefit. Fifty per cent of patients who do not regain the radial pulse will not develop claudication symptoms. A few patients will regain the radial pulse once they warm up and brachial spasm regresses. Overall a lost radial pulse occurs in < 1% of brachial catheterization cases.

A numb hand may occur in the presence of a good radial pulse. This is usually the effect of lignocaine on the median nerve at the catheter site and the sensation returns within 12 hours. Residual median nerve damage is rare and probably due to unnecessary manipulation of the nerve during the catheter procedure.

A loss of the foot pulses following femoral artery catheterization is also rare, but may be transient (24 hours) in children. In adults, however, loss of the foot pulses is usually irreversible and requires femoral thrombectomy.

6 Angina

May occur during or after coronary angiography, or as a result of paroxysmal tachycardia in the ischaemic patient. It usually responds to sublingual nitroglycerine and sedation. The ECG should be checked and if the angina recurs the patient should be monitored. Occasionally i.m. or i.v. diamorphine 2.5–5 mg is required.

In severe cases with recurrent pain, intravenous nitrates should be started (page 158).

If ST-segment elevation occurs, the patient has probably occluded a major coronary artery due to thrombus or dissection following intubation or instrumentation of the coronary artery. Very occasionally it may be due to coronary spasm. In either case treatment with intravenous nitrates is started. The next stage depends on the findings at cardiac catheterization. The patient may be suitable for an immediate angioplasty, or emergency coronary artery bypass surgery may be necessary. If immediate surgery or PTCA is not possible then intra-aortic balloon pumping is considered. This will help maintain coronary flow and reduce infarct size until a more definitive treatment is available. In the elderly, or those who have had a difficult salvage angioplasty, it may be felt that supportive medical treatment is appropriate. (See **5.7**.)

7 Arrhythmias

These are usually transient and dealt with during catheterization. They may occasionally recur on the ward, e.g. paroxysmal AF or SVT, more rarely paroxysmal ventricular tachycardia. Each arrhythmia must be treated on its merits along the lines discussed in **7.12**, page 315.

8 Pericardial tamponade

This should be considered in any patient who becomes hypotensive and anuric following catheterization. It is a very rare complication of routine cardiac catheterization but is a recognized complication of the transseptal puncture procedure or RV biopsy. Diagnosis is confirmed by M-mode and two-dimensional echocardiography. Pericardial aspiration may be required.

Valve area calculation

Calculation of aortic or mitral valve area from cardiac catheter data is possible if the cardiac output is measured together with simultaneous pressures from either side of the aortic or mitral valve. Calculations of tricuspid and pulmonary valve area are perfectly possible but rarely needed.

The calculation of valve area thus depends on:
- the mean valve gradient
- the forward flow across the valve
- a constant.

The range of aortic and mitral valve area in adults

	Aortic (cm^2)	Mitral (cm^2)
Normal	2.5–3.5	4–6
Mild stenosis	1.0–1.5	1.5–2.0
Moderate stenosis	0.5–1.0	1.0–1.5
Severe stenosis	< 0.5	< 1

The constant used derives from the calculations of Gorlin and Gorlin (1951), which has been established by comparing calculated valve area and actual valve area measured at autopsy or at operation. Since the calculation depends on 'forward flow' the method is invalidated in the presence of regurgitation unless angiographic output is used.

The table on page 494 relates to native valves. The method can also be used for prosthetic valves.

The Gorlin formula tends to overestimate the true valve area at high cardiac outputs, and underestimate valve area at low cardiac outputs.

Aortic valve area (same formula for pulmonary valve)

(Figure 12.32)

$$\text{Aortic valve area} = \frac{\text{Aortic valve flow (ml/s)}}{44.5 \sqrt{\text{Mean aortic gradient (mmHg)}}}$$

$$\text{Aortic valve flow} = \frac{\text{Cardiac output (ml/min)}}{\text{Systolic ejection period (s/min)}}$$

44.5 = The Gorlin constant for aortic (or pulmonary) valves.

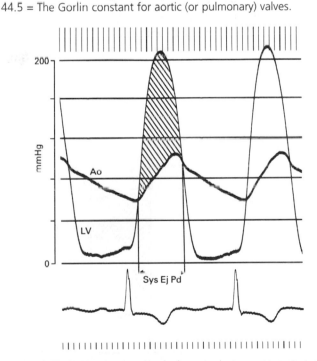

Figure 12.32 Aortic valve area. Hatched area is planimetred for calculation of mean aortic gradient. Sys Ej Pd, systolic ejection period in s/min. Computerized catheter laboratory systems are programmed to calculate valve area automatically.

Mean aortic gradient is calculated by planimetry (5 cycles in sinus rhythm, 10 in atrial fibrillation) of the area shown shaded in Figure 12.32.

Mitral valve area (same formula for tricuspid valve)
(Figure 12.33)

$$\text{Mitral valve area} = \frac{\text{Mitral valve flow (ml/sec)}}{31 \sqrt{\text{(Mean mitral gradient (mmHg))}}}$$

$$\text{Mitral valve flow} = \frac{\text{Cardiac output (ml/min)}}{\text{Diastolic filling period (s/min)}}$$

Mean mitral gradient is calculated by planimetry of the area shown in Figure 12.33; 31 is the Gorlin constant for mitral (or tricuspid) valves (0.7×44.5) in the original calculation where LV mean diastolic pressure was assumed to be 5 mmHg.

With simultaneous measurement of LV and LA (or PAW) pressures the constants 38 or 40 are frequently used.

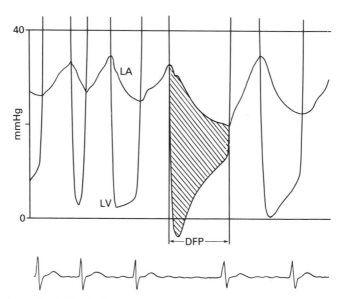

Figure 12.33 Mitral valve area. Hatched area is planimetred for calculation of mitral valve area. Ten consecutive cycles should be measured for patients in AF. DFP, diastolic filling period in s/min.

Angiographic estimation of left ventricular volume

(Figure 12.34)

In spite of the fact that gross assumptions are made about the shape of the LV cavity, that magnification errors may arise and that single-plane cine is usually used, the angiographic assessment of LV volume correlates very closely with ventricular cast measurements or echocardiographic estimations of LV volume.

Although formulae for biplane cineangiography have been produced, most centres use a single-plane 30° RAO projection for the LV cine. Most formulae assume the left ventricular cavity is an ellipsoid of revolution: thus assuming that the minor axes in two planes are identical

$$V = \frac{4\pi}{3} \times \frac{D}{2} \times \frac{D}{2} \times \frac{L}{2} = \frac{\pi}{6} \times D^2 \times L$$

(uncorrected for magnification)

The magnification factor (f) is calculated from filming a marked catheter or grid/ruler of known length (at central chest level). The corrected volume equation becomes:

$$V = \frac{\pi}{6} D^2.L.f^3 = 0.524.D^2.L.f^3 \text{ (Greene formula)}$$

The formula can be modified by calculation of the area (A cm²) and length (L cm) only. The area is measured by planimetry or more usually

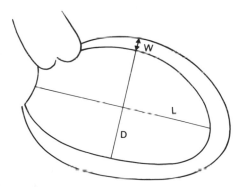

Figure 12.34 Estimation of LV volume by single-plane 30° RAO projection. L, major axis (cm); D, minor axis in two planes (cm); V, ventricular volume (ml); W, wall thickness (cm, see LV mass estimation).

by a programmed computer system. Using this area–length method the minor axis need not be measured as:

$$\frac{D}{2} = \frac{2A}{\pi L}$$

where A = area of LV in cm^2.

Substituting this in the original volume equation we can simplify the equation to:

$$V = \frac{0.849 \times A^2 \times f^3}{L} \text{ (Dodge formula)}$$

Programming this formula into a computer, rapid sequential LV volume analysis is possible.

Formulae for the calculation of right ventricular volume have been derived but each makes assumptions of RV cavity shape that are even more unfounded than the assumption of LV cavity shape.

Angiographic assessment of left ventricular mass

The volume of the left ventricular cavity is subtracted from the volume of cavity and LV wall. Uniform wall thickness is assumed.

If W is the wall thickness at mid-point of intersection of the minor axis, and the specific gravity of heart muscle is 1.05 then:

$$\text{LV mass} = 1.05 \times \left[\frac{4}{3} \pi f^3 \left(\frac{D}{2} + W \right)^2 \left(\frac{L}{2} + W \right) \right] - \left[\frac{\pi}{6} f^3.D^2.L \right]$$

LV wall + cavity volume	Cavity volume

In spite of the obvious invalidity of the assumptions involved in the calculation, this estimate of LV mass has been shown to correlate well with post-mortem measurements.

Normal values for LV angiographic volumes (Kennedy)

LVEDVI	70 + 20 (mean + SD) ml/m^2
LVESVI	24 ± 10 ml/m^2
Ejection fraction	0.67 ± 0.08
LV mass	92 ± 16 g
Wall thickness	10.9 ± 2.0 mm

....

Cardiac output calculations

Direct Fick method
The main difficulty with this method is an accurate measurement of oxygen consumption:

$$\text{Cardiac output} = \frac{\text{Oxygen consumption}}{\text{Arteriovenous oxygen content difference}}$$

$$\text{or CO (l/min)} = \frac{O_2 \text{ consumption (ml/min)}}{(A_0 - PA)\ O_2 \text{ content (ml/100 ml)} \times 10}$$

Oxygen content calculation
The haemoglobin and oxygen saturation must be known.

$$O_2 \text{ content} = (\text{Hb} \times 1.34 \times \%\text{ saturation}) + \text{plasma } O_2 \text{ content}$$

where Hb is haemoglobin; 1.34 is derived from the fact that 1 g Hb when 100% saturated combines with 1.34 ml O_2.

$$\text{Plasma } O_2 \text{ content in 100 ml plasma} = \frac{100 \times 0.0258 \times P_{O_2}}{760}$$

Thus with Hb of 15g/100 ml and 97% saturation, the arterial oxygen content is $(15 \times 1.34 \times 0.97) + 0.3 = 19.65$ ml/100 ml, where 0.3 is the plasma correction factor.

It does not matter from which systemic artery the O_2 content is

Plasma correction factors

Saturation (%)	Correction
97	0.3
96	0.27
94	0.24
92	0.21
90	0.19
85	0.17
80	0.14
75	0.12
70	0.11
60	0.10
50	0.08
40	0.07
30	0.05
20	0.04

calculated. Only the pulmonary artery should be used for mixed venous oxygen content calculation.

Oxygen content can also be measured by specific equipment containing a galvanic fuel cell which releases electrons on absorbing oxygen (Lexington instruments) or by a manometric method (Van Slyke).

Oxygen consumption calculation

Expired air is collected for 3–10 min of steady-state respiration. The method is only really possible or accurate in the basal state. Three methods are available:

- closed circuit spirometer – containing 100% oxygen and expired CO_2 is absorbed by soda-lime canister
- open circuit – with expired air collected in a Douglas bag
- fuel cell technique – with a sample of expired air measured for oxygen concentration using purpose built equipment.

$$\dot{V}_{O_2} = \dot{V}_E STP(F_{IO_2} - F_{EO_2}) \times 10 \text{ ml/min}$$

where $\dot{V}_{O_2}$ = oxygen consumption in ml/min

$\dot{V}_E STP$ = expired volume of air corrected for standard temperature and pressure

F_{IO_2} = concentration of inspired oxygen, in room air this is 20.93% and need not be measured

F_{EO_2} = concentration of expired oxygen

The correction of $\dot{V}_E$ for standard temperature and pressure is:

$$\dot{V}_E STP = \dot{V}_E ATP \times \frac{273}{273 + T} \times \frac{P - W}{P} \times \frac{P}{760}$$

where $V_E ATP$ = measured expired volume at atmospheric temperature and pressure

T = room temperature in °C

P = barometric pressure in the room (mmHg)

W = water vapour pressure (mmHg)

Table of water vapour pressure (W) at various room temperatures

°C	W (mmHg)	°C	W (mmHg)	°C	W (mmHg)
15	12.79	21	18.65	27	26.74
16	13.63	22	19.83	28	28.35
17	14.53	23	21.07	29	30.04
18	15.48	24	22.38	30	31.82
19	16.48	25	23.76	31	33.70
20	17.54	26	25.21	32	35.60

Indirect Fick method

Using the table of estimated oxygen consumption, the direct Fick measurement or an indicator dilution method can be checked. The table is a guide and cannot be comprehensive for all ages at any heart rate.

Mean oxygen consumption in the basal state per body surface area in ml/min/m² (see body surface area nomogram on page 522). Basal state: adults approximately 70 bpm, children approximately 120 bpm

Age	Male	Female	Age	Male	Female
3	185	178	23	129	118
4	180	173	24	129	117
5	177	170	25	127	117
6	174	167	27	127	117
7	169	163	28	127	117
8	166	155	30	125	117
9	162	151	32	125	116
10	158	146	33	124	115
11	153	143	35	124	114
12	150	137	36	123	113
13	147	133	38	123	112
14	143	127	40	122	112
15	140	124	42	119	112
16	137	122	45	118	111
17	135	121	50	117	110
18	134	120	55	115	109
19	132	119	60	114	108
20	131	118	65	113	107
21	130	118	70	112	106
22	130	118	75	110	105

Cardiac output by indicator dilution

Indocyanine green (peak absorption at 800 nm) is injected into the right heart or main pulmonary artery. Downstream sampling is from the aorta, brachial or femoral artery through a densitometer. The Gilford densitometer is often used. It is insensitive to changes in O_2 saturation. Background dye causes a baseline shift.

The disadvantage of the technique is that two catheters are involved and that recirculation occurs. Also a calibration factor (K) must be calculated from known concentrations of green dye in fresh heparinized non smokers' blood.

Then $K = \dfrac{\text{Indicator concentration in mg/l}}{\text{Deflection through densitometer (mm)}}$

Several concentrations of dye in blood must first be prepared (e.g. 1–10 mg/l).

From the Hamilton equation:

$$CO = \frac{I \times 60}{C \times t}$$

where I = amount of green dye injected (mg)

C = mean concentration of dye (mg/l)

t = duration of curve (s)

The product ($C \times t$) is the area under the curve excluding the recirculation component, the primary curve. There are two chief methods for calculation of the area. The most accurate is to reconstruct the primary curve by plotting the time–concentration curve on semi-logarithmic paper with the indicator concentration on the semi-log axis. The straight line on the descending limb is extrapolated and the primary curve reconstructed from the semi-log plot: it is assumed that the decay of the primary curve is exponential (Figure 12.35).

The second type of calculation employs short cuts which ignore the recirculation component and do not involve reconstruction of the primary curve.

1 Reconstruction of the primary curve (Figure 12.35)
Once the primary curve is constructed there are several methods for calculation of the area some of which are discussed below:
• by planimetry (Figure 12.36)
• summation of 1-s interval concentration values (ordinates).
This is easier if the curve is traced on to graph paper (Figure 12.37).

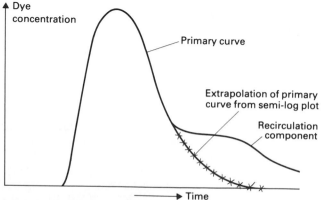

Figure 12.35 Reconstruction of the primary curve.

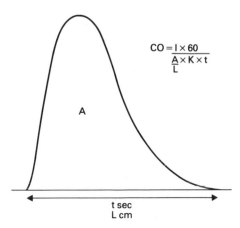

$$CO = \frac{I \times 60}{\frac{A}{L} \times K \times t}$$

Figure 12.36 Calculation of the basic area by planimetry. A, planimetred area of curve (cm²); L, length of baseline (cm), K, calibration factor; t, time of curve (s); I, quantity of dye injected (mg).

2 Short cuts not requiring primary curve reconstruction

These methods are quicker and reconstruction of the primary curve from the dye curve is unnecessary. Several other measurements are required depending on the method used (Figure 12.38), where:

AT = appearance time (s) of dye

BT = build-up time (s) from onset of curve

T_{50} = time at half peak concentration

C_p = peak concentration (mg/l)

PCT = time to peak concentration from dye injection

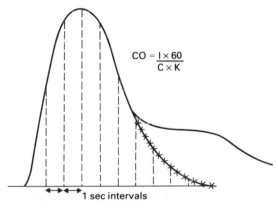

$$CO = \frac{I \times 60}{C \times K}$$

Figure 12.37 Summation of 1-s intervals. C = sum of ordinate values (mm s) at 1-s intervals.

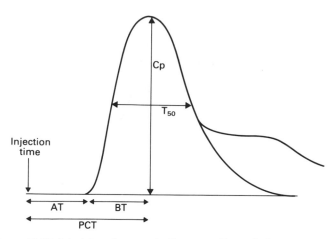

Figure 12.38 Calculation of area under the curve without planimetry.

Dow's formula:

$$Area = \frac{PC \times PCT}{3 - 0.9(PCT/AT)} \text{ mm s}$$

Hetzel *et al.* formula (forward triangle method):

$$CO = \frac{I \times 60 \times K}{BT \times C_p/2}$$

K in this case is an empirical constant (0.37 for central injection, 0.35 for peripheral injection).

Bradley and Barr formula (fore-'n'-aft triangle method):

$$Area = C_p \times T_{50} \text{ mm s}$$

Thermodilution method

This is usually performed using a Swan–Ganz catheter in the right heart. Doses of 5 or 10 ml of 5% dextrose (at either room temperature or 4°C) are injected in the right atrium, and the thermistor at the catheter tip in the pulmonary artery senses the transient fall in temperature as a rise in resistance.

Advantages over green dye measurements are:
- the recirculation curve can be ignored
- only one catheter is needed
- the method can be repeated rapidly following drug intervention and the catheter may be left in the right heart for further assessment of the sick patient.

A variety of cardiac output computers are available that integrate electronically the area under the curve. Several methods are used, all of which assume the downslope of the curve is exponential (Figures 12.39 and 12.40).

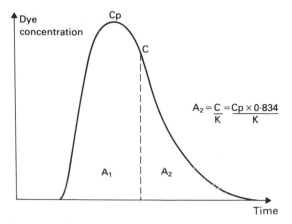

Figure 12.39 Measuring area, where the downslope of the curve is exponential K is the decay constant of the downslope. The exponential decay is assumed to start at 83.4% of peak concentration.

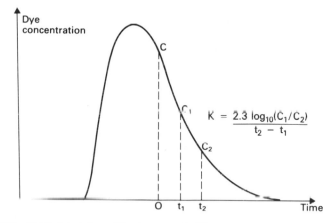

Figure 12.40 Calculation of the decay consta (K).

Shunt quantitation by dye dilution

Shunt quantitation is possible by either dye dilution or oximetry. Dye dilution is more sensitive but more complex. Two types of curve may be produced. The normal curve is superimposed in each case. In both cases peak concentration is less. Early appearance of dye occurs in the

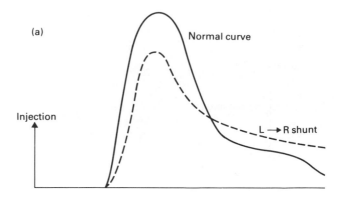

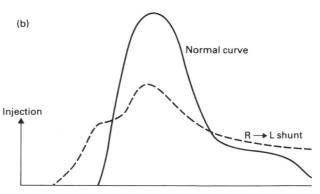

Figure 12.41 Shunt quantitation by dye dilution: (a) left-to-right shunt, (b) right-to-left shunt.

right-to-left shunt and the curve has a double hump, with the unshunted dye forming the second peak (Figure 12.41).

1 Left-to-right shunt (Figures 12.41 and 12.42)

The dye must be injected in the main pulmonary artery and sampled in the descending aorta or more peripherally. If the dye is injected in the left heart distal to the shunt site, the curve will have a normal appearance.

Using the method of Carter et al. for the left-to-right shunts (Figure 12.42):

the ratio of $\dfrac{C_{(p+BT)}}{C_p}$ and $\dfrac{C_{(p+2BT)}}{C_p}$ is calculated

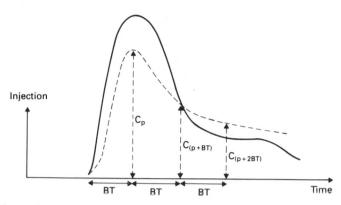

Figure 12.42 Calculation of left-to-right shunt. Where C_p, peak concentration; BT, build-up time; $C_{(p+BT)}$, concentration one build-up time after peak; $C_{(p+2BT)}$, concentration two build-up times after peak.

then:

$$\frac{\text{Left-to-right shunt}}{\text{Pulmonary flow}} \times 100 = 141 \times \frac{C_{(p+BT)}}{C_p} - 42 \text{ (A)}$$

and:

$$= 135 \times \frac{C_{(p+2BT)}}{C_p} - 14 \text{ (B)}$$

A and B are averaged to produce the ratio of shunt to pulmonary flow. (The equations are derived from regression lines of studies by Carter *et al.*)

2 *Right-to-left shunt* (Figures 12.41 and 12.43)
The forward triangle method compares areas under the early and late hump of the curve. The early hump is assumed to be due to the right-to-left shunt only. The later hump is assumed to be due to systemic flow (Figure 12.43). Then:

$$\frac{\text{right-to-left shunt}}{\text{systemic flow}} = \frac{BT_1 \times PC_1}{(BT_1 \times PC_1) + (BT_2 \times PC_2)}$$

Shunt quantitation by oximetry
Oximetry is used to detect shunts rather than quantitate them accurately. Errors in quantitation arise from streaming and sampling in

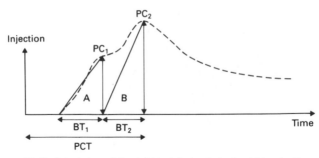

Figure 12.43 Calculation of the right-to-left shunt. A, shunt triangle; B, systemic flow triangle; PC_1, peak concentration of initial hump (shunt) (mg/l) PC_2, peak concentration of second hump (systemic) (mg/l); BT1, build-up time of initial hump (s), BT_2 = build-up time of second hump (sec) (= 0.46 × PCT); PCT, time to peak concentration PC_2.

the wrong place. An estimation of shunt size can be made from saturation measurements during catheterization.

From the Fick equation:

$$\text{Pulmonary flow} = \frac{O_2 \text{ consumption}}{(PV - PA\ O_2 \text{ content})}$$

Pulmonary vein sampling is not possible unless there is an ASD or transseptal catheterization is performed. PV saturation is assumed to be 98%.

The equation becomes:

1 Pulmonary flow =

$$\frac{O_2 \text{ consumption}}{\dfrac{(98 - PA \text{ saturation})}{100} \times Hb \times 1.34 \times 10}\ \text{l/min}$$

Similarly:

2 Systemic flow =

$$\frac{O_2 \text{ consumption}}{\dfrac{(A_o \text{ l/min saturation} - \text{mixed venous saturation})}{100} \times Hb \times 1.34 \times 10}\ \text{l/min}$$

Mixed venous saturation is calculated as:

$$\frac{(3 \times SVC \text{ saturation}) + (1 \times IVC \text{ saturation})}{4}$$

SVC saturation is usually lower than IVC saturation.

Rather than measure O_2 consumption the ratio of pulmonary to systemic flow can be estimated by dividing **1** by **2**, i.e.

$$\frac{\text{Pulmonary}}{\text{Systemic flow}} = \frac{A_o \text{ saturation} - \text{mixed venous saturation}}{98 - \text{PA saturation } \%}$$

True pulmonary vein saturation is substituted for 98% if it is obtained. Small left-to-right shunts may be missed by oximetry and green dye or ascorbate techniques are more sensitive. Oximetry will not usually detect a PDA or small VSD. A primum ASD may be mistaken on oximetry as a VSD with the oxygenated stream being missed in low right atrial sampling.

Nevertheless it provides a useful check during catheterization and an estimate of shunt size. A routine saturation run during catheterization usually involves sampling from:

High SVC	RV inflow
Low SVC	RV body
RA/SVC junction	RV outflow
High RA	Main PA (RPA + LPA)
Mid RA	LA and PV if possible
Low RA	LV
IVC	A_o

Sampling through the right atrium is performed down the lateral RA wall to detect anomalous venous drainage. Bidirectional shunting can be detected but not accurately quantitated using oximetry.

Assessment of left ventricular function

The importance of the assessment of LV function to the cardiologist is in the prognosis following cardiac surgery. To the clinical pharmacologist, the importance lies in the measurement of the effects of drugs and to the physiologist the understanding of the heart as a pump.

The problem remains that there is no single index of LV function that can be used to diagnose early myocardial damage.

Compensatory mechanisms for volume or pressure overload result in many of the indices mentioned below remaining normal even in the presence of some myocardial damage or disease.

Myocardial mechanics is a complex subject, which cannot be covered here. The indices discussed briefly below are those which are most commonly used. None of the contractility indices are entirely independent of preload or afterload.

Compensatory autoregulation mechanisms

1 Frank–Starling effect (heterometric autoregulation). Increasing fibre length results in increased velocity of contraction. Thus an increase in end-diastolic volume results in an increased stroke volume. The descending limb of the curve does not exist in humans.

2 Anrep effect (homeometric autoregulation). Increasing afterload resulting in increased contractility. Possibly due to noradrenaline release from the myocardium.

3 Bowditch effect (inochronic autoregulation). Increasing heart rate resulting in increased contractility. Mediated via calcium flux.

These three mechanisms are independent of the sympathetic or parasympathetic system influences on the heart. During exercise the increase in cardiac output is primarily due to an increase in heart rate (and not stroke volume) mediated via the sympathetic nervous system.

Parameters of ventricular function

1 Angiographic (page 497):

LVEDV	LV mass
LVESV	LV ejection rate
Ejection fraction	

2 Radionuclide:
Ejection fraction

3 Haemodynamic:

Cardiac index	Minute work index
LVEDP	LV power
Stroke work index	Myocardial O_2 consumption and efficiency

4 Pre-ejection/isovolumic phase indices:
Systolic time intervals
Max. dP/dt, min. dP/dt
Derivatives of max. dP/dt correcting for preload, e.g.

$$\frac{\text{max. } dP/dt}{\text{LVEDP}}$$

V_{pm} = maximum measured rate of contractile element shortening from force–velocity loop

V_{max} = maximum rate of contractile element shortening at zero pressure (extrapolated from force–velocity loop)

5 Ejection phase indices (derived from echocardiogram or left ventricular angiogram); e.g. Peak V_{cf}

6 Diastolic indices:

dP/dV (diastolic stiffness) or dV/dP (compliance)

Left ventricular work

Left ventricular work is commonly calculated as the LV stroke work index (LVSWI):

$$LVSWI = LV \times SVI \times 0.0136 \text{ g m/m}^2$$

where LV = mean LV pressure in mmHg during ejection (as in
      calculation of TTI, see Figure 12.45)
    SVI = stroke volume index in ml/m^2/beat (calculated from
      angiogram or from thermodilution cardiac output).

Since planimetring the LV pressure during ejection to derive mean LV pressure is time consuming, provided there is no aortic valve gradient mean aortic pressure may be used. This calculates systolic work.

Net LV work is calculated as:

$$LVSWI = (LV - LVED) \times SVI \times 0.0136$$
$$\text{or} \qquad (A_o - PAW) \times SVI \times 0.0136$$

where A_o = mean aortic pressure
    PAW = mean pulmonary artery wedge pressure
    LVED = LV end-diastolic pressure

LV minute work index

LVMWI is calculated as $LVSWI \times \dfrac{HR}{1000}$ (kg m/m^2/min)

This allows consideration of heart rate in work calculation as HR tends to have an inverse relation with SVI.

Pressure–volume loops (Figure 12.44)

Left ventricular work may be calculated by measuring the area within a pressure–volume loop. Intraventricular pressure is measured during an LV angiogram. By recording ECG timing on cine film, instantaneous LV pressure can be calculated at any LV volume (Figure 12.44).

The pressure–volume loop is used to study LV compliance (dV/dP) and stiffness (dP/dV). There are major problems in the study of LV compliance as in contractility. The slope of the diastolic pressure–volume plot at any instant of volume is a measure of diastolic stiffness. Assumptions from the excised dog's heart that the diastolic

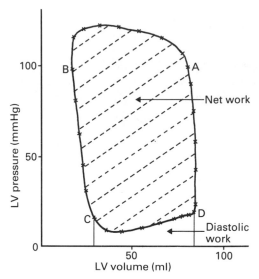

Figure 12.44 Pressure–volume loop to show calculation of net left ventricular work. A, aortic valve opening; B, aortic valve closure; C, mitral valve opening; D, mitral valve closure.

pressure–volume relation is an exponential are not necessarily valid in humans.

Diastolic pressure time index/tension time index (Figure 12.45)
The diastolic pressure time index (DPTI)/tension time index (TTI) ratio is established as a measure of subendocardial ischaemia. The DPTI gives a measurement of myocardial oxygen supply, and the TTI a measure of myocardial oxygen consumption. It is thus a supply/demand ratio (Buckberg and Hoffman).

DPTI = mean LV pressure during diastole × diastolic filling period × heart rate

TTI = mean LV pressure during ejection × systolic ejection period × heart rate

Figure 12.45 shows simultaneous pressure recordings of LV and aorta in a patient with aortic stenosis. The stippled area represents the area planimetred to calculate mean LV pressure in diastole and hence DPTI. The hatched area represents the area planimetred to calculate mean LV pressure in systole and hence TTI. Normal ratio = > 0.7, typical range in aortic stenosis 0.3–0.5. SEjP, systolic ejection period in s/min; DFP, diastolic filling period in s/min.

Common indices of cardiac function

Index	How derived	Normal range
Cardiac index	Cardiac output (CO)/body surface area	2.5–4.0 l/min/m^2
Stroke volume index (SVI)	Stroke volume/body surface area	40–70 ml/m^2
LV stroke work index (LVSWI)	Stroke volume index × 0.0136 × mean arterial – mean wedge pressure	40–80 g m/m^2
LV minute work index (LVMWI)	Stroke work index × heart rate (HR)/1000	4.5–5.5 kg m/m^2/min
Systemic vascular resistance (SVR)	(a) $\dfrac{80\,(\overline{A_O} - \overline{RA})}{CO}$ or (b) $\dfrac{(\overline{A_O} - \overline{RA})}{CO}$	(a) 770–1500 dyn s cm^{-5} (b) 10–20 units
Pulmonary vascular resistance (PVR)	(a) $\dfrac{80\,(\overline{PA} - \overline{PAW})}{CO}$ or (b) $\dfrac{(\overline{PA} - \overline{PAW})}{CO}$	(a) < 200 dyn s cm^{-5} (b) < 2.5 units
Tension time index (TTI)	LV pressure during ejection × HR × systolic ejection period (mmHg s/min)	DPTI/TTI ratio > 0.7
Diastolic pressure time index (DPTI)	LV pressure during diastole × HR × diastolic filling period (mmHg s/min)	
LV dP/dt max	Differentiated LV pressure from micromanometer	Approximately 1000–2400 mmHg/s
V_{max}	$\dfrac{dP/dt}{kP}$	Developed pressure V_{max} Approximately 2.0–3.3/s

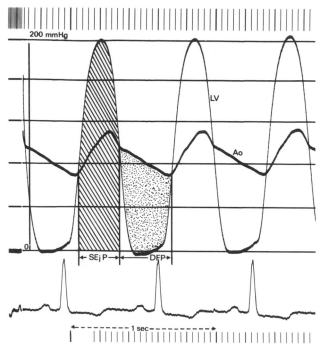

Figure 12.45 Calculation of tension time index and diastolic pressure time index in aortic stenosis.

Inotropes will reduce the ratio by increasing TTI and decreasing DPTI (by shortening diastole with the inevitable chronotropic effect). Beta-blockade will increase the ratio by reducing TTI and by increasing DPTI (longer diastole).

Indices of ventricular contractility

The ideal index of contractility should be easily measurable in the human heart, reproducible and independent of changes in preload or afterload. No ideal index exists. Only two pre-ejection phase indices will be briefly discussed.

1 Max. dP/dt. The maximum rate of rise of LV pressure during the isovolumic phase is recorded via a catheter tip micromanometer in the left ventricle and the pressure differentiated. It is known that max. dP/dt depends not only on the inotropic state of the muscle, but also on preload, afterload and left ventricular volume (end-diastolic fibre length). It is thus not a particularly useful index of contractility.

Attempts to avoid preload dependence by deriving other indices from max. dP/dt (e.g. max. $dP/dt \div$ LVEDP) do not solve the problem. Min. dP/dt (peak negative dP/dt) depends on the inotropic state of the muscle and on end-systolic volume.

2 V_{max} (Figure 12.46). This index is defined as the maximum velocity of contractile element (VCE) shortening at zero load. As with max. dP/dt it is derived from high-fidelity catheter tip manometer recordings of LV pressure. The LV pressure is differentiated and divided by the instantaneous LV pressure. This is plotted on the vertical axis with LV pressure on the horizontal axis. Using numerous assumptions about the left ventricle it can be shown that:

$$VCE = \frac{dP/dt}{KP}$$

The force–velocity loop appears as shown in Figure 12.46.

Conversion of the vertical axis to a log scale allows for a straight-line extrapolation. The extrapolation distance is shorter if 'developed pressure' is used (i.e. LVEDP).

Some workers prefer to express results as KV_{max} since K, the coefficient of series elasticity, has not been calculated in humans. Many of the assumptions used to generate V_{max} are generally agreed to be invalid. It is probably dependent on preload.

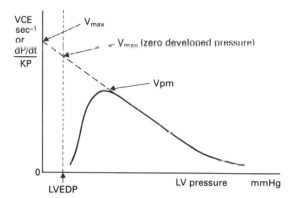

Figure 12.46 Force–velocity loop to show extrapolation of curve to zero developed pressure (LVEDP) to calculate V_{max}. VCE – velocity of contractile element shortening (s^{-1}), dP/dt = rate of rise of LV pressure (mmHg/s), K = coefficient of series elasticity (calculated in dogs as 28, but unknown in humans), P = instantaneous LV pressure – LVEDP, i.e. this is developed LV pressure.

Systolic time intervals

This non-invasive assessment of LV function is mainly used in the study of drugs on LV performance and in the follow up of cardiac disease in a single patient. However, it should not really be used in interpatient comparisons.

Intervals measured (see Figure 12.47):

Q–S_2. Onset of Q wave to onset of aortic valve closure. This is total electromechanical systole.

LVET. LV ejection time. Onset of carotid upstroke to dicrotic notch. This interval has been shown to equal ejection time measured from the same interval in the aortic root.

PEP. Pre-ejection period. This is taken from the onset of Q wave to aortic valve opening. However, unless taken at cardiac catheterization with LV and A_0 pressures recorded the non-invasive measurement is:

$$PEP = Q - S_2 - LVET$$

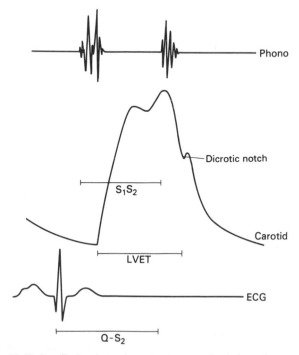

Figure 12.47 Systolic time intervals. Q–S_2, electromechanical systole. LVET, left ventricular ejection time.

There are two components to the PEP:

(a) the electromechanical interval (Q wave to onset of systolic rise of LV pressure);

(b) the isovolumic contraction time (IVCT); onset of rise of LV pressure to aortic valve opening.

IVCT. Isovolumic contraction time = S_1–S_2 interval – LVET. The exact definition of the onset of mitral valve closure from the beginning of S_1 may be difficult. It is not usually measured non-invasively. The indices Q – S_2, PEP and LVET are dependent on heart rate. The ratio PEP/LVET has been widely used to avoid this dependence.

Predicted normals (intervals in ms)

	Male	Female
Q–S_2	546 – 2.1 × HR	549 – 2.0 × HR
LVET	413 – 1.7 × HR	418 – 1.6 × HR
PEP	131 – 0.4 × HR	133 – 0.4 × HR
PEP/LVET	0.35 ± 0.04 (1 SD)	

Range of abnormality of PEP/LVET in LV dysfunction:

Mild	Moderate	Severe
(0.44–0.52)	(0.53–0.6)	(> 0.6)

The ratio increases with a combination of prolonged PEP and shortened LVET. The ratio may also be increased by:

• LBBB (lengthens PEP)

• beta-blockade

• reduction in LV volume, diuretics, haemorrhage.

The ratio decreases (shortening of PEP) if inotropes are given (digoxin or catecholamines). Moderate aortic valve disease also reduces the ratio by lengthening the LVET. As LV function in aortic valve disease deteriorates, the ratio returns towards normal. It is thus not a useful index in aortic valve disease. It has been found useful, however, in assessing prognosis following myocardial infarction.

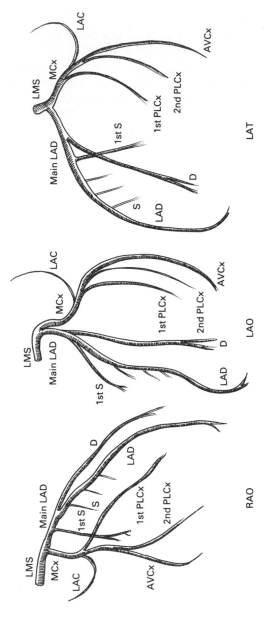

Figure 12.48 Left coronary artery.

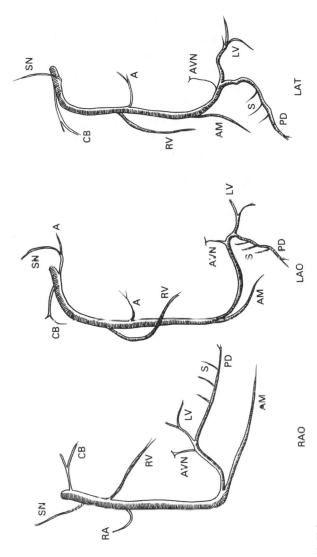

Figure 12.49 Right coronary artery.

Coronary artery nomenclature

Key to coronary artery anatomy, Figures 12.48 and 12.49, as seen at coronary angiography.

A	Atrial branch
AM	Acute marginal artery
AVCx	Atrioventricular groove branch of circumflex
AVN	Atrioventricular node artery
CB	Conus branch
D	Diagonal branch of LAD
LAC	Left atrial circumflex
LAD	Left anterior descending
LAO	30° left anterior oblique projection
LAT	Left lateral projection
LMS	Left main stem
LV	Left ventricular branches
MCx	Main circumflex
PD	Posterior descending
PLCx	Posterolateral circumflex branch (obtuse marginal)
RA	Right atrial branch
RAO	30° right anterior oblique projection
RV	Right ventricular branch
1st S	First septal perforator
S	Septal perforating arteries
SN	Sinus node artery

Appendices

1 Nomogram for body size

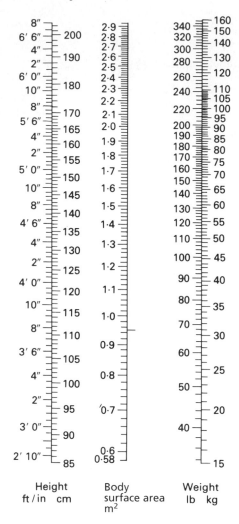

Height
ft / in   cm

Body
surface area
m²

Weight
lb   kg

2 Rate conversion chart

Heart rate	R–R interval (ms)
30	2000
35	1714
40	1500
45	1333
50	1200
52	1154
54	1111
56	1071
58	1034
60	1000
62	968
64	938
66	909
68	882
70	857
72	833
74	811
76	789
78	769
80	750
82	732
84	714
86	698
88	682
90	667
92	652
94	638
96	625
98	612
100	600
110	545
120	500
130	462
140	429
150	400
160	375
170	353
180	330
190	315
200	300

3 Further reading

Bennett D.H. (1993) *Cardiac Arrhythmias.* Butterworth-Heinemann, Oxford.

Braunwald E. (ed.) (1996) *Heart Disease. A Text-Book of Cardiovascular Medicine.* W.B. Saunders, Philadelphia.

Carter S.A., Bajec D.F., Yannicelli, E. & Wood E.M. (1960) Estimation of left-to-right shunt from arterial dilution curves. *J. Lab. Clin.* **55**, 77.

Ellenbogen K.A., Kay N. & Wilkoff B.L. (eds) (1996) *Clinical Cardiac Pacing.* Blackwell Science, Cambridge, Mass.

El Sherif N. & Samet P. (1991) *Cardiac Pacing and Electrophysiology.* W.B. Saunders, Philadelphia.

Feigenbaum H. (1994) *Electrocardiography.* Lea & Febiger, Philadelphia.

Fogoros R.N. (1994) *Electrophysiologic Testing.* Blackwell Science, Oxford.

Grossman W. & Baim D.S. (1996) *Cardiac Catheterization Angiography and Intervention.* Lea & Febiger, Philadelphia.

Hall R.J.C. & Julian D.C. (1989) *Diseases of the Cardiac Valves.* Churchill Livingstone, London.

Houston A.B. & Simpson I. (1988) *Cardiac Doppler Ultrasound. A Clinical Perspective.* Butterworth Scientific, London.

Jefferson K. & Rees S. (1980) *Clinical Cardiac Radiology.* Butterworth, London.

Julian D.G., Camm A.J., Fox K.M., Hall R.J.C. & Poole-Wilson P.A. (1996) *Diseases of the Heart.* Baillière Tindall, London.

Lown B., Calvert A.F., Armington R. & Ryan M. (1975) Monitoring for serious arrhythmias and high risk of sudden death. *Circulation* **52**, 189–198.

Miller G. (1989) *Invasive Investigation of the Heart.* Blackwell Scientific Publications, Oxford.

Opie L.H. (1991) *The Heart. Physiology and Metabolism.* Raven Press, New York.

Opie L.H. (1995) *Drugs for the Heart.* W.B. Saunders, Philadelphia.

Perloff J.K. & Child J.S. (1991) *Congenital Heart Disease in Adults.* W.B. Saunders, Philadelphia.

Reaven G.M. (1988) Role of insulin resistance in human disease. *Diabetes* **37**, 1595–1607.

Redington A., Shore D. & Oldershaw, P. (1994) *Congenital Heart Disease in Adults.* W.B. Saunders, Philadelphia.

Ross D., English T. & McKay R. (1992) *Principles of Cardiac Diagnosis and Treatment – A Surgeons' Guide.* Springer-Verlag, London.

Schamroth L. (1989) *The 12 Lead Electrocardiogram.* Blackwell Scientific Publications, Oxford.

Sokolow M., McIllroy M.B. & Cheitlin M.D. (1993) *Clinical Cardiology.* Lange Medical Publications, Los Altos, Calif.

Uretsky B.F. (1997) *Cardiac Catheterization: Concepts, Techniques and Applications.* Blackwell Science, Malden, Mass.

Ward D.E. & Camm A.J. (1987) *Clinical Electrophysiology of the Heart.* Edward Arnold, London.

Yang S.S., Bentivoglio L.G., Maranhao V. & Goldberg H. (1978) *From Cardiac Catheterisation Data to Haemodynamic Parameters.* F.A. Davis, Philadelphia.

Zipes D.M. & Jalife J. (1995) *Cardiac Electrophysiology.* W.B. Saunders, Philadelphia.

4 References of important trials or papers quoted in the text

Hyperlipidaemia
CARE study. Efficacy of pravastatin on coronary events after myocardial infarction in patients with average cholesterol levels
Five-year follow up of patients with starting cholesterol < 6.2 mmol/l treated with pravastatin. Sacks F.M., Pfeffer M.A., Moye L.A. *et al. New Eng. J. Med.*, **335**, 1001 (1996).

CHAOS trial. Cambridge Heart Antioxidant Study. Randomised controlled trial of vitamin E in patients with coronary disease
Reduction in non-fatal MI (but not cardiovascular death) in patients receiving vitamin E. Stephens N.G., Parsons A., Schofield P.M., Kelly F., Cheesman K., Mitchinson M.J., and Brown M. *Lancet*, **347**, 781 (1996).

FATS study. Familial atherosclerosis treatment study
Regression of coronary artery disease as a result of intensive lipid lowering therapy in men with high levels of apolipoprotein B. Brown G.B., Albers J.J., Fisher L.B. *et al. New Eng. J. Med.*, **323**, 1289 (1990).

POSCH study. Program on the surgical control of the hyperlipidaemias
Effect of partial ileal by-pass surgery on the mortality and morbidity from coronary heart disease in patients with hypercholesterolaemia. Report of the program on the surgical control of hyperlipidaemias. Buchwald H., Varco R.L., Matts P.J. *et al. New Eng. J. Med.*, **323**, 946 (1990).

4S study. Randomised trial of cholesterol lowering in 4444 patients with coronary heart disease: the Scandinavian Simvastatin Survival Study (4S)
Secondary prevention trial of simvastatin in patients with hypercholesterolaemia followed for a median of 5.4 years. Scandinavian Simvastatin Survival Sudy Group. *Lancet*, **344**, 1383 (1994).

WOSCOPS study. Prevention of coronary heart disease with pravastatin in men with hypercholesterolaemia
West of Scotland primary prevention trial in men followed for 4.9 years treated with pravastatin. Shepherd J., Cobbe S.M., Ford I. *et al. New Eng. J. Med.*, **333**, 1301 (1995).

Catheter ablation
Catheter technique for closed-chest ablation of the atrio-ventricular conduction system. Gallagher J.J., Svenson R.H., Kasell J.H. *et al. New Eng. J. Med.*, **306**, 194 (1982).

Catheter ablation of accessory atrio-ventricular pathways (Wolff–Parkinson–White syndrome) by radiofrequency current. Jackman W.M., Wang X., Friday K. *et al. New Eng. J. Med.*, **324**, 1605 (1991).

Arrhythmias
CAMIAT trial. Randomised trial of outcome after myocardial infarction in patients with frequent or repetitive ventricular premature depolarisations

Amiodarone reduced arrhythmic death. The Canadian amiodarone myocardial infarction arrhythmia trial investigators. *Lancet*, **349**, 675 (1997).

CAST study. The cardiac arrhythmia suppression trial
Mortality and morbidity in patients receiving encainide, flecainide or placebo. Echt D.S., Liebson P.R., Mitchell B. *et al. New Eng. J. Med.*, **324**, 781 (1991).

EMIAT trial. Randomised trial of effect of amiodarone on mortality in patients with left ventricular dysfunction after recent mycardial infarction
Amiodarone reduced arrhythmic deaths but not overall mortality. Julian D.G. *et al.* for the European myocardial infarct amiodarone trial investigators. *Lancet*, **349**, 667 (1997).

PROMISE trial. Prospective randomised milrinone survival evaluation
Effect of oral milrinone on mortality in severe chronic heart failure. Packer M., Carver J.R., Rodeheffer R.J. *et al. New Eng. J. Med.*, **325**, 1468 (1991).

ESVEM trial. Electrophysiologic study versus electrocardiographic monitoring
A comparison of electrophysiologic testing with Holter monitoring to predict anti-arrhythmic drug efficacy for ventricular tachyarrhythmias. Mason J.M. for the ESVEM investigators. *New Eng. J. Med.*, **329**, 445 (1993).

MADIT trial. Improved survival with an implanted defibrillator in patients with coronary disease at high risk for ventricular tachycardia
The ICD reduced mortality over a 5-year period, but drug therapy did not influence mortality. *New Eng. J. Med.*, **335**, 1933 (1996).

Coronary angioplasty
ACME study. Angioplasty compared to medicine
A comparison of angioplasty with medical therapy in the treatment of single-vessel coronary disease. Parisi A.F., Folland E.D., Hartigan P. *et al. New Eng. J. Med.*, **326**, 10 (1992).

BENESTENT study. A comparison of balloon expandable stent implantation with balloon angioplasty in patients with coronary artery disease
Stent implantation compared with balloon dilatation alone reduced restenosis rate in arteries of 3.0 mm or more from 32% to 20% at 7 months. Serruys P.W., de Jaegere P., Kiemeneij F. *et al. New Eng. J. Med.*, **331**, 489 (1994).

EPIC trial. Randomised trial of coronary intervention with antibody against platelet IIb/IIIa intergrin for reduction of clinical restenosis: result at 6 months
Evaluation of c7E3 for the prevention of ischaemic complications. c7E3 reduced acute events following PTCA and also the need for revascularization at 6 months. Topol E.J., Califf R.M., Weisman H.F *et al. Lancet*, **343**, 881 (1994).

RITA trial. Randomised intervention treatment of angina
Coronary angioplasty versus coronary artery by-pass surgery. RITA trial participants. *Lancet*, **341**, 573 (1993).

PRAMI trial. Primary angioplasty in myocardial infarction study group
A comparison of immediate angioplasty with thrombolytic therapy for acute

....

myocardial infarction. Grines C.L., Browne K.F., Marco J. *et al. New Eng. J. Med.*, **328**, 673 (1993).

CAVEAT study. Coronary angioplasty versus excisional atherectomy
A comparison of directional atherectomy with coronary angioplasty in patients with coronary artery disease. Topol E.J., Leya F., Pinkerton C.A. *et al. New Eng. J. Med.*, **329**, 221 (1993).

CCAT study. Canadian coronary atherectomy trial
A comparison of directional atherectomy with balloon angioplasty for lesions of the left anterior descending coronary artery. Adelman A.G., Cohen E.A., Kimball B.P. *et al. New Eng. J. Med.*, **329**, 228 (1993).

STRESS trial. Stent restenosis study. A randomised comparison of coronary stent placement and balloon angioplasty in the treatment of coronary artery disease
Fischman D.L., Leon M.B., Baim D.S., *et al. New Eng. J. Med.*, **331**, 496 (1994).

Myocardial infarction and thrombolysis
GISSI 1 trial. Gruppo Italiano per lo studio della streptochinasi nell'infarto miocardico
Effectiveness of intravenous thrombolytic treatment in acute myocardial infarction. *Lancet*, **1**, 397 (1986).

ISIS 2 trial. Second international study of infarct survival
Randomised trial of intravenous streptokinase, oral aspirin, both or neither among 17 187 cases of suspected acute myocardial infarction. Collaborative group. *Lancet*, **2**, 349 (1988).

ASSET study. Anglo-Scandinavian study of early thrombolysis
Trial of tissue plasminogen activator for mortality reduction in acute myocardial infarction. Wilcox R.G., von der Lippe G., Olsson C.G. *et al. Lancet*, **2**, 525 (1988).

TIMI II. Thrombolysis in myocardial infarction. Phase II trial
Comparison of invasive and conservative strategies after treatment with intravenous tissue plasminogen activator in acute myocardial infarction. *New Eng. J. Med.*, **320**, 618 (1989).

AIMS trial. APSAC intervention mortality study
Long-term effects of intravenous anistreplase in acute myocardial infarction: final report of the AIMS study. *Lancet*, **427**, (1990).

GISSI 2 trial
A factorial randomised trial of alteplase versus streptokinase and heparin versus no heparin among 12 490 patients with acute myocardial infarction. *Lancet*, **336**, 65 (1990).

DAVITT II trial. Danish study group on verapamil in myocardial infarction
Effect of verapamil on mortality and major events after an acute myocardial infarction. *Am. J. Cardiol.*, **66**, 779 (1990).

SWIFT trial. Should we intervene following thrombolysis?
SWIFT trial of delayed elective intervention vs. conservative treatment after thrombolysis with anistreplase in acute myocardial infarction. *Brit. Med. J.*, **302**, 555 (1991).

ISIS 3. Third international study of infarct survival
A randomised comparison of streptokinase vs. tissue plasminogen activator vs. anistreplase and of aspirin plus heparin vs. aspirin alone among 41 299 cases of suspected acute myocardial infarction. *Lancet*, **339**, 753 (1992).

LIMIT 2 trial. Leicester intravenous magnesium intervention
Intravenous magnesium sulphate in suspected acute myocardial infarction: results of the second Leicester intravenous magnesium intervention LIMIT 2 trial. *Lancet*, **339**, 1553 (1992).

GUSTO trial. Global utilisation of streptokinase and tissue plasminogen activator for occluded coronary arteries
An international randomised trial comparing four thrombolytic strategies for acute myocardial infarction. The GUSTO investigators. *New Eng. J. Med.*, **329**, 673 (1993).

Heart failure
CONSENSUS I. The cooperative North Scandinavian enalapril survival study
Effects of enalapril on mortality in severe congestive heart failure: results of the North Scandinavian enalapril survival study. The CONSENSUS trial study group. *New Eng. J. Med.*, **316**, 1429 (1987).

DIG trial. The effect of digoxin on mortality and morbidity in patients with heart failure
Digoxin did not reduce mortality in chronic CCF but did reduce hospital admissions for heart failure. The Digitalis Investigation Group. *New Eng. J. Med.*, **336**, 525 (1997).

ELITE trial. Randomised trial of losartan versus captopril in patients over 65 with heart failure. (Evaluation of losartan in the elderly study, ELITE)
Lower mortality in patients treated with losartan compared to captopril. Pitt B., Segal R., Martinez F.A. *et al. Lancet*, **349**, 747 (1997).

PRAISE trial. The effect of amlodipine on morbidity and mortality in severe chronic heart failure
Amlodipine did not increase mortality in severe chronic CCF and possibly reduced it in dilated cardiomyopathy. Packer M., O'Connor C.M., Ghali J.K. *et al. New Eng. J. Med.*, **335**, 1107 (1996).

SAVE trial. Survival and ventricular enlargement trial
Effect of captopril on mortality and morbidity in patients with left ventricular dysfunction after myocardial infarction. Pfeffer M., Braunwald E., Moye L.A. *et al. New Eng. J. Med.*, **327**, 669 (1992).

CONSENSUS II. The cooperative new Scandinavian enalapril survival study
Effects of the early administration of enalapril on mortality in patients with acute

....

myocardial infarction. Swedberg K., Held P., Kjekshus J., *et al. New Eng. J. Med.*, **327**, 678 (1992).

The SOLVD study. Studies of left ventricular dysfunction
Effects of enalapril on mortality and the development of heart failure in asymptomatic patients with reduced left ventricular ejection fractions. The SOLVD investigators. *New Eng. J. Med.*, **327**, 685 (1992).

Unstable angina

FRISC trial. Low molecular weight heparin during instability in coronary artery disease
Fragmin reduced myocardial infarcts and deaths in patients on aspirin in unstable angina. Fragmin during instability in coronary artery disease (FRISC) study group. *Lancet*, **347**, 561 (1996).

ESSENCE trial. A comparison of low molecular weight heparin with unfractionated heparin for unstable coronary artery disease.
Enoxaparin was more effective than unfractionated heparin (both with aspirin) at reducing ischaemic events in unstable angina. ESSENCE study group. *New Eng. J. Med.* **337**, 447 (1997).

5 Useful addresses

British Heart Foundation, 14 Fitzhardinge Street, London W1H 4DH. *Tel*: 0171-935-0185

British Cardiac Society, 9 Fitzroy Square, London W1P 5AH. *Tel*: 0171-383-3887

British Cardiac Intervention Society (BCIS)
British Pacing and Electrophysiology Group (BPEG)
British Society of Echocardiography   } As for British
British Nuclear Cardiology Group   Cardiac Society
Heart (formerly British Heart Journal)
Cardiovascular Research

European Heart Journal (Journal of the European Society of Cardiology), Academic Press (London), 24–28 Oval Road, London NW1 7DX or Academic Press Inc, 111 Fifth Avenue, New York, NY 10003

American College of Cardiology, Heart House, 9111 Old Georgetown Road, Bethesda, MD 20814

American Heart Association or Circulation, 7320 Greenville Avenue, Dallas, TX 75231

America Heart Journal, C.V. Mosby Co, 11830 Westline Industrial Drive, St Louis, MO 63141

American Journal of Cardiology, 875 Third Avenue, New York, NY 10022

Journal of the American College of Cardiology, Elsevier Science Publishing Co Inc, 52 Vanderbilt Avenue, New York, NY 10017

NASPE, North American Society of Pacing and Electrophysiology, 13 Eaton Court, Wellesley Hills, MA 02181. *Tel*: (617) 237-1866

6 Fitness to drive in the UK and heart disease

Vocational driving licence

Revised guidelines 1996 for drivers of buses, lorries and other professional drivers, (formerly heavy goods vehicles (HGV) and public service vehicles (PSV). The standards are necessarily strict.

Patients with any of the following conditions may not hold a licence, should notify the DVLC, and should stop driving their vehicle. A patient should not have a disqualifying condition from any section. Applicants with arterial disease (coronary or peripheral) who are successfully relicensed will have to have a satisfactory annual medical report and a repeat assessment every 3 years.

Coronary heart disease

- Angina. On or off treatment.
- Heart failure. On or off treatment.
- Within 3 months of a myocardial infarct, any episode of unstable angina, CABG or PTCA.

Applicants will then have to be able to complete three stages of the standard Bruce treadmill protocol without symptoms or signs of cardiac dysfunction, with no ST-segment change, malignant arrhythmia or claudication. Blood pressure response should be normal. The test must be completed off all anti-anginal therapy, but ACE inhibitors are allowed.

Coronary arteriography is not required. However if requested by the DVLA the licence will be refused or revoked if it shows:

- LV ejection fraction impaired (< 40%)
- left main stem stenosis of > 30%
- main LAD stenosis (proximal to first septal) of > 50%
- two or more vessel disease.

ECG abnormality

- Pathological Q waves in three or more leads.
- LBBB.

Relicensing may be possible if the criteria above are satisfied.

Disease of other arteries

- Aortic aneurysm > 5 cm in diameter. Either thoracic or abdominal, unless repaired satisfactorily and there is no evidence of myocardial ischaemia.
- Aortic dissection.
- Peripheral vascular disease with evidence of myocardial ischaemia. (If there is peripheral vascular disease but no evidence of myocardial ischaemia applicants may be relicensed.)

Hypertension

- Casual blood pressure > 200 systolic or 110 diastolic.
- Established hypertension > 180/100.
- Drug treatment causing symptoms affecting driving ability.

Arrhythmias

Any significant arrhythmia in the last 5 years. This includes AV block (congenital or acquired), sinus node disease, any supraventricular, junctional or ventricular tachycardia. Includes AF and atrial flutter. It does not include isolated VPBs in the presence of a normal heart.

Relicensing may be allowed if:
• in the last two years the arrhythmia has not caused any sudden impairment of consciousness or distraction to the driver and is not thought likely to do so
• the echocardiogram is normal
• the treadmill test is successfully completed as in the coronary disease section above. Patients may remain on their anti-arrhythmic therapy for this test.

At 3 months after successful RF ablation of an accessory pathway, relicensing may be allowed if:
• there has been no recurrence of the arrhythmia
• anti-arrhythmic therapy is no longer required
• there is no other disqualifying condition.

Permanent pacemaker
Relicensing will normally be allowed provided the unit was implanted for bradycardia, and there is regular pacemaker follow up at least annually.

Malignant vasovagal syndrome
Relicensing will also be considered if:
• patient has been symptom free for 6 months on treatment
• exercise testing and echocardiography have excluded ischaemic heart disease
• repeat tilt testing has failed to provoke symptoms.

Implantable cardioverter defibrillator
This is usually an absolute bar to relicensing. If the device has only ever been used for antitachycardia pacing relicensing may be possible.

Valve disease
History in the last 5 years of:
• cerebral ischaemic event
• systemic embolism
• persisting LV or RV hypertrophy or dilatation
• associated arrhythmia.
Anticoagulation is not a bar to relicensing. Atrial fibrillation persisting for > 3 months after valve replacement is also not a bar provided none of the above have occurred and the patient is anticoagulated.

Cardiomyopathy
• Established cardiomyopathy: HCM, DCM or restrictive.
• Heart or heart–lung transplantation.

Congenital heart disease
Relicensing will be considered for simpler congenital heart disease which has been repaired surgically: i.e. ASD, small VSD, mild aortic or pulmonary stenosis, PDA, coarctation of the aorta with mild gradient and no systemic hypertension, and anomalous pulmonary venous drainage. Patients with:
• complex cyanotic congenital heat disease
• persisting pulmonary hypertension
• aortic root dilatation (e.g. Marfan)
are unlikely to qualify.

   More information can be obtained from: The Medical Advisor, Drivers' medical group, DVLA, Swansea. SA99 1TU.

7 List of abbreviations

ACE	Angiotensin-converting enzyme
AF	Atrial fibrillation
AML	Anterior mitral leaflet
ANF	Antinuclear factor
AP	Aortopulmonary
APD	Action potential duration
APSAC	Anisoylated plasminogen streptokinase activator complex
APTT	Activated partial thromboplastin time
APVD	Anomalous pulmonary venous drainage
AR	Aortic regurgitation
AS	Aortic stenosis
ASD	Atrial septal defect
ASO	Antistreptolysin-O titre
AV	Atrioventricular
AVD	Aortic valve disease
AVR	Aortic valve replacement
BCR	British corrected ratio
CABG	Coronary artery bypass grafting
CAD	Coronary artery disease
CCF	Congestive cardiac failure
CFT	Complement fixation test
CPK-MB	Creatine phosphokinase isoenzyme of cardiac muscle
CPR	Cardiopulmonary resuscitation
CRP	C-reactive protein
CVA	Cerebrovascular accident
CVP	Central venous pressure
CVS	Cardiovascular system
CW	Continuous wave
CXR	Chest X-ray
DC	Direct current
DCM	Dilated cardiomyopathy
Dd	Diastolic dimension
DFP	Diastolic filling period
DOLV	Double-outlet left ventricle
DORV	Double-outlet right ventricle
DPTI	Diastolic pressure time index
DTPA	Diethylenetriamine penta-acetic acid
DXT	Deep X-ray therapy
EDM	Early diastolic murmur
EFE	Endocardial fibroelastosis
EP	Electrophysiological
ERP	Effective refractory period
ESR	Erythrocyte sedimentation rate
FBC	Full blood count

533

FDPs	Fibrin degradation products
FEV_1	Forced expiratory volume in 1 second
FFA	Free fatty acids
GTN	Glyceryl trinitrate
HBD	Hydroxybutyrate dehydrogenase
HMG	Hydroxymethylglutaryl
HR	Heart rate
HCM	Hypertrophic cardiomyopathy
HRAE	High right atrial electrogram
H–V	His–ventricular
IABP	Intra-aortic balloon pumping
ICD	Implantable cardioverter defibrillator
INR	International normalized ratio
ISA	Intrinsic sympathomimetic activity
ITU	Intensive therapy unit
IVC	Inferior vena cava
IVS	Interventricular septum
IVU	Intravenous urogram
JVP	Jugular venous pulse
LA	Left atrium
LAD	Left axis deviation. Left anterior descending
LAHB	Left anterior hemiblock
LAID	Left atrial internal dimension
LAO	Left anterior oblique
LAT	Lateral
LBBB	Left bundle branch block
LDH	Lactic dehydrogenase
LFT	Liver function test
LPHB	Left posterior hemiblock
LSE	Left sternal edge
LV	Left ventricle
LVEDP	Left ventricular end-diastolic pressure
LVEDV	Left ventricular end-diastolic volume
LVEF	Left ventricular ejection fraction
LVESV	Left ventricular end-systolic volume
LVET	Left ventricular ejection time
LVF	Left ventricular failure
LVFP	Left ventricular filling pressure
LVIDd	Left ventricular internal dimension at end diastole
LVIDs	Left ventricular internal dimension at end systole
LVMWI	Left ventricular minute work index
LVOTO	Left ventricular outflow tract obstruction
LVSWI	Left ventricular stroke work index
MAOIs	Monoamine oxidase inhibitors
METS	Metabolic equivalents

MIC	Minimum inhibitory concentration
MR	Mitral regurgitation
MS	Mitral stenosis
MUGA	Multiple gated acquisition
MV	Mitral valve
MVR	Mitral valve replacement
NYHA	New York Heart Association
PA	Pulmonary artery
PAEDP	Pulmonary artery end-diastolic pressure
PATB	Paroxysmal atrial tachycardia with varying block
PAW	Pulmonary artery wedge
PDA	Patent ductus arteriosus
PE	Pulmonary embolism
PEP	Pre-ejection period
PFO	Patent foramen ovale
PGE_2	Prostaglandin E_2
PGI_2	Prostaglandin I_2 (prostacyclin)
PHT	Pulmonary hypertension
PLVW	Posterior left ventricular wall
PND	Paroxysmal nocturnal dyspnoea
PR	Pulmonary regurgitation
PS	Pulmonary stenosis
PTCA	Percutaneous transluminal coronary angioplasty
PV	Pulmonary vein
PVC	Premature ventricular contraction
PVR	Pulmonary vascular resistance
PW	Pulsed wave
PXE	Pseudoxanthoma elasticum
RA	Right atrium
RAD	Right axis deviation
RAO	Right anterior oblique
RBBB	Right bundle branch block
REM	Rapid eye movement
RF	Radio frequency
rt-PA	Recombinant tissue plasminogen activator
RV	Right ventricle
RVEDP	Right ventricular end-diastolic pressure
RVF	Right ventricular failure
RVID	Right ventricular internal dimension
RVOT	Right ventricular outflow tract
SACT	Sino-atrial conduction time
SAM	Systolic anterior movement of the mitral valve
SBE	Subacute bacterial endocarditis
SEJP	Systolic ejection period
SLE	Systemic lupus erythematosus
SNRT	Sinus node recovery time
SR	Sinus rhythm

SSS   Sick sinus syndrome
SV   Stroke volume
SVC   Superior vena cava
S$\dot{\text{V}}$O$_2$ Mixed venous oxygen saturation
SVR   Systemic vascular resistance
SVT   Supraventricular tachycardia

TAPVD   Total anomalous pulmonary venous drainage
TGA   Transposition of the great arteries
TOE   Transoesophageal echocardiography
tPA   Tissue plasminogen activator
TPHA   Treponema pallidum haemagglutination
TR   Tricuspid regurgitation
TS   Tricuspid stenosis
TSH   Thyroid stimulating hormone
TTI   Tension time index
TV   Tricuspid valve
TXA$_2$ Thromboxane A$_2$

U and E   Urea and electrolytes

VCE   Velocity of contractile element shortening
VCF   Velocity of circumferential fibre shortening
VF   Ventricular fibrillation
VDRL   Venereal disease reference laboratory
VPB   Ventricular premature beats
VSD   Ventricular septal defect
VT   Ventricular tachycardia

WPW   Wolff–Parkinson–White
WT   Wall thickness

Index

Page numbers in *italics* refer to figures, those in **bold** refer to tables.

Index

Index

....